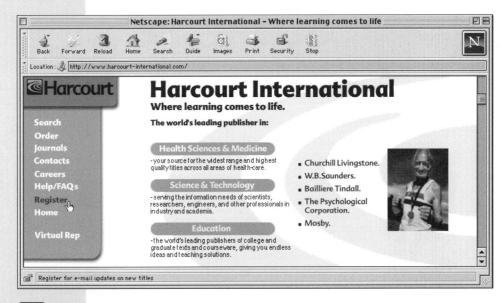
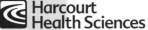

WITHDRAWN

Forensic Mental Health

Dedication

During the development of this book, two pioneers of forensic psychiatric nursing, Tony Hillis and John Parry, died. We would like to dedicate this book to their memory.

For Baillière Tindall:

Senior Commissioning Editor: Jacqueline Curthoys
Project Development Manager: Dinah Thom
Project Manager: Jane Shanks
Design Direction: George Ajayi

Forensic Mental Health
Issues in Practice

Edited by

Colin Dale MA RN DipN(Lond) CertEd RNT CertCouns DipMS
Nurse Consultant, Merseyside, UK

Tony Thompson RMN RNMH DipN(Lond) CertEd RNT BEd(Hons) MA
Director of Practice Development, Ashworth Centre, Ashworth Hospital Authority, Liverpool, UK

Phil Woods PhD DipHCResearch CertResearch RMN
Lecturer, School of Nursing, Midwifery and Health Visiting, University of Manchester, Manchester, UK

Foreword by

Malcolm Rae RMN RGN OBE ENB770
Nursing Officer, Department of Health, London, UK

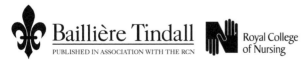

Baillière Tindall
PUBLISHED IN ASSOCIATION WITH THE RCN

Royal College of Nursing

Edinburgh London New York Philadelphia St Louis Sydney Toronto 2001

BAILLIÈRE TINDALL
An imprint of Harcourt Publishers Limited

First published 2001

ISBN 0 7020 2441 4

British Library Cataloguing in Publication Data
A catalogue record for this book is available from the British Library.

Library of Congress Cataloging in Publication Data
A catalog record for this book is available from the Library of
Congress.

Note
Medical knowledge is constantly changing. As new information
becomes available, changes in treatment, procedures, equipment and
the use of drugs become necessary. The editors, contributors and
publishers have taken care to ensure that the information given in this
text is accurate and up to date. However, readers are strongly advised
to confirm that the information, especially with regard to drug usage,
complies with the latest legislation and standards of practice.

The
publisher's
policy is to use
**paper manufactured
from sustainable forests**

Printed in China

Contents

Contributors

Pat Abbott
Consultant Psychiatrist, Ashworth Hospital
Authority, Liverpool, UK

Fran Aiken
Lecturer/Practitioner, Ashworth Hospital
Authority, Liverpool, UK

Richard Backhouse
Head of Social Work Practice, Ashworth
Hospital Authority, Liverpool, UK

Maggie Clifton
Research and Clinical Effectiveness Coordinator,
Ashworth Hospital Authority, Liverpool, UK

Colin Dale
Nurse Consultant, Merseyside, UK

David Duffy
Nurse Consultant, Mental Health Services of
Salford NHS Trust, Manchester, UK

Helen Edment
Senior Nurse, Outreach Services, Directorate of
Forensic Mental Health, Greater Glasgow
Primary Care NHS Trust, Glasgow, UK

Jim Gardner
Senior Nurse Manager, North Wales Forensic
Psychiatric Service, Bryn-y-Neuadd Hospital,
Llanfairfechan, Gwynedd, UK

Alan Gilmour
Nursing Services Manager, Directorate of
Forensic Mental Health, Greater Glasgow
Primary Care NHS Trust, Glasgow, UK

Ros Harvey
Training and Development Advisor, Ashworth
Hospital Authority, Liverpool, UK

Les Jennings
Lecturer/Practitioner, Ashworth Hospital
Authority, Liverpool, UK

Nicola Lees
Clinical Nurse Manager, Adult Forensic Services,
Edenfield Centre, Mental Health Services of
Salford NHS Trust, Manchester, UK

John McGinley
Director of Psychology, State Hospital, Carstairs,
Lanark, UK

Debbie Murdock
Manager, Women's Services, Rampton Hospital
Authority, Retford, UK

Mike Musker
Ward Manager, Ashworth Hospital Authority,
Liverpool, UK

Chris Skelly
Ward Manager, Ashworth Hospital Authority,
Liverpool, UK

Peter Snowden
Consultant Forensic Psychiatrist,
Mental Health Services of Salford NHS Trust,
Manchester, UK

Les Storey
Senior Lecturer, Faculty of Health, University of
Central Lancashire, Ormslairls Campus, UK

Tony Thompson
Director Practice Development, Ashworth
Hospital Authority, Liverpool, UK

Paul Williams
Lecturer in Social Work, Department of
Professional Education in Community Studies,
University of Reading, Reading, UK

Jeff Withington
Project Nurse, Mental Health Services of Salford
NHS Trust, Manchester, UK

Phil Woods
Lecturer, University of Manchester, School of
Nursing, Midwifery and Health Visiting,
Manchester, UK

Foreword

Forensic psychiatry has awakened as a sleeping giant into public and professional consciousness in recent years. Media and political interest has been fuelled by inquiries and exposés which have made the challenges for those involved within the services all the more complex and difficult to respond to in measured ways, while attempting to satisfy the seemingly competing demands of therapy and security.

Texts such as this one can only help those professionals within the services, or those contemplating joining them, to reach a clearer understanding of the issues involved and how they can best be responded to. The evidence base in this speciality is still emerging and we continue to be reliant on 'expert opinion' in the main for best practice. I am sure that our agenda should be to ensure that the research base continues to grow, to help to validate and underpin the views of leaders and opinion formers in the speciality.

The past year has seen no fewer than four new texts covering aspects of this subject area, together with the UKCC study on *Nursing in Secure Environments*, which has in turn been a catalyst for further work into developing guidance on the use of therapeutic management of violence and aggression, competency work and evidence-based approaches to policies and protocols in the prison service in England and Wales, and guidance on therapeutic nurse–patient relationships for people with a personality disorder. This is clearly heartening from a national perspective and the speciality is to be applauded for its response to the challenges presented.

Forensic services will continue to stretch professionals, being at the outer edge of our understanding of complex problems and needs and at the interface between NHS, local authority and criminal justice systems. The patients and staff within these services deserve our compassion, understanding and support in ensuring that they are not discriminated against and in some instances demonized or marginalized in their striving for better and improved services.

Those professionals who have taken the time and effort to share their knowledge and insights in this text should be applauded and thanked by those who follow them.

Malcolm Rae

Preface

There can be little doubt that the detailed and specific practice of providing forensic care is sometimes misunderstood or underestimated, even by those who hold associated interests in general mental health care. This situation is often not helped by the sensationalizing of the services and the people being cared for within them by hostile media. The delivery of forensic care does not fall neatly within a series of policies or procedures, nor do forensic services occur in a specific building or centre. Critical to successful practice is the willingness of professionals to adapt roles and functions making good use of their knowledge and experience of practice, their expertise and their ability, and to transfer knowledge and associated authority to the client.

Practising forensic care and providing services, particularly for mentally disordered offenders, is demanding intellectual, physical and psychological work. Those people and services that do this best have self-confidence and yet continually seek to advance their knowledge and skills within demanding clinical situations. They must do so with enthusiasm, balanced with objectivity. It has been the editors' intention to review areas of service provision within the forensic field that reflect the diversity of such services and at the same time identify the common threads which make the practice somewhat unique. Workers in this field have to be prepared to adapt to the expectations of society and the legal, social and institutional environments within which they function. We have been fortunate, we feel, in being able to identify contributors to this text who set the context of care within operational systems. The authors are authorities in their fields; they have worked fastidiously to provide examples of their expertise in affecting practice and to disseminate this information in an unselfish way.

It has been a major aim to stimulate and provide information, to promote further study of this important field and to help colleagues be selective and critical in the application of practice in an area where difficulties are compounded by conflicting expectations and demands.

This textbook is aimed at building on and developing partnerships with those who provide opportunities for people who work in the specialist area to impart their knowledge and also benefit from others' expertise. It is generally hoped that if the aims are met we will encourage people to look at the national workforce that is available to this client group as being part of teams of highly skilled practitioners rather than different tribes of people. The editors wish to thank all those people who have contributed and of course those who work in the background to ensure that the book was able to come to fruition. It is through these people that we can aim to transform forensic services and to deliver our practice through systems that are respected by society.

Merseyside
Liverpool
Manchester
2000

Colin Dale
Tony Thompson
Phil Woods

Chapter One

Overview

Colin Dale   Phil Woods   Tony Thompson

MENTAL HEALTH POLICY DEVELOPMENT AND ITS IMPACT ON FORENSIC MENTAL HEALTH SERVICES

Government policy changes dating back to the 1960s have led to major changes in the configuration of services, with the process of deinstitutionalization leading to large reductions in the traditional inpatient populations in mental health and learning disabilities. Inpatient care now largely takes place in the wards of district general hospital mental health units and hospital admissions tend to be of a shorter duration. Many patients who used to be treated in hospital are now treated in the community, leading to higher levels of acuity in the hospital inpatient population, now largely composed of people with serious and enduring mental illness, such as schizophrenia and mood disorder.

The current government legislative framework includes *The new NHS: modern, dependable* (DoH 1997) which spells out the need for health services to tackle the root causes of ill health and

ensure high standards of health care and quicker treatment. *Modernising social services* (DoH 1998a) highlights three priorities for personal social services: promoting independence, improving protection and raising standards. Both the NHS and Social Services are charged to work more in partnership, to provide integrated services which will improve the quality of life for the population.

In *Modernising mental health services: safe, sound and supportive* (DoH 1998b) the government sets out its strategy for mental health services in England for the new millennium (the policy frameworks for Scotland, Wales and Northern Ireland are set out in separate papers but have fundamentally similar aims and objectives).

Care in the community has been seen to have partially failed because, while it improved the treatment of many people who were mentally ill, it left far too many walking the streets, often at risk to themselves and a nuisance to others. A small but significant minority has been a threat to themselves or others.

The laws on mental health are currently under review (DoH 1999a) and there is no doubt that the current Mental Health Act 1983 reflects a

1

bygone age and is not in tune with modern service delivery. Present legislation is hospital orientated and consequently dated as modern treatment and care arrangements, quite rightly, enable more people who are mentally ill to live in their own homes or community settings rather than in the confines of a hospital ward. Proposals have a particular emphasis on ensuring that who might otherwise be a danger to themselves and others are no longer allowed to refuse to comply with the treatment they need.

Specific developments include 24-hour crisis teams to respond to emergencies, more acute mental health beds, more hostels and supported accommodation, more home treatment teams, more training for all involved in dealing with patients who are mentally ill and access to NHS Direct for 24-hour help and advice. NHS Direct, the 24-hour nurse helpline, already covers 60% of the population and by the end of 2000 the whole of England will have access and be able to receive information on local mental health services (NHS Direct will provide first-line advice about mental health concerns, and, for those who need it, connect to local crisis services or other helplines).

The National Institute for Clinical Excellence and the Clinical Standards Advisory Group were implemented in autumn 1999 to ensure that clear and authoritative guidance is available on the most effective drugs and therapies, together with the development of a National Service Framework for Mental Health (DoH 1999b).

The government has acknowledged that unacceptable variations in performance and practice continue. People with mental health problems often have complex needs which cross traditional organizational boundaries, and substance misuse and/or personality disorder make treatment of mental illness more difficult.

The government strategy seeks to address the issue of bed shortage by ensuring that there are enough beds of the right kind in the right place. This will include 'the whole range including 24-hour staffed beds, acute beds, and secure beds to make sure that pressures do not build up in any one part of the system' (DoH 1998b: 4.14). Over £14.5 million is being made available for an extra

221 secure places in mental health, more than twice the number anticipated in 1999 when initial targets were set.

The government strategy states that patients who present a risk to others sometimes need to be looked after in secure accommodation where they can receive the care and help they need. A shortage of locally available secure beds can mean that some patients are cared for in acute psychiatric wards, further adding to pressures in the system. The government proposes to provide extra secure places to ensure that the whole care system works together to provide 'the right care in the right place at the right time' (DoH 1998b: 4.17).

The government feels that at present, there are too many cases where people who need secure care cannot be found a bed and sometimes remain inappropriately placed in secure wards or prisons for far too long. It believes that the situation is partly a consequence of the continued separation of both commissioning and provision of high security services from the arrangements that apply to other NHS secure mental health services (DoH 1998b: 4.22).

The government has put forward proposals to improve the way that people with a severe personality disorder are managed, particularly in cases where they present a grave risk to the public. Most people in this group who are convicted of offences are sentenced to a term of imprisonment. Some are admitted to a psychiatric hospital if their personality disorder is recognized and judged to be treatable. But the law as it stands means that people with a severe personality disorder may be released at the end of a prison sentence or discharged from hospital even though they still present a significant risk.

There is also a small group of people with severe personality disorder who present a genuine risk but who have not been involved in any criminal offence. This group may benefit from a range of interventions intended to reduce risk but not all are suitable for treatment as patients in hospital settings. These people fall outside the scope of the Mental Health Act 1983 and cannot be detained or required to comply with supervision (Home Office & DoH 1999).

The government is therefore considering proposals to create a new form of reviewable detention where:

◆ the safety of the public is of prime concern
◆ admission to the new regime will not be dependent upon the person having committed an offence, nor whether they are treatable under the terms of the current Mental Health Act
◆ release into the community will depend upon a rigorous assessment that the person no longer poses a grave risk to the public
◆ the regime will comply with the government's obligations under the European Court of Human Rights.

The proposals are likely to require the development of specialist programmes under conditions providing both appropriate security and interventions designed to reduce and manage risk.

The 1999 Health Act (DoH 1999c) has made it legal for health and social services to pool budgets to enable greater partnership in planning and delivering mental health services. In the National Priorities Guidance (DoH 1998c), which is issued to health and local authorities, mental health has for the past 2 years been a shared priority for health and local authorities.

Saving lives: our healthier nation strategy focuses on social inclusion, employment, education, housing and transport. This recognizes the wider social and economic factors of ill health. Mental health has been identified as one of four priority areas for action. It is estimated that 4000 lives could be saved by meeting the national target to reduce deaths from suicide by 20% by 2010 (DoH 1999d).

The Mental Health National Service Framework (DoH 1999b) is one of the government's key initiatives for modernizing mental health services, aimed at helping them to meet the targets in *Our healthier nation* (DoH 1999d). The framework aims to drive up quality and reduce variations by setting national standards to ensure that people with mental health problems receive the services they need regardless of who they are or where they live. Progress will be monitored by NHS regional offices, their social care regional

colleagues and the newly established Commission for Health Improvement.

The National Service Framework (DoH 1999b) is underpinned by a number of central programmes including: information and clinical decision support systems; the NHS research and development programme; initiatives to improve recruitment, retention, training and education of the workforce.

Revised guidance has recently been issued on the streamlined care programme approach as a response to concerns expressed by mental health professionals and requires the integration of the care programme approach and care management (DoH 2000).

The recently introduced Beacons initiative (DoH 1999e), which aims to spotlight leading examples of practice in mental health, primary care and health improvement, has 35 mental health programmes listed although only one forensic initiative. The NHS Beacon services programme aims to celebrate success and spread best practice.

In future, prison health care will be delivered through a formal partnership between the NHS and the Prison Service. The aim will be to provide health-care services to standards comparable to those received in the wider community. The Prison Service will continue to provide primary care in prisons whilst responsibility for secondary and specialist care will rest with the NHS. To reinforce the partnership, a new Prison Health Care Policy Unit and Task Force, jointly accountable to both the Prison Service and the Department of Health, is being established (HM Prison Service & NHSE 1999).

With the shift of responsibility for commissioning of mental health secure services from the High Security Psychiatric Service Commissioning Board to district health authorities, a greater integration of forensic mental health services at all levels is being planned. Each regional health authority was required by April 2000 to have arrangements in place for the commissioning of both medium and high security services. Their strategy must ensure integration of forensic mental health services with general mental health services in a whole-systems approach, to ensure sufficient facilities are provided to enable the smooth progression of patients through the appropriate levels of security. In the longer term this is likely to mean changes in the provision of high security care in particular, as a greater spread of new services is commissioned to meet assessed needs (NHSE 1999).

MULTIDISCIPLINARY TEAMWORK

A fundamental prerequisite for work within forensic services is the availability of effective teamwork at all levels of the service. Successful teamwork, particularly at the level of patient care team, is frequently the difference between effective and ineffective services. Teamwork implies working together with the desirable benefits of cooperation, continuity and a sense of purpose. The work of the team is conducted by a group of people who possess individual expertise, who are responsible for making individual decisions, who hold a common purpose and who meet together to communicate, share and consolidate knowledge on which plans are made, future decisions are influenced and action determined.

Teamwork requires that each member of that team has equal opportunity to influence the work of the team. It may well be that in certain circumstances, an individual's professional responsibility may involve making decisions which affect the work of colleagues.

Successful care and rehabilitation needs to take a broad and comprehensive view of patients' problems. All members of the team have an active role in making the best use of resources available as members will have skills and attributes that go beyond the professional core functions.

The disciplines of medicine, psychology, nursing and social work are seen as core members of the patient care team but the role of other disciplines, who at various times may have significant impact on a patient's care and treatment, should be clarified. Consideration should be given to coopting those disciplines on to a patient care team. The successful operation of a multidisciplinary team depends upon the acceptance of divergent views amongst its members, at the same time resolving them into a broad-based coherent plan of action. Role clarification is a key element in this.

Decision making should be based upon a clear process. It should accept that consensus may not always be possible and that the outcome of this process may depend on a number of variables, such as expertise or professional responsibilities. The decision-making process must be open with all key decisions having multidisciplinary involvement, allowances being made for dissenting voices to be heard and recorded. Each team member's professional practice should be open to challenge and there must be some mechanism whereby an alternative opinion may be sought.

BACKGROUND AND RATIONALE TO THIS TEXT

The critical basis for practice within forensic mental health services has been subjected to particular focus in recent policy initiatives, as well as addressing the many issues in the wake of major inquiries. There is a tremendous increase in initiatives associated with expanding the speciality, including specialist forums, consultant nurses and research activity. The definition of forensic care is sufficiently wide to encompass work in a variety of settings, including the community, with very vulnerable adults who are at risk of becoming involved with the criminal justice system. It therefore requires a high level of complex skills and knowledge, not least in the realm of assessment, planning and management of care.

This sensitive and often high-risk work is undertaken by nurses and others in a complex and rapidly changing context of legislative, governmental and social policy developments. Care of this client group also has a high public and political profile.

The few texts that currently exist on forensic topics tend to take a more theoretical/academic approach to this area. It is felt that a practice-based text, which is grounded in empirical forensic application, will provide clear guidance on tackling core issues in relation to the care and management of this particular client population. Staff and services taxed with providing service delivery systems for this group currently struggle with the paucity of pragmatic advice and direction and it is felt that this text will go some way to fulfilling this particular need.

OVERALL APPROACH

All the chapters draw on available research and evidence and seek to encourage evidence-based practice as a guide to enhancing forensic services. The chapters outline the underlying policy framework, where relevant, as well as reflecting the organizational context for forensic care practice. The practical approach and accessibility of material are intended to allow people to transfer approaches and underpinning knowledge to their own practice arenas.

The text recognizes that practical development of competence in the professions associated with forensic work can be guided and directed by sharing the views of known experts and competent practitioners. One of the text's key strengths is that people who are managing services, and those people who work within them, will be able to recognize the context of everyday work demands.

Chapter Two addresses medicine. Peter Snowden outlines the changing role of the responsible medical officer in the context of interdisciplinary working and compares general and forensic psychiatry. Attributes possessed by forensic psychiatrists are discussed, together with an evaluation of secure units and contemporary trends.

Chapter Three addresses nursing. Colin Dale, Phil Woods and Tony Thompson stress that nurses spend almost all their practice in direct patient contact. They point out that the history of forensic nursing is not well described and that no theoretical framework exists at present which accommodates the core skills and role of the forensic mental health nurse. The authors argue that forensic mental health nursing requires a particular knowledge base, centring on risk management, offending behaviour and the interface with mental disorder.

Chapter Four addresses clinical psychology. John McGinley describes how clinical psychologists have an ethical responsibility to use, where possible, one of the growing number of psychological treatment interventions with proven efficacy. The psychological contributions to the assessment and treatment of personality disorders, anger management, fire-setting, sex offending, addictions, services for women, people with learning disabilities and people with schizophrenia are covered in some detail.

Chapter Five addresses social work. Richard Backhouse discusses how forensic social work is a relatively new profession with its components involving the establishment of a clear social history, involvement with inpatient care planning, keeping patients in contact, predischarge care planning and interagency liaison. Within a forensic setting social workers are engaged in more therapeutic intervention owing to the longer term nature of the patient group.

Chapter Six addresses clinical governance: a framework for quality in forensic mental health care. David Duffy outlines the historical development of quality initiatives in the NHS, culminating in the current government's policy of clinical governance. Details of the policy framework for governance are outlined and a specific example of its application to suicide prevention is detailed. A useful description of one mental health trust's approach to clinical governance is provided.

Chapter Seven addresses evidence-based practice and clinical monitoring. Maggie Clifton and Ros Harvey describe the place of R&D within the NHS, with particular emphasis on clinical interventions and the development of generalizable knowledge for dissemination and public scrutiny. The authors emphasize the need for support systems to maintain the R&D focus and describe how clinicians can discover and apply evidence in practice.

Chapter Eight addresses education and training developments in the context of clinical governance. Tony Thompson, Fran Aiken and Ros Harvey stress that knowledge and skills for clinical governance are about linking the process of learning to the clinical workplace. A high standard of education and training encourages staff to appreciate a greater moral and practical value in their efforts to work with a difficult client group. Organizations have to consider the context of education and training, the goals or intended outcomes of this training and the policies which are affecting the delivery of interprofessional teaching within forensic mental health services.

Chapter Nine addresses risk assessment and management. Phil Woods describes how the assessment and management of risk is an ongoing and evaluative process and risk assessment should incorporate both an actuarial or statistical approach and a clinical approach. A six-point organizational risk management strategy, encompassing organizational, cultural, clinical, employee, environmental and incident-reporting issues, could reduce the chance of potential harm and litigation.

Chapter Ten addresses the reporting and management of incidents. Phil Woods stresses that incidents are important factors, not only when considering the risk an individual poses in the short term but also in the long term. They are also fundamental components of evaluating the service's risk assessment and management strategies. It is vitally important that incident monitoring is maintained on a regular basis and placed within the context of key situational, environmental and demographic variables.

Chapter Eleven addresses the involvement of service users. Nicola Lees and Jeff Withington consider that referral to advocacy does not mean the mental health worker is wrong; on the contrary, the involvement of advocacy lends more power to the therapeutic approach. The greater the involvement, the greater the response and the better the outcome for the patient. The vast majority of professionals have been unwitting contributors to stigma and there is a need to make discrimination against people with mental illness an offence.

Chapter Twelve addresses interpersonal relationships: staff development, awareness and monitoring issues. Colin Dale describes how the development and maintenance of positive interpersonal relationships are critical in the care of patients in forensic psychiatry. Given the psychopathologies and disordered development of many forensic patients, nursing staff in these services are at particular risk of being drawn into damaging relationships. The maintenance of professional boundaries is a key component of the forensic practitioner's role with education and supervision playing a critical role in helping to prepare the staff member and ensure a safe physical and psychological environment.

Chapter Thirteen addresses the application of values in working with patients in forensic mental health settings. Paul Williams and Colin Dale describe the application of six professional values and general positive cultural values to enhance the life experiences of people at risk of poor or negative experiences in forensic services. Examples of the possibilities for the pursuit of social role valorization in forensic mental health settings are discussed and how patients' own values can be divided into those that are positive and should be respected and those that are unacceptable and should not be colluded with. A model is suggested for planning and sustaining professional work in forensic mental health settings that applies a range of values-led approaches.

Chapter Fourteen addresses mental illness. Mike Musker, Phil Woods and Colin Dale discuss how those with mental illnesses are the largest group within forensic mental health services. They have severe and enduring mental illness, are often treatment resistive, and their care and treatment are complex, time consuming and expensive. Psychosocial interventions are proving successful in treating this patient group.

Chapter Fifteen addresses learning disability. Mike Musker describes how there has been a marked reduction in the learning disability population in secure care although there is a continued but reduced need for medium/maximum secure care. There is a high incidence of mental illness and personality disorders amongst those with learning disabilities in forensic services, together with challenging behaviour. The key issues for the future development for this population include local care provision and training

Chapter Sixteen addresses personality disorders. Phil Woods identifies that a high proportion of any forensic mental health population will have a diagnosable personality disorder. There is little evidence, however, of what treatments are effective although current thinking suggests that a focus on interpersonal deficits and behavioural repertoires may be productive. Assessment and treatment have to focus on the reduction of risk and dangerousness in the long term.

Chapter Seventeen addresses women in secure care. Les Storey and Debbie Murdock examine the issues surrounding the care and treatment of women in forensic mental health care. Concerns about the appropriateness of services available to women and dissatisfaction with provision of services in secure environments are described. The criminal justice system, when applied to women who have offended or behaved in a disturbed fashion, appears to use different standards for assessing women from those applied to men. As a result, women often receive harsher sentences for similar offences.

Chapter Eighteen addresses dual diagnosis. Colin Dale discusses the complex interaction between psychopathology and substance use disorders with the incidence of substance abuse amongst forensic populations being especially high. He describes how those with dual diagnosis have higher rates of clinical and social problems including relapse, violence, communicable diseases, hopelessness and non-compliance with treatment. Research amassed over the past 10 years supports a shift to treatment that combines interventions directed simultaneously to both conditions.

Chapter Nineteen addresses clinical supervision. Les Jennings outlines the practice of clinical supervision and describes its purpose. The benefits of supervision to the forensic mental health practitioner are stressed and the various models and key elements of supervision described. The concept of supervision as providing the basis for effective practice is proposed.

Chapter Twenty addresses rehabilitation in practice. Pat Abbott discusses how rehabilitation approaches make an important contribution to the comprehensive treatment and care of those people with serious mental health problems who come into contact with forensic mental health services. A range of approaches is available, although most of the research and practice base is focused upon the needs of people with severe

and enduring mental illness. Rehabilitation approaches are highly compatible with these systematic processes and should be actively integrated into all forensic services, from high security through to the community.

Chapter Twenty One addresses the transition from higher to lower levels of security. Chris Skelly describes how most patients detained in high security hospitals will be discharged via lower levels of security rather than straight into the community. Transfer to lower levels of security often fails and the patient is readmitted to the high security hospital. High security patients have considerable rehabilitation needs, some of which are difficult to address in a high security environment. A number of innovative schemes to assist in the transition to lower levels of security have been developed in high security hospitals, with aftercare and support being beneficial in maintaining the patient at a lower level of security.

Chapter Twenty Two addresses the supervision of the rehabilitated patient in the community. Alan Gilmour and Helen Edment describe the variable services available to meet the diverse needs of mentally disordered offenders in the community. There needs to be considerable coordination of effort within and between agencies to ensure comprehensive support for this population. The care programme approach provides the framework for the systematic planning of community services to support individuals in danger of relapse or recidivism. Supervised discharge and supervision registers provide useful mechanisms for ensuring compliance with treatment. Risk assessment and management, crisis intervention and relapse prevention, assertive follow-up, compliance and engagement are highlighted.

Chapter Twenty Three addresses maintaining a safe environment: security in forensic environments, strategic and operational issues. Colin Dale and Jim Gardner describe how there is a paucity of research and published material informing forensic mental health services on issues of security, with ethical issues being of key importance in any consideration. Security can be achieved in a forensic mental health service by two means: dynamic and passive measures. The role of supervision and monitoring is vital to ensuring that policies and procedures are adhered to whilst clarifying the powers of staff in exercising control over patients.

REFERENCES

Department of Health 1997 The new NHS: modern, dependable. Cm 3807. HMSO, London

Department of Health 1998a Modernising social services: promoting independence, promoting protection, raising standards. Stationery Office, London

Department of Health 1998b Modernising mental health services: safe, sound and supportive. HMSO, London

Department of Health 1998c Modernising health and social services: national priorities guidance, 1999\00–2001\02. HSC1998\159. Department of Health, London

Department of Health 1999a Reform of the Mental Health Act 1983: proposals for consultation. Cm 4480. Stationery Office, London

Department of Health 1999b Mental health national service framework: modern standards and service models. Stationery Office, London

Department of Health 1999c The Health Act. Stationery Office, London

Department of Health 1999d Saving lives: our healthier nation. Stationery Office, London

Department of Health 1999e Beacon learning activity. Stationery Office, London

Department of Health 2000 Effective care co-ordination in mental health services: modernizing the care programme approach: a policy booklet. Stationery Office, London

Her Majesty's Prison Service, National Health Service Executive 1999 The future organisation of prison health care. Stationery Office, London

Home Office, Department of Health 1999 Managing dangerous people with severe personality disorder: proposals for policy development. Stationery Office, London

National Health Service Executive 1999 Specialised commissioning – high and medium security psychiatric services. HSC 99\141. HMSO, London

FURTHER READING

Department of Health 1998 Modernising mental health services: safe, sound and supportive. HMSO, London

Department of Health 1999 Reform of the Mental Health Act 1983: proposals for consultation. Cm 4480. Stationery Office, London

Department of Health 1999 Mental health national service framework: modern standards and service models. Stationery Office, London

Nolan P 1993 A history of mental health nursing. Chapman and Hall, London

Chapter Two

Medicine

Peter Snowden

INTRODUCTION

This chapter explores the professional contribution of the forensic psychiatrist within the multidisciplinary team. The development of the forensic psychiatrist's role, from the Prison Service to the medium secure services, training and the role of the Responsible Medical Officer all form components of the discussion.

The work of a forensic psychiatrist is, in many ways, not that different from that of a psychiatrist in other branches of psychiatry, working as part of a multiprofessional team to meet wide-ranging patient needs. Psychiatrists are generally required to be leaders of these teams, yet it is vital that they value the contribution of other professions, whatever the level of experience. In essence, the task of the psychiatrist is to provide proper diagnosis, appropriate treatment and, when ready, rehabilitation of the patient back into the community.

There are, of course, differences between forensic and general psychiatry practice, the former having a particular focus on the risk of harm to others. A balance needs to be struck between security and therapy in order to protect the patient, other patients and the public (which includes members of staff). Whilst primarily this task is undertaken by nurses working in the secure units, the forensic psychiatrist has a part to play in fine-tuning this process. The correct setting of the therapy and security tasks is difficult to achieve, as it is a dynamic process influenced by both internal forces (i.e. patient mix, staffing issues) and external expectations. Moreover, medical team members spend more time off the wards and outside the secure hospital unit. Therefore, by 'looking in' from outside, the forensic psychiatrist should be robust in questioning security practices.

THE FORENSIC PSYCHIATRIST

Forensic psychiatrists work predominantly within medium secure units and the high security (special) hospitals (Chiswick & Cope 1995). Medical services in high security hospitals are primarily inpatient based; there is a mixture of forensic psychiatrists and others who have special skills to meet the particular needs of the patient group, such as consultants in rehabilitation psychiatry or learning disability. Those based in medium secure units, although providing inpatient treatment, also hold outpatient clinics in hospitals, prisons and in some cases probation offices. The majority of patients are seen after referral by the courts, lawyers, the Probation Service or prison doctors. Patients are also referred by other psychiatrists, sometimes general practitioners, and also by other agencies, such as Social Services.

Forensic psychiatrists spend a considerable amount of their time in prisons, assessing remand and convicted prisoners. Requests may be for assessment from the prison doctor, advice in relation to a prisoner posing management problems or for reports to court and parole boards. The most common diagnoses of patients admitted to secure units are schizophrenia, delusional disorders and personality disorders. Many have had prior contact with mental health services.

Chiswick (1995), in the introduction to his book on practical forensic psychiatry, described eight personal attributes that a successful forensic psychiatrist needs.

◆ Good clinical skills
◆ Natural curiosity
◆ Tolerance for difficult patients
◆ Balanced attitudes towards offenders
◆ Clear thinking and clear speaking
◆ Attention to detail
◆ Capacity to lead a clinical team
◆ Good self-organization and energy.

Forensic psychiatrist training

The training of psychiatrists at basic senior house officer level may include a placement in a secure unit but there is no basic requirement for all doctors at this training grade to have experience in forensic psychiatry. After successful membership examination of the Royal College of Psychiatrists, those who wish to train in forensic psychiatry apply for a speciality registrar post on a forensic psychiatry training scheme. Most training schemes offer experience in medium and high security units; some also provide experience in adolescent forensic psychiatry, rehabilitation psychiatry and psychotherapy.

The trained forensic psychiatrist should:

◆ be able to take on the full clinical and managerial charge of forensic clinical services in several settings, including outpatients, inpatients, security and juvenile services
◆ have expert knowledge of all the relevant literature
◆ be able to teach the skills of forensic psychiatry to medical and other professional staff
◆ be able to conduct research.

Of course, there is always the danger that, having such a wide variety of tasks, one achieves none in a satisfactory manner.

DEVELOPMENT OF SERVICES AND THE MEDICAL CONTRIBUTION

The first purpose-built hospital unit for offenders opened in 1816 at the Bethlem Hospital. In 1863 Broadmoor Hospital opened to deal with overcrowding in various asylums, including Bethlem Hospital. By the 1930s there were three special hospitals to serve England and Wales: Broadmoor, Rampton and Moss Side. However, the speciality of forensic psychiatry did not exist at this time. The influential pioneers in criminological psychiatry, as it was then known, worked in the Prison Service.

The determinists, influenced by psychoanalytical thinking, argued that punishment was not an adequate response to crime. Dr Hamblin Smith, a prison medical officer, argued that psychoanalysis could provide both understanding and treatment (Bowden 1990). Forensic psychotherapy reached a peak during this period with the opening of a psychopathic clinic in central London, the forerunner of the Portman Clinic. However, until recently there has been little development of this important speciality outside the Portman Clinic. Within the Prison Service the situation was similar. In the 1930s Dr de Bargue Hubert, a hospital psychiatrist with experience working in prisons, suggested that special prison units should be developed to provide psychotherapy for selected prisoners. There was little enthusiasm for this and Grendon Prison did not open until 1962.

In 1951, Dr Trevor Gibben was the first forensic psychiatry academic appointment; based at the Maudsley Hospital, he was important in the development of forensic psychiatry. Many notable individuals based in this department, such as Dr Peter Scott and Professor John Gunn, went on to train many of the forensic psychiatrists in practice today.

Until the mid 1970s the treatment and management of mentally disordered offenders were undertaken in prisons or high security hospitals. However, a service gap had begun to appear by this time between the prisons and the high security hospitals, as many psychiatric hospitals were opening their secure wards. Moreover, Bowden (1975) showed that hospitals without a locked ward were less likely to admit offenders. Thus the system became blocked and mentally abnormal offenders were wrongly paced within the prisons and high security hospitals. To help deal with this, in the mid 1960s the Government reviewed the prison health-care system, recommending the establishment of joint appointed consultant forensic psychiatrists between the NHS and the prisons. Eventually there were eight such appointments and amongst this group were the medical leaders who developed the medium secure forensic services of today.

Eventually forensic psychiatry developed in response to the tragedies perpetrated by mentally disordered offenders. Modern forensic psychiatry services owe a great deal to the notorious case of Graham Young. As a schoolboy he was detained in Broadmoor, following conviction for the administration of noxious substances to family members and a school acquaintance. His supervision was poor after discharge from Broadmoor and he reoffended in a similar manner, this time with fatal consequences. Following the public outcry and on the day of his conviction for these crimes, the Home Secretary announced the establishment of two committees. The first was a working party under the chairmanship of Sir Carl Aarvold, the Recorder of London. This group reviewed the discharge and supervision of restricted patients (section 65 of the 1959 Mental Health Act). One of the recommendations was the establishment of a non-statutory, non-executive body to give advice to the Minister of State in cases where it is difficult to predict the likelihood of serious offending. The Advisory Board, as it is now known, is chaired by a judge. On the Board there is a Director of Social Services, Chief Probation Officer, a lawyer, two forensic psychiatrists and two members with a criminal justice system background, currently an ex-senior police officer and a parole board member. No other mental health professional is involved in the work of this group.

The second committee was chaired by Lord Bulter of Saffron Walden. This distinguished committee reviewed mental health services for mentally disordered offenders. The Butler Report (Home Office & DHSS 1975) recommended the setting up of regional secure units which were to be the base of new forensic psychiatry services; they would link with the high security hospitals, other psychiatric facilities, prisons and Probation Service. This was just what the small group of jointly appointed forensic psychiatrists had been waiting for. Outside the prisons they had no secure inpatient hospital base. It was through the enthusiasm and energy of this group of product champions that forensic psychiatry developed from the mid 1970s (Snowden 1985).

Most health regions opened converted hospital wards as interim secure units, whilst the purpose-built medium secure units were developed. From the outset a different model developed from that which existed in the high security hospitals. These early charismatic medical leaders realized that a multidisciplinary approach was essential. Thus, a health-based staffing model was chosen, with nurses, occupational therapists, psychologists and social workers. These were innovative services and managing offenders in a local secure environment was a new endeavour. The strategies and approaches were unclear, as by this period many of the skills of managing difficult and violent patients in locked wards had been lost. It became evident that for interim secure units to function effectively, there had to be close links with the Probation Service, the Prison Service and the courts.

Because of the nature and risks of some of these cases, many when discharged would need to be followed up by the forensic service. This required a dedicated forensic community team to be developed, with a community psychiatric nurse, social worker and consultant. The experience gained in running these units was helpful in highlighting and solving the problems surrounding the referral and assessment process, admission criteria, ward policy (in particular the balance between security and therapy) and discharge. There was an informal networking arrangement between these first medium secure units, which led to a similar approach being adopted in these new services.

One of the most significant changes in practice exemplified by these units was the assessment process, which was undertaken by the team which at a minimum comprised a doctor and nurse. The nurse lead on the appropriateness of admission to the interim secure unit in terms of security, risk, patient mix and ward milieu whilst the doctor focused on diagnosis, classification in terms of the mental health legislation, the link between offending and the crime and the need for inpatient hospital treatment.

Most of those referred were offenders on prison remand. There was a second small group of offenders, referred by the high security hospitals for rehabilitation at lower levels of security, and some difficult-to-manage non-offenders who were inpatients in open psychiatric facilities. This team-based admission approach was in stark contrast to that which existed in general psychiatry, where the consultant would telephone the ward to inform nurses of an impending admission! This team approach was further developed with inpatients, though not surprisingly there were tensions from time to time in relation to the management of individual cases. For example, there could be disagreements over continuation of the inpatient stay, i.e. the consultant disagreeing with nurses over the return of a patient to prison, or the degree of leave that a patient should be granted. These disputes arose out of the role of the consultant as a clinician and member of a clinical team and the responsibilities inherent in the status of Responsible Medical Officer (RMO), as almost all patients are detained.

THE RESPONSIBLE MEDICAL OFFICER

In relation to a patient detained under part II (civil) or part III (criminal) of the 1983 Mental Health Act, the Responsible Medical Officer (RMO) is the registered medical practitioner in charge of the patient. This is usually the patient's consultant but the Mental Health Act 1983 does not specify that it must be the consultant and, for example, the RMO could be an associate specialist.

Specific powers and duties are set out under the Mental Health Act 1983 which include the power to grant and revoke leave of absence for certain patients (such as offenders detained under a hospital order – section 37), make statutory reports for the renewal of detention in hospital and bar the discharge of certain patients. The functions of the RMO in relation to patient treatment are not specified in the Mental Health Act 1983. The RMO is described as the doctor 'in charge of the treatment of the patient' and 'medical treatment' includes care, habilitation and rehabilitation 'under medical supervision' (section 145(1)).

Gostin (1986) was cautious in his interpretation of the RMO role. He suggested that it was never intended that the role conferred any specific powers outside the powers and accountability expressly provided in the Mental Health Act 1983. Gostin also highlighted the separate duty of care owed by each individual providing the treatment, including non-medical professionals. Nevertheless, even though there is nothing in the Mental Health Act 1983 which specifies where responsibility for the patient primarily resides or in whom accountability for every treatment is vested, in practice it is seen as resting on the shoulders of the RMO. It is not possible for anyone other than a doctor to take on the RMO role within current legislation. In part because of the inherent leadership qualities of the original product champions but also because of the RMO responsibilities, the early multidisciplinary teams were led by the forensic consultant.

The report of the Committee of Inquiry into the personality disorder unit at Ashworth Hospital (DoH 1999: 326), chaired by Peter Fallon QC, gives the most up-to-date review of the status of the RMO and the position of the consultant in a multidisciplinary team. It states:

> *The consultant in charge of the patients' care should be the leader of the clinical team, even though he delegates the chair at meetings from time to time to another member of the team. As a consultant and RMO, he has the responsibility for the patient. We recognize that RMOs exercise very considerable powers over patients' lives. Some psychiatrists exercise their powers and duties in a very personal manner. Others effectively share with colleagues in their multidisciplinary team, although they retain the personal accountability for treatment. The principle that one person is in ultimate clinical charge of an individual patient, even if care is provided by a multidisciplinary team, is well rooted in the NHS, and is sound.*

In forensic psychiatry, the role of the RMO means that the consultant is expected to take ultimate responsibility for decisions regarding greater freedom for the patient, transfer to lower levels of security or recommendations for discharge. For mental health review tribunals the RMO must provide a report, which should be informed by the views of other disciplines and where there is

disagreement, the report should cover this. The RMO must write to the Home Office Mental Health Unit for any request for transfer, leave or discharge of a restricted patient, but this should be supplemented by reports from other disciplines and team meeting minutes.

RESPONSIBILITIES OF THE CONSULTANT

The first responsibility of any consultant is as a doctor to his or her patient, in a confidential relationship within the limitations defined by law and guidance on practice, such as that issued by the General Medical Council as part of its statutory function under the 1983 Medical Act (UK). Within this framework the Royal College of Psychiatrists (1996a) issued a council report setting out the responsibilities of the consultant psychiatrist. It states:

> *Good communication and listening skills are essential, and consultants must ensure that their patients are encouraged to talk openly, kept informed about salient features of their illness, and are made fully aware of the benefits of and any disadvantages or potentially harmful effects inherent in the proposed treatment.*

This report goes on to list a number of other responsibilities.

Confidentiality

Consultants must preserve the confidentiality of personal information but clearly, within a multi-professional team approach, information will be shared. It is important for the doctor to make the boundaries of information sharing clear to the patient.

Ethical standards

Consultants must maintain the ethical standards of the profession as agreed by the appropriate professional bodies which have the power to discipline professional misbehaviour.

Appropriate and effective treatment

Consultants must at all times act according to their professional conscience and, in their opinion, in the best interests of the patient and undertake to deliver the most appropriate and effective evidence-based treatment currently available. Though some treatments do not at this stage have a sufficient evidence base, their use is supported by informed clinical opinion.

Management of resources

If it can be justified, it is the duty of a consultant to challenge the level of available resources. Conflict may arise in relation to use of resources, particularly with regard to medical staff.

Autonomy of patient care

The Medical Act 1983 gives registered medical practitioners legal powers to provide the public with a professional service. The view of such practitioners is the ultimate medical opinion. Consultants are responsible to their employers in all matters except clinical professional standards and responsibilities, the clinical needs of the patient and the appropriate care required. The consultant can delegate to other professionals the responsibilities of diagnosis and treatment but these responsibilities cannot be abrogated.

Responsibility for care

Consultants should work within the care programme approach framework, as part of a team, and should ensure that all other appropriate agencies are involved. Effective treatment requires a well-functioning multidisciplinary team. This implies the consultant contributing to the leadership of the team dealing with clinical problems and accepting the responsibilities of leadership. For forensic psychiatry, leadership should not be viewed as a right; it should be earned and

consistently worked on. Effective multidisciplinary work cannot be undertaken where there are unresolved issues around leadership.

MULTIDISCIPLINARY FUNCTIONING

The multidisciplinary team (MDT) has been described as 'a group of colleagues acknowledging a common involvement in the care and treatment of a particular patient' (Royal Commission 1979). Cordess, in an introduction to the MDT in his book on forensic psychotherapy, states:

> *The subject of the MDT is not necessarily one which generates wide enthusiasm or excitement; rather, dissatisfaction is frequently expressed about how teams operate and a range of criticisms are to be heard. The issues raised by interdisciplinary and multidisciplinary work are, indeed, frequently, painful and potentially divisive, involving as they do our place within an ensemble or group. Matters of hierarchy, status, leadership, and power – and its abuse – and the necessary demarcation and maintenance of personal and professional boundaries are not easy: they require much thought, effort, and continuing vigilance if the team is to function as an integrated whole. (Cordess 1996: 97–8)*

Multidisciplinary functioning has lacked clarity and has been liable to different interpretation, depending on the perspective of the particular discipline. Teamwork between disciplines in managerial teams should not be confused with clinical team functioning. It should be possible for management issues to be resolved jointly through discussion between disciplines, if of equal standing. The same system cannot be applied in clinical matters. Effective teamwork requires a commitment from all involved in the interest of the patient. Although one cannot legislate on how different disciplines relate to each other, perhaps disputes have arisen because there has not been an investment in the development of open and transparent 'rules of engagement', through operational policies. Many secure units now have agreed policy documents on multidisciplinary functioning so that tensions and difficulties are faced and dealt with.

The Royal College of Psychiatrists (1996a) states:

> *The consultant represents ultimate medical authority within the hospital service for patients in his or her care. There are no senior medical opinions that can override a medical opinion held at this level (with the exception of a Second Opinion doctor appointed by the Mental Health Act Commission) ... each doctor (consultant) must formulate his or her own opinion, whether assisted in this process by others or not, and the legal, ethical, diagnostic and prescriptive responsibilities of the medical profession cannot be delegated to a multidisciplinary group when treating the patient. Multidisciplinary functioning in this context, from the medical point of view, is a process of consultation, the final decision resting with the consultant on matters where he or she has the ultimate responsibility, including the prescription of medication ... in addition, it is likely that the consultant will be the most long-standing and permanent member of the team, and as such, will be able to ensure continuity of care, and offer a long term view of the patient.*

However, leadership should be viewed as specific to the task and leadership roles can move to other members of the team, when appropriate to the work in hand. In the care programme approach process, each qualified member of the team is allocated responsibilities. The key worker role means that in a healthy team the leadership tasks may shift from one person to another as different issues are discussed. This sort of approach should prevent medical and diagnostic issues taking precedence over personal and social matters. The consultant here is facilitator, coordinator and progress chaser.

Good communication within the team is essential for high-quality patient care and this is a requirement for all disciplines, including the consultant. An autocratic style of leadership will not encourage good communication and will discourage the valuable contributions of the other professions. Time should be set aside for sharing and pooling information. True clinical multidisciplinary working is the most effective and efficient method of providing appropriate treatment and care of the patient.

ASSESSMENT AND CLINICAL MANAGEMENT OF RISK OF HARM TO OTHERS

There is no clinical matter that exemplifies the importance of teamwork and interagency cooperation more than the assessment and management of risk. In forensic psychiatry the assessment of risk to others and its management is an integral part of clinical practice (Royal College of Psychiatrists 1996b). Risk assessment is not a task for one person alone. Each discipline has a role and responsibility to collect the information against which risk is assessed. Information must be shared, as must the outcome of the assessment, and all members of the team will need to be clear about their role in managing risk.

Some forensic cases, because of the nature of the risks, can be very worrying and stressful to manage. Teamwork in these cases requires professionals to look after each other, in terms of support and advice, and to protect team members so that they are not themselves put at risk. A properly functioning team that cares for the patient should care for the team members too.

COMMUNITY MANAGEMENT OF HIGH-RISK PATIENTS

The majority of medium secure units follow up some of the high-risk patients discharged to the community. Usually these are the high-risk patients subject to a restriction order (section 37/41 of the 1983 Mental Health Act), who are discharged into the community. These forensic community teams include the forensic consultant and other members of the medical team: the community forensic nurse and often a forensic social worker or sometimes a local authority social worker or probation officer.

For conditionally discharged patients there are statutory responsibilities for medical and social supervision. Though community psychiatric nurses play an important part in the management of these cases in the community, they have no statutory responsibilities. However, it is important for the medical supervisor to include information from the community psychiatric nurse when reporting to the Home Office Mental Health Unit.

The difficulties in managing such patients in the community are highlighted in the Luke Warm Luke Mental Health Inquiry (Baroness Scotland of Asthal et al 1998). The staff involved in managing and supervising such cases must meet together, have adequate experience and training and be clear about their respective tasks. Prins (1990) describes the intrusive style of management necessary to safely supervise such patients. He suggests that (medical and social) supervisors (and this is equally true for community psychiatric nurses) should be prepared to ask the uncomfortable questions and should consider the following.

◆ Have past precipitants and stresses been removed?
◆ How accurately can the offender patient's current capacity for coping with provocation be assessed?
◆ For sex offenders in particular, what clues are available as to the offender patient's self-image?
◆ Are the circumstances of the index offence understood and can trigger factors and precipitants be recognized?
◆ Are the risks general or specific?
◆ Is the patient complying with treatment?
◆ Is use of alcohol and illicit drugs an issue?

THE BLAME CULTURE

All psychiatrists, but in particular forensic psychiatrists, are becoming increasingly bound by guidelines and codes of practice, many of which are central government responses to tragedies perpetrated by patients. The tiered care programme approach, supervision register, supervised discharge and the debate about compulsory treatment in the community are all responses to such catastrophes.

The Zito Trust was established in 1994 followed the killing of Jonathan Zito by Christopher Clunis. Many psychiatrists sympathize with the concerns expressed by the Zito Trust in relation to homicides perpetrated by mentally disordered individuals. However, the focus on tragedies, rather than successes, coupled with mandatory homicide inquiries in every case of killing perpetrated by such individuals who are in contact with mental health services, has thrown forensic psychiatry into the spotlight. Clinical risks can never be reduced to zero and mistakes are bound to occur. The lessons of the homicide inquiries are already clear (Amos et al 1999).

◆ Non-compliance and inappropriate treatment environments
◆ Poor communication between members of the multidisciplinary team and between other agencies and family members
◆ Not seeing enough of the patient
◆ Inadeqate risk assessment
◆ Inadequate knowledge of the Mental Health Act 1983

However, the media attention paid to violence by the mentally disordered stigmatizes the mentally ill and those who work with them. This working environment encourages defensive practice, particularly for consultant decision making. It is hoped that there will be a change in the mandatory nature of inquiries into serious untoward incidents. The most recent report by the National Confidential Inquiry into Suicide and Homicide by People with Mental Illness (Appleby et al 1999) suggests that mandatory inquiries are not the best vehicle from which to learn lessons. The report recommends a new universal and simple system of documentation to be used for:

◆ clinical risk assessment
◆ allocation to care under the care programme approach according to level of risk
◆ transfer of information between services.

CONCLUSION

This chapter has highlighted the fact that the role and function of the forensic psychiatrist are changing. The changes are making demands on the way in which psychiatrists are being prepared and upon expectations associated with public and professional accountability.

The evolution of service developments has been discussed and this has shown how recent developments have their roots in past endeavours. The advent of clinical governance has meant that the responsibilities placed upon clinical specialists are being reinforced. The role of medical leadership is now seen in the light of national standards and a clear evidence base for their practice. The importance of interdisciplinary working has been recognized but also its limitations if not undertaken with clarity of role contribution.

Risk management once again forms the anchor which ties the individual contribution of the forensic psychiatrist to the overall competence of the care team. The potential of the care management approach, seen in the light of transfer of information between services, should help services to avoid adverse reports, reviews and inquiries.

REFERENCES

Amos T, Appleby L, Shaw J 1999 Homicide and mental disorder. Risk Management February: 20–22

Appleby L, Shaw J, Amos T, McDonnell R 1999 Safer services: national confidential inquiry into suicide and homicide by people with mental illness. Department of Health, London

Baroness Scotland of Asthal, Kelly H, Devaux M 1998 The report of the Luke Warm Luke mental health inquiry. Lambeth, Southwark and Lewisham Health Authority, London

Bowden P 1975 Liberty and psychiatry. British Medical Journal ii: 94–96

Bowden P 1990 Pioneers in forensic psychiatry. Maurice Hamblin Smith: the psychoanalytic panacea. Journal of Forensic Psychiatry 1(1): 103–113

Chiswick D 1995 Introduction. In: Chiswick D, Cope R (eds) Practical forensic psychiatry. Gaskell, London, ch 1, pp 1–13

Chiswick D, Cope R (eds) 1995 Practical forensic psychiatry. Gaskell, London

Cordess C 1996 The multi-disciplinary team. In: Cordess C, Cox M (eds) Forensic psychotherapy: crime, psychodynamics and the offender patient. Jessica Kingsley, London

Department of Health 1999 Report of the committee of inquiry into the personality disorder unit, Ashworth Hospital. Volume 1. Cm 4194-II. Stationery Office, London

Gostin L 1986 Mental health services: law and practice. Shaw & Sons, London

Home Office & Department of Health and Social Security 1975 Report of the committee on mentally abnormal offenders (Butler Report). Cm 6244. HMSO, London

Prins H 1990 Some observations on the supervision of dangerous offender patients. British Journal of Psychiatry 156: 157–162

Royal College of Psychiatrists 1996a The responsibilities of consultant psychiatrists: revised statement. Council report CR 51. Royal College of Psychiatrists, London

Royal College of Psychiatrists 1996b Assessment and clinical management of risk of harm to other people. Council report CR 53. Royal College of Psychiatrists, London

Royal Commission 1979 Royal commission on the National Health Service. HMSO, London

Snowden P 1985 A survey of the regional secure unit programme. British Journal of Psychiatry 147: 499–507

FURTHER READING

Chiswick D, Cope R (eds) 1995 Practical forensic psychiatry. Gaskell, London

Cordess C, Cox M (eds) 1996 Forensic psychotherapy: crime, psychodynamics and the offender patient. Jessica Kingsley, London

Chapter Three

Nursing

Colin Dale   Phil Woods   Tony Thompson

INTRODUCTION

Forensic mental health nursing occurs within a broad range of forensic mental health settings from the community through medium secure units to high security hospitals and prisons, court liaison schemes, forensic learning disability and adolescent services. Nurses are the people who spend almost all their practice in direct patient contact. Apart from the risk of violence from some patients, they are also subject to an overwhelming emotional burden as a consequence of the intensity of nurse–patient interaction. Cordess (1996) indicates that the time has clearly come for due recognition of the crucially important, if not primary place that forensic mental health nursing plays in good forensic mental health care.

Beds specializing in secure care for mentally disordered offenders have increased significantly over the past 10 years (DoH 1999) and consequently nursing in secure care is likely to be a significant and constant feature of provision for these groups.

The Secure Environments Project (UKCC & University of Central Lancashire 1999) found that caring for those deemed dangerously mentally disordered is a long-standing public policy problem and that the problems in secure care are exacerbated by lack of flow in general psychiatric services.

Nurses working in secure environments continue to care for a predominantly young male population, where the majority of patients are diagnosed as having a mental illness, with personality disorders being another significant group (DoH 1999). Amongst current admissions, the largest single group are those with histories of violence against the person whilst patients with sexual offences have increased threefold in the past 10 years. Maden et al (1995) found that it was difficult to distinguish between the range of clinical problems and treatment needs of individuals with different diagnoses and different levels of security. Patients in these populations have extremely complex health, social, psychological and forensic backgrounds, all of which directly impact on their nursing care on a day-to-day basis.

The history of nursing within these services is not well described during its early period and has led some authors (McCourt 1999, Topping-Morris 1992) to suggest a history which only dates back as far as the mid 1980s, coinciding with the introduction of the regional secure unit programme. It is suggested here, however, that there were three phases of development: an initial inert stage, when the work largely took place within large high security hospitals that were shrouded in secrecy (1863–1985); a stage of awakening, that commenced with new services being developed and nurses being eager to share their experiences in a descriptive way (1985–95); and a more recent empirical stage, when evidence is beginning to emerge from individual research endeavours from PhDs and organizational examination in terms of evidence-based practice and clinical governance (1995 to date).

Forensic mental health nursing, although not a specific title, has a history intrinsically linked with generic mental health nursing. Care has been provided by nurses in controlled environments since Bedlam (Tarbuck 1994). Its history has been traced as a unique thread through the developments of Broadmoor, Rampton and Ashworth special hospitals, through to the foundation of the regional secure unit (Topping-Morris 1992).

No theoretical framework exists at present which accommodates the core skills and role of the forensic mental health nurse but there is extensive work ongoing to try to understand this. According to Aiyegbusi (1998), a coherent theoretical framework necessarily needs definition, in light of the psychically complex and disturbing situations nurses can find themselves in when attempting to work therapeutically with patients whose internal working models for relationships may be grossly disturbed, on account of their formative developmental experiences. The feelings, attitudes and behaviour of nurses risk compromise by the very nature of the interpersonal transactions that are currently inherent in their role functions.

Killian & Clark (1996) began to explore some of the more complex interpersonal issues associated with nursing in forensic mental health services. These authors describe the challenges associated with applying humanistic interventions, instead of more mechanistic ones, in forensic mental health nursing:

The exchange of physical boundaries for the security provided by relationships that patients develop with nurses places a large demand upon nursing staff. They have to provide emotional and practical (physical) containment whilst allowing at the same time for optimum conditions of therapeutic interaction.

Further, they observe that mainly, nurses have to find the right balance between their custodial and more clinical roles for themselves. Kitchener et al (1992) identified that conflict and ambiguity associated with forensic nurses' therapeutic and controlling roles were common problems. This chapter will bring together key aspects of this literature.

DEMOGRAPHY

Within the health sector, no central statistics are held on the numbers of nurses employed to work specifically within secure environments. Indeed, the actual number of units operating as secure environments is not known, as the number of low secure units varies considerably from definition and function and the same unit can be variously described as an intensive care unit, a high dependency unit or a low security unit, depending on who is asked the question and who does the questioning. A possible determinant could be whether the nursing staff receive the lead payment available to staff who work in secure settings; another approach could be to determine whether patients are held at the unit under sections of the 1983 Mental Health Act and are therefore not allowed to leave the unit.

The UKCC & University of Central Lancashire (1999) Secure Environments Project identified four high security hospitals in the UK, 38 medium secure units and 96 low secure units. The high security and medium secure services can be relied upon, with some confidence, and this is verified by publications such as the Rampton *Forensic directory* (Rampton Hospital Authority 1998). The number for low secure units is less reliable and was achieved by personal contact with the eight regional offices of the NHSE and health departments of Wales, Scotland and Northern Ireland.

Rough 'guestimates' of nurse staffing would therefore be approximately 3000 nurses in high security (1800 qualified, 1200 unqualified); 2280 in medium secure, based on an average of 60 nurses per unit (1368 qualified, 912 unqualified); and 3840 in low secure, based on an average of 40 nurses per unit (2304 qualified, 1536 unqualified). This would give a total of 9120 nurses (5472 qualified, 3648 unqualified). All figures are estimated on a grade mix of 60% qualified staff and 40% unqualified staff.

In the 161 prisons in England and Wales there are known to be 879 (53.2%) registered nurses, 288 (17.4%) registered nurses employed as health care officers and 486 (29.4%) non-nurse qualified health care officers employed within the various health centres. Scotland employs a 100% registered nurse workforce (161) in its 18 prisons and Northern Ireland 20 (64.5%) registered nurses and 11 (35.5%) non-nurse qualified health care officers (UKCC & University of Central Lancashire 1999).

DEFINITIONS

Petryshen (1981: 26) defined forensic mental health nursing as the 'application of psychiatric knowledge to the provision of mental health care to the mentally disordered offender'. Later Morrison & Burnard (1992) described it as 'a specialist branch of psychiatric nursing'. Peternelj-Taylor & Hufft (1997: 772) define the speciality as:

> ... the integration of mental health nursing philosophy and practice, within a socio-cultural context that includes the criminal justice system, to provide comprehensive care to individual clients, their families, and their communities.

ROLE

According to Kettles & Robinson (2000), little has been written on the nature and role of the

forensic mental health nurse, apart from speculative accounts lacking any empirical basis. Within their text (Robinson & Kettles 2000) they bring together an international literature on the research and empirical base on the role of the forensic mental health nurse. To date, this is the most comprehensive text on this topic and the reader is directed to this.

McCourt (1999) presents five concepts that represent one impression of current thinking on the role of the forensic mental health nurse: risk management; the use of self; the therapeutic appreciation of control in nursing; nursing interventions; and social balance.

Nurses have the role of regular and random searching of a patient's personal, living and working environment; the control of visitors (family and professional); escorting patients; random urinalysis for illicit substances; and constant observation of patients deemed a risk to themselves or others. Watson & Kirby (2000) indicate that nurses must develop a range of interpersonal skills which enable them to carry out these procedures in a caring, professional way. Consequently role conflict in mental health nursing is brought into stark relief when considering issues in secure care.

SKILLS

Aiyegbusi (1998) suggests that forensic mental health nursing is predominantly concerned with interpersonal relationships with patients and has its primary base in their social environment. It is for these reasons that the patients' developmental experiences are of such immediate concern to nursing. It is noted that nurses are the most likely targets of interpersonal violence by patients, followed by fellow patients, and this is consistently reported in research studies about risk, violence and assaultiveness. The ability to establish a therapeutic relationship is one of the most important competencies, as the nurse–patient relationship affects every aspect of the nursing process and the quality of care given. Swinton (2000: 113) states that:

> In order to offer effective care which is re-humanising rather than de-humanising, it is crucial that forensic

nurses have a clear perception as to the full extent of their role. ... Forensic nurses are called upon to care for people who have committed acts that are often horrific, frightening, repulsive and extremely difficult for most people to understand or identify with. They are frequently called upon to offer care to patients whose aggressive and unpredictable behaviour means that the primary therapeutic goal may be to develop and maintain some kind of workable equilibrium.

Swinton & Boyd (2000: 136) indicate that forensic mental health nurses are caught in a dilemma:

On the one hand, they are faced with the difficult reality of having to respect the personhood of individuals who show little respect for themselves or for others; who are frequently aggressive and violent, sometimes dishonest, often deceitful; and who may appear to have little or no remorse for the antisocial acts they may have perpetrated. On the other hand, their professional role means that it is not possible for them to offer any kind of meaningful nursing care if they do not or cannot respect the personhood of the other.

The balance between security and therapy, often referred to as 'custody and caring', is a particular concern and dominant theme within the forensic mental health nursing literature and is covered in some detail in Chapter 23.

Niskala (1986) identified 13 core skills required by forensic mental health nurses. Of these, the most important were: maintaining security; communicating effectively; performing the nursing process; and maintaining the professional role. The least important were thought to be: administration; research skills; and the ability to teach. The remaining skills were: maintaining records; counselling; planning and participating in groups; planning and participating in programmes; diagnostic and treatment procedures; and psychiatric nursing approaches. Peternelj-Taylor (2000) describes the characteristics of the forensic mental health nurse as being:

◆ respect and dignity for another human being, no matter how horrific the crime
◆ role modelling by teaching prosocial values

◆ excellent listening and assessment skills
◆ being flexible and being able to adapt therapy to the individual
◆ believing people can change
◆ self-awareness of one's own values and belief systems
◆ confidence in one's own abilities
◆ enriched understanding of subcultures
◆ excellent report-writing skills
◆ being able to recognize one's limitations
◆ ability to motivate change
◆ assertiveness
◆ non-judgemental attitude
◆ maturity
◆ life experiences.

The State Hospital at Carstairs has developed competences for maintaining a safe environment, utilized for all grades of nurses (C Watson, unpublished work, 1999), which have been validated as S/NVQ units by SCOTVEC. The areas covered by the competences include:

◆ fire searching, escorting, visitor control
◆ risk assessment and management
◆ assessment and management of dangerousness
◆ prevention and management of aggression
◆ observation, communication
◆ management of hostage and other security breaches.

Occupational standards have also been developed for delivering care and treatment, including:

◆ anger management
◆ offence-related work
◆ reasoning and rehabilitation/moral reasoning and empathy
◆ social skills training
◆ psychoeducation
◆ psychotherapies, counselling, psychosocial interventions.

The UKCC & University of Central Lancashire (1999) Secure Environments Project used a variety of methods (focus groups, interviews and questionnaires) to identify a number of key skills for staff. These were primarily attributed to relationships, boundaries, communication and counselling and more specifically:

- safety and security
- assessment and observation, including risk assessment and management
- management of violence and aggression, control and restraint, deescalation techniques
- therapies and treatments, including cognitive-behavioural therapy and psychosocial interventions
- knowledge of offending behaviour and appropriate legislation
- report writing
- jail craft
- practical skills, including primary health care, first aid and practice nursing.

The UKCC & University of Central Lancashire (1999) Secure Environments Project found that competences required for nurses working in these environments are not clearly articulated by their employers. The report states that:

> In the significant majority of cases the job descriptions for nursing posts describe the main components of the job, including line of responsibility, but do not identify specific competences. The job descriptions reviewed as part of the scoping exercise could be described as being generic, they could apply to a wide range of posts in acute or secure settings. (p. 58)

The report goes on to suggest that a clearer understanding of expectations from both employee and employer could emerge from the introduction of competence-based job descriptions which could also contribute to training needs analysis and individual performance review and provide a basis for developing continuing education packages that meet the needs of the service and individual employees.

The UKCC & University of Central Lancashire (1999) Secure Environments Project used these themes, together with the published material and standards developed for staff working with personality disorder (University of Central Lancashire & Ashworth Hospital Authority, unpublished work, 1997), to develop a framework of nursing competences that met both the mental and physical health needs of clients.

The interventions were clustered into five key areas:

1. Promote and implement principles which underpin effective, quality practice.
2. Assess, develop, implement, evaluate and improve programmes of care for individuals.
3. Develop, implement, evaluate and improve environments and relationships which promote therapeutic goals and limit risks.
4. Provide and improve resources and services which facilitate organizational functioning.
5. Develop the knowledge, competence and practice of self and others (Storey & Dale 1998).

The UKCC & University of Central Lancashire (1999) study reported a high level of agreement amongst over 700 nurses in criminal justice and secure health settings in support of the competence framework. The framework could enable the sectors, it suggests, to identify the competences needed to meet the demands of the service and when negotiating with education providers, as well as to develop education and training tailored to the needs of the service. In particular, the competence framework would not be dependent on classroom-based programmes but could utilize existing open and distance learning packages or further develop others.

The study suggests that the benefits of this type of approach are that modular programmes can be undertaken over a period of time and can, therefore, be more cost effective for participants. They can be multidisciplinary in nature, covering aspects of roles common to a range of health-care professionals, and multisectoral, providing for the needs of health care, social care and the Prison Service. They also allow progression that will enable participants to undertake appropriate modules, achieve accreditation for completed modules and have multiple entry and exit points, again meeting the needs of individuals and employers. This approach acknowledges previous experience and qualifications and is flexible and can thus be modified to meet changing needs.

TRAINING

Forensic mental health nursing requires a particular knowledge base, usually centring on risk management, offending behaviour and specific sections of the Mental Health Act 1983. Furthermore, the internal tensions and conflicts within this field of specialist mental health care raise questions about the kinds of treatment and care that should be provided and about the balance between care and punishment, custody and containment, empowerment and control (McCann 1999). Few opportunities exist for specific certificates or degrees in forensic mental health nursing.

The Reed Review (DoH & Home Office 1992) recommended that training courses for community psychiatric nurses include consideration of forensic mental health nursing issues, opportunities for placement in forensic settings and for the English National Board to consider the future need for Project 2000 training in forensic mental health nursing, including opportunities for suitable placements. The review also recommended that prisons continue to forge closer links with local hospitals, colleges of nursing and others who can assist in the development of nurse education. The review also felt that it was likely that Project 2000 students would receive less specialized training than their RMN and RNMH predecessors, with opportunities for practical experience of the range of problems found amongst psychiatric inpatients being increasingly limited, owing to the provision of services away from hospitals. Project 2000 graduates would therefore require some additional education in forensic mental health issues (DoH & Home Office 1992).

The English National Board guidance to education providers, *Creating lifelong learners: partnership for care*, highlights the need for students:

> ... to develop their skills and to gain the necessary confidence, they need to have experience of caring for people with a variety of mental illnesses across the age range. Examples include mentally disordered offenders, people who abuse substances ... people with challenging behaviour. (ENB 1994)

The UKCC & University of Central Lancashire (1999) Secure Environments Project surveyed all education providers for pre- and postregistration nurse training for mental health and learning disabilities in the UK, discovering a variance in this guidance being applied. Some education institutions provide an opportunity for students to undertake a 13-week elective experience in a secure environment, others include a shorter placement as an integral part of the mental health or learning disabilities branch programme, whilst some institutions only provide a single lecture on the subject. The project identified that there were a number of problems with existing preregistration nurse training programmes including: time constraints; availability and access of placements; poor curriculum design; weakness of tutorial staff; poor research programmes; disagreement concerning inclusion of the topic at all. As a consequence of this, it was felt that students emerge from preregistration programmes without the appropriate competences to undertake the role of a registered practitioner in a secure environment and that service needs and cost constraints preclude effective preceptorship for newly qualified nurses.

In relation to postregistration training the study found that there was a considerable resource available for training and development, within both prisons and secure mental health services. However, this was described as 'an ad hoc arrangement', lacking in a strategic approach, which consequently meant the workforce were inadequately prepared to meet patient and organizational needs. Despite the fact that the study identified a wide range of validated courses available to staff working in secure care and the Prison Service, there was insufficient evidence to state whether any postregistration courses improve competency for working in secure environments. The only examples cited of competence being enhanced were in relation to cognitive-behavioural therapy and psychosocial intervention programmes.

CARE AND TREATMENT ISSUES

The majority of research into assessment of the treatment needs of mentally disordered offenders limits itself to an analysis of the level of security that the individuals require (Maden et al 1995, Murray et al 1994, Shaw et al 1994a, b, Thompson et al 1997). In summary, this research indicated that between 50% and 75% of patients in high security care do not require that level of security and remain there because other care settings, more appropriate to their needs, are not currently available (McCann 1999). Forensic mental health nursing over the past few years has developed more specialist responses to address the combination of patients' mental health, criminogenic and social needs; for example, cognitive-behavioural therapy (Guy & Hume 1998, Rogers & Gronow 1997) and psychosocial interventions (McCann & McKeown 1995). Tarbuck (1994) suggested a wide range of knowledge and skills that can facilitate positive interventions, including counselling, behaviour modification, the management of dangerousness and the therapeutic use of security.

The UKCC & University of Central Lancashire (1999) Secure Environments Project report notes the absence of evidence-based practice from the literature to guide nursing practice. The majority of the literature that does exist is described as anecdotal and based on opinion and/or experience and has not been subjected to a systematic evaluation. Closed environments, the report suggests, are:

> ... motivated, at least by part, by a reliance on 'routines, rituals and regimes', evidence based practice appears to have difficulty penetrating this from a dynamic and social perspective rather than an intellectual one. (p. 83)

The report found that much practice emerges as the result of a serious incident, which causes changes in practice in order to prevent a recurrence. Consequently, the report goes on to use the terms 'incident-based practice' and 'inquiry-based practice'. Further, the report identified a number of practice standards for care and treatment which had been suggested by the registered nurses participating in focus groups. These included:

◆ hepatitis A, B and C
◆ detoxification protocols covering both drug and alcohol withdrawal

◆ suicide and self-harm
◆ security and risk assessment/management systems
◆ the provision of women's services
◆ chronic disease management, including asthma, diabetes and epilepsy
◆ management of communicable diseases including HIV, AIDS and hepatitis
◆ seclusion and special observations
◆ non-prescription medications.

Hunt (1981) suggests the five following reasons why nurses do not use the standards or research findings in practice.

1. They do not know about them.
2. They do not understand them.
3. They do not believe them.
4. They do not know how to apply them.
5. They are not allowed to use them.

Tarbuck (1996) describes the development of a needs assessment tool consisting of 22 fields of enquiry and containing 280 items associated with the primary nurses' perceptions of patients' nursing needs. He acknowledges the limitations of the tool and the problems of interrater reliability of those applying it. Nonetheless, it represents a serious attempt at identifying the nursing needs of forensic patients in a high security setting. The information obtained reflected the views and professional opinions of 10 nurse educators, 19 ward managers and charge nurses and 38 primary nurses about their perceptions of the nursing needs of 389 patients within their care. Of the patients, the primary nurses said:

◆ 34.2% could benefit from counselling
◆ 21.9% could benefit from group psychotherapy
◆ 21.1% could benefit from social skills training
◆ 15.1% could benefit from anger management training
◆ 14.9% could benefit from behaviour therapy
◆ 13.9% could benefit from psychodynamic counselling
◆ 13.6% could benefit from reality therapy
◆ 11.8% could benefit from cognitive-behavioural therapy
◆ 11.6% could benefit from relaxation therapies
◆ 8.7% could benefit from drama therapy.

Tarbuck's stated aim was to use this information to develop a programme of training and development for staff which was more closely geared to the needs of patients, as he had come to appreciate that, despite strenuous efforts and no shortage of courses at the Ashworth Hospital training department, there was clear evidence from the Blom-Cooper report (DoH 1992a) that this was making very little impact on the service. He had realized that traditional methods of asking line managers to identify training needs had been a dramatic failure.

MULTIDISCIPLINARY ISSUES

Aiyegbusi (1998) suggests that forensic mental health nurses feel isolated and without sufficient gravitas to influence multiprofessional teamwork or control their own working lives and appropriately contribute to their patients' cases. Peternelj-Taylor (2000) found that forensic mental health nurses contribute to the multidisciplinary team in a number of ways.

◆ General contributions
◆ Psychosocial evaluation and assessment
◆ Individual therapy
◆ Crisis intervention
◆ Short-term supportive therapy
◆ Group therapy
◆ Advocacy
◆ Case management
◆ Liaison with community and other agencies

The primary aspect of the role may seem obvious at first but is worthy of emphasis. It is that nurses are the sole professional group who have direct contact with patients on a 24-hour, 7 days a week basis. They therefore enjoy a unique relationship with patients. The only comparison can be that of a close relative or friend who may share their lives with an individual in a community setting. Nurses are often seen as the eyes and ears for other professional groups and will give these professionals valuable insight and feedback on the efficiency of their therapeutic interventions. However, as well as providing this valuable partnership with other professional groups,

nurses themselves would lay claim to a base model and philosophy of practice and treatment interventions of their own.

One way for nurses to achieve parity in the multidisciplinary team is by participating in the team's active shaping of its place in its organization's institutional map. Thus, the role of the mental health nurse in the multidisciplinary clinical team can be seen as:

◆ using accurately recorded observations to structure a bias-free assessment of an individual's mental health
◆ negotiating with individuals to resolve problems defined during assessment
◆ measuring and comparing the cost or outcome, or both, of all alternative nursing interventions
◆ collaborating with other health-care professionals to implement the interventions required to assist individuals to behave in ways which promote their mental health
◆ collaborating with other health-care professionals to define their team's procedures and systems of work and participating in review and evaluation (Dale & Rae, unpublished work, 1993).

CURRENT RESEARCH AND DEVELOPMENT

Local and national research priorities for forensic services have been well documented (DoH 1992b, 1993a, b, DoH & Home Office 1992, Grubin & Gunn 1991, Rae 1994, Reed & Robinson 1992, Taylor 1991). What is less clear is the extent to which nursing will play a part in their development and implementation. Nursing remains a minority interest in research terms and is a poor relation in terms of resources allocated in comparison with the disciplines of medicine and psychology. Indeed, nursing struggles to be taken seriously in the debates surrounding research and it feels at times that nursing receives the 'crumbs from the table' in allocations and priorities.

The Institute of Psychiatry has created an international register of forensic research (Grubin &

Gunn 1991), with a view to publishing a yearly update. However, to date this publication has carried little concerning nursing research. The International Forensic Psychiatric Database (Robinson 1999) has been created to promote the dissemination of research findings and enhance practice. The recent development of this database to identify programmes for dissemination has resulted in an international initiative allowing more sharing of and access to knowledge. Many nursing programmes are described; the criticism that must be made, however, is that the database is a mixture of research activities, individuals' interests and project work. No attempt has been made to evaluate the list's contributors, in terms of quality of the listing or project described. It is best to consider this as a contact database and as such, it is a useful addition to the material.

The National Forensic Nurses' Research and Development Group evolved from the research and development forum and was developed by nurses engaged in research in the three English high security hospitals and the State Hospital, Carstairs, Scotland. The original group's brief was directed towards promoting research and development within the high security hospitals. It has developed to integrate its activities within the wider NHS and now enjoys representation from all branches of forensic mental health nursing involved in research and related research activities. The group has fostered strong links with universities and academic programmes and included three PhD holders within the inaugural group's membership (Robinson 1999). The aims and objectives of the group are:

◆ to promote the contribution of nursing in the research and development of forensic mental health care in a wider multidisciplinary context
◆ to establish and contribute to a body of knowledge to inform practice.

The past 5 years have seen a growth in nursing research programmes within forensic mental health services. Within high security services, there have been over 70 studies carried out at various levels (i.e. diploma, first degree, Master's and PhD). In addition, there are many examples of good practice and innovation that could be the seeds of research and development programmes.

CONCLUSION

The ultimate challenge for forensic mental health nurses is to develop a research agenda which will produce a unique nursing body of knowledge. Forensic mental health nursing is viewed as an evolving nursing speciality from which new theory and models of health-care delivery will emerge. The challenge for forensic mental health nurses is how to ensure that evidence-based judgements inform their management of risk as this will contribute to improving practice (Hollin 1997). Forensic mental health nursing has to incorporate both legal and physical boundaries of therapeutic yet custodial detention.

Educational providers, both pre- and postregistration, need to work more closely with service providers to ensure that programmes meet the needs of the nursing staff to work in these challenging and complex services. A competency-based approach offers some hope of a framework, which is both flexible and adaptable, to encompass many of the aspects under consideration. Full use should be made of existing programmes in the health, social and criminal justice sector as well as encouraging the formulation of more focused programmes.

Forensic nursing is emerging from a fledgling service to a new-found confidence in its ability to make a significant contribution to the multidisciplinary agenda as an equal partner and contributor to the care and treatment process.

REFERENCES

Aiyegbusi A 1998 Personality disorder and nursing at Ashworth Hospital: a position paper. Evidence to the inquiry into the personality disorder unit at Ashworth Hospital Authority. Unpublished

Cordess C 1996 The multi-disciplinary team. In: Cordess C, Cox M (eds) Forensic psychotherapy: crime, psychodynamics and the offender patient. Jessica Kingsley, London

Department of Health 1992a Report of the Committee of Inquiry into complaints about Ashworth Hospital. HMSO, London

Department of Health 1992b Ministerial review: draft action plan for 1992–3 (7th revision). Department of Health, London

Department of Health 1993a A vision of the future: the nursing and health visiting contribution to health care. Department of Health, London

Department of Health 1993b Report of the taskforce on the strategy for research in nursing, midwifery and health visiting. HMSO, London

Department of Health 1999 Inpatients formally detained in hospitals under the Mental Health Act 1983 and other legislation. Department of Health, Statistics Division, London

Department of Health & Home Office 1992 Review of health and social services for mentally disordered offenders and others requiring similar services: final summary report. Cm 2088. HMSO, London

English National Board 1994 Creating lifelong learners: partnership for care. English National Board, London

Grubin D, Gunn J 1991 Report on the register of research relating to the mentally disordered offender. Mental Health Foundation, London

Guy S, Hume A 1998 A CBT strategy for offenders with a personality disorder, Part 1. Mental Health Practice 2(4): 12–16

Hollin C 1997 Assessing and managing forensic risk. Psychiatric Care 4(5): 212–215

Hunt J 1981 Indicators for nursing practice: the use of research findings. Journal of Advanced Nursing 6: 189–194

Kettles AM, Robinson D 2000 Overview and contemporary issues in the role of the forensic nurse in the UK. In: Robinson D, Kettles A (eds) Forensic nursing and multidisciplinary care of the mentally disordered offender. Jessica Kingsley, London

Killian M, Clark N 1996 The multidisciplinary team – the nurse. In: Cordess C, Cox M (eds) Forensic psychotherapy: crime, psychodynamics and the offender patient: part II mainly practice. Jessica Kingsley, London, pp 101–106

Kitchener N, Wright I, Topping-Morris B 1992 The role of the forensic psychiatric nurse. Nursing Times 91(25): 11–12

Maden T, Curle C, Meux C, Burrow S, Gunn J 1995 Treatment and security needs of special hospital patients. Whurr, London

McCann G 1999 Care of mentally disordered offenders. Mental Health and Learning Disabilities Care 3(2): 65–67

McCann G, McKeown M 1995 Applying psychosocial interventions: Thorn initiative in forensic settings. Psychiatric Care 2(4): 133–136

McCourt M 1999 Five concepts for the expanded role of the forensic mental health nurse. In: Tarbuck P,

Topping-Morris B, Burnard P (eds) Forensic mental health nursing: policy, strategy and implementation. Whurr, London

Morrison P, Burnard P 1992 Introduction. In: Morrison P, Burnard P (eds) Aspects of forensic psychiatric nursing. Avebury, Aldershot

Murray K, Rudge S, Lack S, Dolan R 1994 How many high security beds are needed? Implications from an audit of one region's special hospital patients. Journal of Forensic Psychiatry 5: 487–499

Niskala H 1986 Competencies and skills required by nurses working in forensic areas. Western Journal of Nursing Research 8(4): 178–181

Peternelj-Taylor C 2000 The role of the forensic nurse in Canada. In: Robinson D, Kettles A (eds) Forensic nursing and multidisciplinary care of the mentally disordered offender. Jessica Kingsley, London

Peternelj-Taylor CA, Hufft AG 1997 Forensic psychiatric nursing. In: Johnson BS (ed) Psychiatric-mental health nursing: adaptation and growth. Lippincott, Philadelphia

Petryshen P 1981 Nursing the mentally disordered offender. Canadian Nurse 77(6): 26–28

Rae MA 1994 Freedom to care. Ashworth Hospital, Liverpool

Rampton Hospital Authority 1998 The forensic directory: national health and private forensic facilities in the UK, 3rd edn. Rampton Hospital Authority Social Work Department, Retford

Reed V, Robinson DK 1992 The Rampton Hospital community liaison nursing service: achievements and opportunities. Special Hospitals Service Authority, London

Robinson D 1999 Developing the contribution of research in nursing: accessing the state-of-the-art in technology and information. In: Tarbuck P, Topping-Morris B, Burnard P (eds) Forensic mental health nursing: policy, strategy and implementation. Whurr, London, ch 16, pp 190–216

Robinson D, Kettles A (eds) 2000 Forensic nursing and multidisciplinary care of the mentally disordered offender. Jessica Kingsley, London

Rogers P, Gronow T 1997 Turn down the heat … anger management. Nursing Times 93(43): 26–29

Shaw J, McKenna J, Snowden P, Boyd C, McMahon D, Kilshaw J 1994a The north-west region. I: clinical features and placement needs of patients detained in special hospitals. Journal of Forensic Psychiatry 5(1): 93–105

Shaw J, McKenna J, Snowden P, Boyd C, McMahon D, Kilshaw J 1994b The north-west region. II: patient characteristics in the research panel's recommended placement groups. Journal of Forensic Psychiatry 5(1): 107–122

Storey L, Dale C 1998 Meeting the needs of patients with severe personality disorders. Mental Health Practice 1(5): 20–26

Swinton J 2000 Reclaiming the soul: a spiritual perspective on forensic nursing. In: Robinson D, Kettles A (eds) Forensic nursing and multidisciplinary care of the mentally disordered offender. Jessica Kingsley, London

Swinton J, Boyd J 2000 Autonomy and personhood: the forensic nurse as moral agent. In: Robinson D, Kettles A (eds) Forensic nursing and multidisciplinary care of the mentally disordered offender. Jessica Kingsley, London

Tarbuck P 1994 The therapeutic use of security: a model for forensic nursing. In: Thompson T, Mathias P (eds) Lyttle's mental health and mental disorder, 2nd edn. Churchill Livingstone, London

Tarbuck P 1996 Rolling back the years: developing the practice of nursing after a public enquiry. In: Sandford T, Gournay K (eds) Perspectives in mental health nursing. Baillière Tindall, London

Taylor P 1991 Research strategy for the special hospitals. Special Hospitals Service Authority, London

Thompson L, Bogue J, Humphreys M, Owens D, Johnstone E 1997 The State Hospital survey: a description of psychiatric patients in conditions of special security in Scotland. Journal of Forensic Psychiatry 8(2): 263–284

Topping-Morris B 1992 An historical and personal view of forensic nursing services. In: Morrison P, Burnard P (eds) Aspects of forensic psychiatric nursing. Avebury, Aldershot

United Kingdom Central Council for Nursing, Midwifery and Health Visiting & University of Central Lancashire 1999 Nursing in secure environments. United Kingdom Central Council, London

Watson C, Kirby S 2000 A two nation perspective on issues of practice and provision for professionals caring for mentally disordered offenders. In: Robinson D, Kettles A (eds) Forensic nursing and multidisciplinary care of the mentally disordered offender. Jessica Kingsley, London

FURTHER READING

Chaloner C, Coffey M (eds) 2000 Forensic mental health nursing: current approaches. Blackwell Science, Oxford

Mercer D, Mason T, McKeown M, McCann G (eds) 2000 Forensic mental health care: a case study approach. Churchill Livingstone, Edinburgh

Morrison P, Burnard P (eds) 1992 Aspects of forensic psychiatric nursing. Avebury, Aldershot

Robinson D, Kettles A (eds) 2000 Forensic nursing and multidisciplinary care of the mentally disordered offender. Jessica Kingsley, London

Tarbuck P, Topping-Morris B, Burnard P (eds) 1999 Forensic mental health nursing: policy, strategy and implementation. Whurr, London

Chapter Four

Clinical psychology

John D. McGinley

INTRODUCTION

This chapter outlines the professional contribution that clinical psychology makes to the multidisciplinary effort within forensic mental health services, in meeting the complex needs of mentally disordered offenders. No single profession can effectively meet the demands. Successful treatment outcome requires the development of joint clinical strategies, ensuring a collective, collaborative and integrated delivery of services. Organizations must identify their own internal obstacles and sources of resistance that impede the development and delivery of integrated treatment programmes (Laws 1974). With an organizational philosophy and culture in place, the parameters of policy become clearer and practice becomes increasingly purposeful (Hollin 1999).

CLINICAL PSYCHOLOGY

Whilst the standards that govern individual practice are contained in the British Psychological Society (1991a) *Code of conduct* and its *Professional practice guidelines* (BPS 1995), the philosophy of a clinical psychology service is contained in its *Guidelines for clinical psychology services* (BPS 1998), which states:

> *The work of clinical psychologists is based on the fundamental acknowledgement that all people have the same human value and the right to be treated as unique individuals. Clinical psychologists will, therefore, treat all clients and colleagues with dignity and respect, and work with them as equal partners towards the achievement of mutually agreed goals.*
> *(p. 11)*

In the forensic mental health setting, this requires balancing patient needs with public safety needs. Psychologists will strive to maintain rapport and acceptance whilst confronting issues of concern. Whilst they have a duty to complete assessment and treatment, they will take appropriate steps to ensure personal safety (BPS 1998). The need for supervision cannot be overemphasized. It is a means of ensuring professional integrity and personal safety.

Clinical psychologists have an ethical responsibility to use, where possible, treatments that work (Chambless et al 1996), that have benefits beyond those attributable to the passage of time, minimal interventions or social support (Lambert & Bergin 1994). Although psychological interventions have demonstrably been effective for engendering behavioural and personal change in individuals, they are not guaranteed to work all the time or with everyone. However, a consensus appears to be emerging that psychological treatments do work, although the precise nature of the treatment, the patient's presenting problems and the interaction between patient and therapist complicate the picture dramatically (Dobson & Craig 1998).

Unacceptable variations in performance and practice cannot be tolerated. Better guidance is needed on what works for patients and what doesn't. This is an agenda that concentrates on improving standards, efficiency, openness and accountability, life-long learning (continued professional development) and professional self-regulation. It requires the development of evidence-based guidelines to set standards of care. It demands the monitoring of care delivery by objective, independent peer review to ensure that such guidelines are implemented. Variations and innovations in practice can only be justified in meeting patients' needs when they represent good practice, are derived from clinical expertise and patient reference, conform to basic ethical standards and professional guidelines and incorporate clearly defined, reliable procedures to measure effectiveness (Geddes et al 1998).

TREATMENT INTERVENTIONS

Roth & Fonaghy (1996), in reviewing what works for whom, state that the criteria for treatment to be considered effective will always be to some degree arbitrary and identified the following criteria as important:

◆ replicated demonstration of superiority to a control condition or a single high-quality randomized control trial
◆ the availability of a clear description of the therapeutic method (preferably in the form of a manual) of sufficient clarity to be useable as the basis for training
◆ a clear description of the patient group to whom the treatment was applied
◆ research effort indicating some evidence of efficacy.

On the basis of such criteria, the authors identified the following psychological conditions as having treatments that are effective or promising: depression, anxiety, obsessive-compulsive disorders, posttraumatic stress disorder, eating disorders, schizophrenia, personality disorders, alcohol abuse, sexual dysfunctions, contingency management and treatment of undesirable behaviours in pervasive developmental disorders, childhood disorders and reality orientation. This list is not exhaustive and conforms to the list of treatments considered empirically validated by the American Psychological Association (1993).

It has been proposed that psychological treatments with mentally disordered offenders should be no different from those interventions used with offenders in general. There is no list of empirically validated treatments. Forensic clinical psychology must apply the following principles to its practice. It must:

◆ be needs led
◆ be protocol driven
◆ be evidence based
◆ be derived from best practice
◆ be clinically effective
◆ restore self-respect
◆ reduce the risk of further offending to manageable proportions.

The development of psychological programmes to address the needs of mentally disordered offenders has advanced in the following areas: personality disorders, anger, sex offending, fire setting, self-harm, substance misuse. Psychosocial interventions are being developed to address schizophrenia. The applications of these programmes require adaptation to meet the differing needs of men and women, gender orientations, cultural diversities and cognitive, emotional and spiritual variations.

To refer to 'treatment' in relation to psychological approaches to meeting the needs of mentally disordered offenders runs the risk of medicalizing what are basically social issues. Many factors contribute to offending behaviour, including poor housing, socioeconomic factors and unemployment. The key finding of the STOP Project (1998) was that basic skills were lacking in offenders, including a 31% dyslexic rate and a 90% truanting rate, which greatly contributes to extremely poor self-image and social exclusion. Forensic clinical psychology and the other forensic professions are in danger of compartmentalizing the individual in their attempt to apply their discrete skills to rehabilitating the mentally disordered person. The contribution of any mental health profession must be weighed against the expressed needs of the citizen – client, patient or prisoner.

CLINICAL PSYCHOLOGICAL APPROACHES TO ASSESSMENT AND INTERVENTION

Personality disorders

The intolerable risk of recidivism by dangerous people with severe personality disorder (DSPD) has recently emerged as a major concern for public safety and political scrutiny. There is no question here about a condition or illness that is amenable to medical treatment but about how people with severe and enduring psychological difficulties may behave in ways which present risk of harm to themselves and others. The intention is to reduce the risk of such individuals harming themselves and others.

It is the declared opinion of the BPS that the skills needed to design and develop these interventions lie mainly within the related professions of clinical and forensic psychology. Structured psychological interventions should be used in specialist programmes with DSPD people, administered by both psychologists and appropriately trained personnel from other disciplines.

A review of the literature (Benjamin 1997) suggests that the only approaches specific to the treatment of personality disorder are behavioural, cognitive-behavioural or psychopharmacological. Mediators of antisocial behaviours need to be identified, targeted and influenced by appropriate treatment approaches (Blackburn 1993).

The most effective interventions are structured and focused (Lipsey 1995). An important element in the treatment of antisocial personality and the reduction of offending behaviours can be the teaching of cognitive skills as well as behavioural methods to help individuals deal less impulsively with difficult situations. The work involves helping offenders, mentally disordered or otherwise, to face up to the consequences of their actions, to understand their motives and to develop new ways of controlling their behaviour. The Reasoning and Rehabilitation programme is a multimodal programme on the teaching of cognitive skills which may have significant impact on offending behaviour (Ross et al 1989). Such programmes are generally more successful than techniques such as group and individual counselling and non-directive psychological therapies.

Benjamin argues that Linehan's dialectical behavioural treatment for borderline personality disorder and self-harm (Linehan 1993) is the most successful approach to the disorder. For many, self-harm is a positive strategy for survival and it is unreasonable to expect people to stop self-harming without putting equally effective strategies in place. Cognitive therapy showed the greatest reduction in abnormal traits, especially in schizotypal, narcissistic, borderline and compulsive categories of personality disorder (Black et al 1996). Certainly the cognitive-behavioural approaches are reflected in the current offender treatment literature although many programmes are multimodal and include a number of the more successful methods for dealing with particular behavioural problems such as anger management, social skills and problem solving.

McMurran (1996) emphasizes the importance of two findings from research on working with offenders:

1. treatment programmes based on a conceptual model are more likely to be effective
2. individual criminogenic needs must be addressed.

However, it is argued that these relatively brief treatments are aimed simply at symptom change and may not address the underlying nature of personality disorder. Losel (1998) suggests that cognitive-behavioural programmes, multimodal treatment, a structured therapeutic community and social therapy are indicated for personality disordered and serious offenders. The success of intervention programmes depends on a constructive and productive therapeutic milieu in which basic human values are the bedrock on which the safe rehabilitation of disordered citizens is built. It will be oxygenated by a realistic optimism that positive change is possible.

Anger and aggression

Anger is a particularly important subject for professionals who work in forensic mental healthcare settings because it is a significant activator of violent behaviour. Clinically, anger is a neglected area. There are a number of studies on anger treatment with offenders, although there has been considerable variability in the content and process of the treatment. Most applications have been based broadly on the cognitive-behavioural approach of Novaco (1975, 1977), which utilizes the stress inoculation paradigm (Meichenbaum 1985). At the heart of the stress inoculation approach to anger treatment is a focus on emotional dysregulation and a progressive acquisition of self-control coping skills.

The State Hospital Anger Project has been the first systematic attempt to apply Novaco's cognitive-behavioural anger therapy to psychiatric patients with long-standing difficulties associated with an inability to control their anger. However, it should be noted that anger is often part of a much wider spectrum of problems. Although this work has proved complex and difficult, the results achieved have been encouraging (Renwick et al 1997). There is good evidence that anger interventions based on the Novaco approach are effective. Blackburn (1993) concluded that training in anger management has indeed been shown to reduce aggression, at least in the short term, and its usefulness in maintaining order in institutions has been established. Evidence of long-term success is inconclusive, indicating that issues such as offender heterogeneity, effective treatment components and treatment intensity have yet to be addressed (Blackburn 1993).

Fire setting

Although there are numerous descriptive studies and case reports on the topic of adult and juvenile fire raising, there is a dearth of quality treatment research (Bogue 1998). This is often attributed to the heterogeneity of fire raisers in terms of motivation and psychopathology. Historically, the research literature has given an undue degree of prominence to pyromaniacal or fetishistic fire raisers although it is widely acknowledged that such individuals are exceedingly rare and are diagnostically equivocal in any case (Koson & Dvoskin 1982).

Fire raising in the broadest sense represents a form of behaviour in which motivation can vary in different contexts and can be secondary to the mental state of the individual where psychiatric conditions and intellectual impairment may be of particular significance. Jackson et al (1987) describe a useful model in which fire-raising behaviour is viewed as a function of antecedents or stimuli and consequences or reinforcers. Essentially, fire raisers are viewed as a disadvantaged group lacking the skills to change undesired situations in appropriate ways. In the short term, fire raising and its consequences provide a means of influencing events and improving self-esteem. However, the long-term consequences exacerbate the initial difficulties.

Although the Jackson et al (1987) approach is described as a 'functional analysis model' it has a cognitive-behavioural underpinning in the sense that it outlines the hypothetical role of cognitions in maintaining fire-raising behaviour and can be incorporated into an extended cognitive-behavioural framework with ease, adding to its flexibility and applicability.

Sex offending

Reduction of the assessed risk of reoffending is the main aim of psychological treatment programmes for sex offenders (Marshall 1996). Approaches based on a combination of cognitive-behavioural and relapse prevention models have been demonstrated as the most effective (Laws & O'Donohue 1997, Perkins et al 1998). The most common treatment approach is that of cognitive restructuring, involving the discussion and confrontation of distorted attitudes (cognitive component) but also creating discomfort for the client by focusing on victims' responses (affective component). Treatment and assessment will necessarily involve establishing the relationship between motive, personality traits, the biological, behavioural, cognitive and historical facets of the sexual behaviour and assessing the influence of correlated factors such as alcohol abuse or anger (Marshall et al 1990). Treatment is about training individuals to reduce their exposure to risk situations, to develop alternative and more appropriate responses, to alter certain perceptions and beliefs and to provide the skills to implement alternative responses.

A modular approach is recommended that allows the clinical team to tailor the programme to meet the individual profile of the patient and could involve effective protocols for social skills training (Seidman et al 1994), cognitive distortions about sex between adults and children (Abel et al 1989), self-esteem as a necessary prerequisite to productive engagement in treatment (Marshall & Mazzucco 1995), victim empathy and victim harm (Hudson et al 1995), denial and minimization (Barbaree 1991).

It is assumed that the modification of deviant sexual fantasies and arousal patterns is necessary in the successful treatment of sex offenders. The most common treatment approaches in this particular area follow a standard classical conditioning paradigm and their aim is either to decrease deviant arousal or increase appropriate arousal. The treatments used include covert sensitization aversion therapy. There is increasing evidence that the likelihood of engaging in sexually aggressive behaviour is greater among those who are more impulsive (Prentky 1997). Consequently, most treatment programmes include self-control and impulsivity management modules. The main aim of treatment is to develop a self-management system to interrupt the chain of events that lead to a particular behaviour occurring.

There is limited positive evidence for the efficacy of treatment programmes for sex offenders. At one extreme, Barbaree (1999) stated at an American Psychological Association meeting that there was no convincing evidence that sexual offending treatment leads to reductions in the rate of recidivism of sex offenders. He concludes that the estimate of risk should not be lowered by any consideration of the beneficial effects of treatment on recidivism.

Too few studies focus on particular types of sex offenders to permit any conclusions about the effectiveness of programmes for different sex offender typologies (Polizzi et al 1999). Psychology faces an ethical dilemma of deciding how to respond to political and legal dictates demanding that sex offenders undergo treatment with limited efficacy. There is cautious optimism that Hall's metaanalysis highlights the need to integrate clinical and economic benefits of group-based interventions, as in the UK Prison Sex Offender Treatment programme (SOTP), with treatments that address important individual differences between sex offenders' risk factors and treatment needs (Perkins et al 1998). A therapeutically oriented milieu could combine expectations of behaviour change with personal support and multidisciplinary oversight, monitoring and management of individual treatment plans, together with a combination of group-based, cognitive-behavioural interventions addressing criminogenic and personality factors relevant to participating offenders, with individual therapy as required (e.g. the modification of deviant sexual arousal) and including antilibidinal medication as a potential element of the treatment plan.

Addictions

Clinical psychologists question the disease concept of addiction that underpinned Wilson's approach in developing the Alcoholics Anonymous (AA) movement in 1935 because scientific research was not available to support its efficacy (Margolis & Zweben 1998). They developed other approaches to addictions with positive results, such as relapse prevention (McLellan et al 1994) and motivational enhancement. Marlatt & Gordon (1985) developed a set of interventions based on the premise that the behaviours necessary to initiate abstinence are different from those needed to maintain it.

The abstinence violation effect was an excellent conceptual and clinical contribution, describing the impact on the individual of having failed to keep a behavioural commitment. Eating disorders, gambling, compulsive sexual behaviour and crime itself are areas in which disturbed patterns resemble addiction so closely that the addiction treatment model has been applied to develop intervention strategies.

Studies have shown successful application of cognitive-behavioural techniques to reducing alcohol or drug intake without measuring the impact on reoffending (Husband & Platt 1993). McMurran's (1996) review of the literature on alcohol, drugs and crime confirmed that there is insufficient research evidence to permit conclusions about precisely what combinations of cognitive, behavioural and skills elements are necessary for successful intervention, measured in terms of substance intake reduction and reduced recidivism.

Services for women

The provision of mental health services that meet the needs of women is a major challenge (Owen et al 1997). There is a dearth of research concerning the needs of women with long-term mental health problems. Within high security settings, there is a high prevalence of emotional problems (anger/depression), behavioural disturbance, auditory hallucinations and self-harm (McMurran et al 1996). 'Given the time scale of the damaging experiences many of the women have undergone,

it is unrealistic to expect magic recovery over a short time' (Dolan & Bland 1996: 38).

There remains considerable uncertainty about which forms of psychosocial and physical treatments are most effective for patients who self-harm. The two psychological interventions offering promising results were problem-solving therapy (Hawton & Kirk 1989) and dialectical behaviour therapy (Linehan 1993). As the latter intervention is intensive, development of a shorter form of this treatment is required and investigation of its efficacy in men is needed (Hawton et al 1998). If women with a biological disposition to finding their emotions difficult to handle experience an invalidating environment 'within which they have inappropriate, erratic or insensitive responses to their thoughts, beliefs, feelings and sensations, they will find it difficult to regulate the way they react' (Smith et al 1998).

Habilitation of patients with learning disabilities

The British Psychological Society (1991b) document *Definition of learning disabilities* provides the criteria which guide psychologists in the classification of 'mental handicap' (Mental Health (Scotland) Act 1984) and 'mental impairment and severe mental impairment' (Mental Health (England and Wales) Act 1983) and is currently being revised. *Clinical practice guidelines: psychological interventions for challenging behaviour* (BPS 1997) have been produced in draft form by the BPS Special Interest Group in Learning Disabilities.

Cognitive therapy with people with a learning disability is still a developing area. Basic cognitive approaches, such as learning to label and express emotions appropriately, practising self-monitoring skills, examining alternative hypotheses provided by the therapist, are a common part of psychological intervention. The more structured cognitive-behavioural therapy approach using homework tasks that require the client to elicit thinking errors and generate alternative interpretations require focused concentration and the ability to read and write. Such an approach is often too sophisticated for the learning disabled person who is often operating at concrete developmental level rather than via abstract logical thought. A habilitative treatment focus of teaching social/coping skills in conjunction with external management procedures is promising.

To achieve meaningful therapeutic results, the treatment programme should be diagnostically based and needs led, reflect a competency enhancement model (habilitation) and place major emphasis on teaching personal responsibility for one's actions (Gardner et al 1998). Collaborative work in extending anger protocols is being developed at the State Hospital by Novaco and Ramm in collaboration with the Learning Disabilities Service.

There are few evaluations of the effectiveness of psychotherapy with offenders. Carnie (1977) suggested that whilst therapy did not change a personality, it achieved control over violent behaviour. Beail (1995) indicated that there were no well-established methods and measures in the field of learning disabilities as there are in the field of adult mental health for outcome research.

Whilst a clear model for intervention has been devised (i.e. the use of applied behavioural analysis), a number of studies have indicated difficulties in interventions being applied in practice. Hastings & Remington (1994) refer to lack of available resources, lack of support for staff, lack of communication between staff groups and shifts, intrusive programmes which are inflexible or involve technical language and which rely on second-order behavioural modification as hindrances to effective implementation of programmes.

Psychosocial interventions for schizophrenia

Psychological treatments have utility in relieving the symptoms and distress associated with schizophrenia, improving skills, continuing supportive family contact and reducing relapse. Interventions that focus on specific cognitive deficits in schizophrenia may be of great benefit to individual patients since available medication has only limited impact on core cognitive deficits. Innovative attempts to change these cognitive abnormalities are critically needed (Bentall et al 1991). However, more data on the effects and effectiveness of individual therapies are required.

Until the specific therapeutic effects of these treatments can be defined it is unlikely that they will be widely disseminated. Clinical psychologists in the main are arguing that the cluster of symptoms associated with schizophrenia do not represent evidence for a single diagnostic entity and therefore theories should be developed to explain individual symptoms rather than explain the development of the syndrome as a whole.

Evaluation of cognitive-behavioural therapy in schizophrenia is still in its early phases but positive results are emerging from controlled studies (Kingdom & Turkington 1994). The research endeavour should shift from deciding which is the most efficacious treatment to the identification of factors which will predict the acceptability of treatment to a particular client.

CONCLUSION

At the heart of the clinical psychology role in forensic mental health care is the psychological assessment of mood, thoughts, feelings, behaviour and personality functioning. Furthermore, clinical psychologists are extensively involved in the management and treatment of behavioural disorder. They have at the heart of their practice risk assessment and management and through their psychological interventions they aim to reduce risk and thus the chance of relapse.

There is a growing and impressive array of interventions with demonstrable efficacy which can be applied in forensic services. The challenge ahead requires the detailed 'codifying' of these interventions to facilitate their replication whilst further research is undertaken on the application of these interventions in other settings to demonstrate their generalizability.

Further work is required with regard to longitudinal work and whether the skills developed in one setting are generalizable and transferable to other settings, particularly more open and community settings which present the greatest risk to the general public.

It should also be acknowledged that psychology remains a scarce resource in all mental health services and in forensic services in particular. Increasingly, psychologists are required to work through 'third parties', particularly nurses, in the gathering of data and the application of many psychological interventions and this is where effective teamwork and good working relationships between all professionals involved in the patient's care are paramount.

REFERENCES

Abel GG, Gore DK, Holland CL, Camp N 1989 The measurement of the cognitive distortions of child molesters. Annals of Sex Research 2(2): 135–152

American Psychological Association 1993 Task Force on Promotion and Dissemination of Psychological Procedures. Division 12, APA, Washington

Barbaree HE 1991 Denial and minimisation among sex offenders: assessment and treatment outcome. Forum on Corrections Research 3: 300–333

Barbaree HE 1999 Efficacy of sex offender treatment. American Psychological Association Conference, APA CE Office, Washington

Beail N 1995 Outcome of psychoanalysis, psychoanalytical and psychological psychotherapy with people with intellectual disabilities: a review. Change 13: 186–191

Benjamin LS 1997 Personality disorders: models for treatment and strategies for treatment development. Journal of Personality Disorders 11(4): 307–324

Bentall RP, Kaney S, Dewey ME 1991 Persecutory delusions: an attribution theory. British Journal of Clinical Psychology 30: 13–23

Black DW, Monahan P, Wesner R, Gabel J, Bowers W 1996 The effect of fluvoxamine, cognitive therapy, and placebo on abnormal personality traits in 44 patients with panic disorder. Journal of Personality Disorders 10: 185–194

Blackburn R 1993 The psychology of criminal conduct: theory, research and practice. Wiley, Chichester

Bogue J 1998 Fire-setting treatment programme: position paper of forensic clinical psychology service. State Hospital, Carstairs, Lanark

British Psychological Society 1991a Code of conduct. BPS Publications, Leicester

British Psychological Society 1991b Definition of learning disabilities. BPS Publications, Leicester

British Psychological Society 1995 Professional practice guidelines. BPS Publications, Leicester

British Psychological Society 1997 Clinical practice guidelines: psychological interventions for challenging behaviour. BPS Publications, Leicester

British Psychological Society 1998 Guidelines for clinical psychology services: division of clinical psychology. BPS Publications, Leicester

Carnie FL 1977 Outpatient treatment of the aggressive offender. American Journal of Psychotherapy 31: 265–274

Chambless DL, Sanderson WC, Shohan V et al 1996 An update on empirically validated therapies. Clinical Psychologist 49: 5–18

Dobson KS, Craig KD (eds) 1998 Empirically supported therapies: best practice in professional psychology. Sage, London

Dolan B, Bland J 1996 Who are the women in special hospitals? In: Hemingway C (ed) Special women? The experience of women in the special hospital system. Avebury, Aldershot

Gardner WI, Graeber JL, Machkovitz SJ 1998 Treatment of offenders with mental retardation. In: Wettstein RM et al (eds) Treatment of offenders with mental disorders. Guilford Press, New York, ch 7, pp 329–364

Geddes J, Reynolds S, Streiner D, Szatmari P, Haynes B 1998 Evidence-based practice in mental health. Evidence-Based Mental Health 1(1): 3–4

Hastings R, Remington B 1994 Staff behaviour and its implications for people with learning disabilities and challenging behaviours. British Journal of Clinical Psychology 33: 423–428

Hawton K, Kirk J 1989 Problem-solving. In: Hawton K, Salkovkis P, Kirk J, Clark DM (eds) Cognitive behaviour therapy for psychiatric problems: a practitioner guide. Oxford University Press, Oxford

Hawton K, Arensman E, Townsend E et al 1998 Deliberate self harm: systematic review of efficacy of psychosocial and pharmacological treatments in preventing repetition. British Medical Journal 317(7156): 441–447

Hollin CR 1999 Treatment programs for offenders: meta-analysis, 'what works', and beyond. International Journal of Law and Psychiatry 22(33–34): 361–372

Hudson SM, Marshall WL, Ward T, Johnston PW, Jones RL 1995 Kia Marama: a cognitive-behavioural program for incarcerated child molesters. Behaviour Change 12(2): 69–80

Husband SD, Platt JJ 1993 The cognitive skills component in substance abuse treatment in correctional settings: a brief review. Journal of Drug Issues 23(1): 31–45

Jackson H, Glass C, Hope S 1987 A functional analysis of recidivistic arson. British Journal of Clinical Psychology 26: 175–185

Kingdom DG, Turkington D 1994 Cognitive-behavioural therapy of schizophrenia. Guilford Press, New York

Koson DF, Dvoskin J 1982 Arson: a diagnostic survey. Bulletin of the American Academy of Psychiatry and the Law 10(1): 39–49

Lambert MJ, Bergin AE 1994 The effectiveness of psychotherapy. In: Bergin AE, Garfield SL et al (eds) Handbook of psychotherapy and behavior change, 4th edn. Wiley, New York, pp 143–189

Laws DR 1974 The failure of a token economy. Federal Probation 38: 33–38

Laws DR, O'Donohue W (eds) 1997 Sexual deviance: theory, assessment and treatment. Guilford Press, New York

Linehan MM 1993 Cognitive behavioural treatment of borderline personality disorder. Guilford Press, London

Lipsey MW 1995 What do we learn from 400 research studies on the effectiveness of treatment with juvenile delinquents? In: McGuire J (ed) What works? Reducing reoffending: guidelines from research and practice. Wiley, Chichester

Losel F 1998 Treatment and management of psychopaths. In: Cooke DJ, Forth AE, Hare RD (eds) Psychopathy: theory, research and implications for society. Kluwer, Amsterdam, pp 303–354

Margolis RD, Zweben J 1998 Treating patients with alcohol and other drug problems: an integrated approach. American Psychological Society, Washington

Marlatt GA, Gordon JR (eds) 1985 Relapse prevention: maintenance strategies in the treatment of addictive behaviors. Guilford Press, New York

Marshall WL 1996 Assessment, treatment, and theorizing about sex offenders: developments during the past twenty years and future directions. Criminal Justice and Behavior 23(1): 162–199

Marshall WL, Mazzucco A 1995 Self-esteem and parental attachments in child molesters. Sexual Abuse: Journal of Research and Treatment 7: 279–285

Marshall WL, Laws DR, Barbaree HE 1990 Handbook of sexual assault: issues, theories, and treatment of the offender. Plenum, New York

McLellan AT, Alterman AI, Metzzger DS et al 1994 Similarity of outcome predictors across opiate, cocaine, and alcohol treatments: role of treatment services. Journal of Consulting and Clinical Psychology 62: 1141–1158

McMurran M 1996 Alcohol, drugs and criminal behaviour. In: Hollin CR (ed) Working with offenders: psychological practice in offender rehabilitation. Wiley, Chichester, pp 211–242

McMurran M, Clerkin P, Rosenberg H 1996 Problems of female patients in a secure psychiatric hospital. Psychology, Crime and Law 3(1): 15–19

Meichenbaum D 1985 Stress inoculation training. Pergamon Press, New York

Novaco RW 1975 Anger control: the development and evaluation of an experimental treatment. Heath, Lexington

Novaco RW 1977 Stress inoculation: a cognitive therapy for anger and its application to a case of depression. Journal of Consulting and Clinical Psychology 45: 600–608

Owen S, Repper J, Perkins R, Robinson J 1997 Services for women with long term mental health problems. Department of Nursing and Midwifery Studies, University of Nottingham and Trent Regional Health Authority

Perkins DE, Hammond S, Coles D, Bishopp D 1998 Review of sex offender treatment programmes. High Security Psychiatric Services Commissioning Board, London

Polizzi DM, MacKenzie DL, Hickman LJ 1999 What works in adult sex offender treatment? A review of prison and non-prison-based treatment programs. International Journal of Offender Therapy and Comparative Criminology 43(3): 357–374

Prentky RA 1997 A rationale for the treatment of sex offenders. In: McGuire J (ed) What works? Reducing reoffending: guidelines from research and practice. Wiley, Chichester

Renwick SJ, Black L, Ramm M 1997 Anger treatment with forensic hospital patients. Legal and Criminological Psychology 2(1): 103–116

Ross RR, Fabiano EA, Ross B 1989 Reasoning and rehabilitation: a handbook for teaching cognitive skills. The Cognitive Centre, Ottawa

Roth A, Fonaghy P 1996 What works for whom? A critical review of psychotherapy research. Guilford Press, New York

Seidman BT, Marshall WL, Hudson SM, Robertson PJ 1994 An examination of intimacy and loneliness in sex offenders. Journal of Interpersonal Violence 9(4): 518–534

Smith G, Cox D, Saradjian J 1998 Women and self-harm. The Women's Press, London

STOP Project 1998 Specific training for offenders on probation. Shropshire Chamber of Commerce, Training and Enterprise, Trevithick House, Stafford

Chapter Five

Social work

Richard Backhouse

INTRODUCTION

Social work is essentially a statutory activity which
is underpinned by a framework of social care legislation, which requires the practitioner to intervene
in a range of situations according to prescribed
criteria. The social work contribution to mental
health service provision is principally defined by
the statutory role of the Approved Social Worker
within the Mental Health Act 1983 section 145
and the Code of Practice (DoH & Welsh Office
1999). The Approved Social Worker has an
autonomous personal decision-making authority
on the forced detention of mentally disordered
persons. The task of social work in mental health is
also substantially defined by the National Health
Service and Community Care Act 1990 as: 'the
requirement on Local Authority Social Services
Departments to carry out needs assessments in
respect of people who have mental health problems', which has led to the mental health social
worker taking on the brokerage responsibilities of
the care manager in addition to the more specific
statutory duties of the Approved Social Worker.

It is a peculiar paradox of forensic mental
health social work that as one goes further from
mainstream community-based mental health
services towards specialist medium and high security service provision, the role of the social worker
becomes less clearly defined by statute and thus
potentially more equivocal. This is largely owing
to the anomaly within the 1983 Mental Health
Act that the statutory duty of the Approved Social
Worker to assess, which is so central to detention
under part II of the Act, is entirely absent in
respect of patients detained under part III.
Similarly, the care manager role under the NHS
and Community Care Act 1990 is less directly
attributable to social workers based in a regional
or supraregional forensic setting. Thus, social
workers in a high security hospital, for example,
who are not employed by local authorities, do not

41

fulfil the function of either Approved Social Worker or care manager.

The question which needs to be addressed is therefore: 'What is the role and professional contribution of social work in a forensic mental health setting?'. In recent years, considerable work has been undertaken within the high security forensic social work services, leading to the development of a comprehensive framework for the practical delivery of social work and social care.

In August 1994 the Special Hospitals Service Authority produced a statement of principles on the role of social work entitled *Beyond care? Social work in the special hospitals* which described the social work process as:

> *Social work within the special hospitals addresses our patients' needs within their social context. Appreciation of social context is essential to explaining patients' past behaviour, to understanding their current functioning, and to planning safe future placements. (Special Hospitals Social Work Service 1994)*

The Central Council for Education and Training in Social Work (1995) outlined the key purpose of forensic social work as:

> *To hold in balance the protection of the public and the promotion of the quality of life of individuals and by working in partnership with relevant others to: identify, assess and manage risk; identify and challenge discriminatory structures and practices; engage effectively with mentally disordered offenders and other people with similar needs; identify, develop and implement strategies.*

Any model of forensic social work practice must be focused on the goal of safe and successful social care outcomes. The social worker in forensic mental health has to work with complex extended client systems, which can include not only the patient and the patient's family but also victims and others who might be at risk from the patient. Social care outcomes, both short and long term, must be safe and successful from the viewpoint of all those involved or potentially involved. Within this context, high priority must always be given to ensuring that outcomes are planned with adequate regard to the protection of children.

Having acknowledged the paramount importance of safe practice, it is also essential that forensic social work adopts a strong value base in applying principles of antidiscriminatory practice in its approach to patient care. Within the closed environment of long-stay forensic psychiatric facilities, there is a danger that discriminatory practices, such as institutionalized racism, will evolve (see Chapter 6 of the Stephen Lawrence Inquiry for a full debate of this concept; DoH 1999a). Forensic social work practitioners must therefore be proactive in addressing the needs of individual patients with due regard to race, ethnicity, religion, gender, etc. Despite this awareness throughout forensic mental health care services and the wider psychiatric provision, it can still be demonstrated through the 2nd National Visit of the Mental Health Act Commission (Mental Health Act Commission 2000: 6) that two-thirds of the 104 units visited had no policy on training in race equality and antidiscriminatory practice for staff.

In April 1995, to translate these principles into a practical framework for forensic social work practice, the social work services at Ashworth, Broadmoor and Rampton hospitals developed the 'Special Hospital Social Work Service Specification'. Compiled by social work managers and practitioners, the service specification drew on statutory guidance, as well as on existing best practice, to identify the unidisciplinary contribution of social work within a multidisciplinary/multiagency approach to patient care. Revised and updated annually, the service specification underpins the professional contribution of social work to patient care within the three high security hospitals. The chronological approach described below is derived from the service specification.

A CHRONOLOGICAL APPROACH TO SOCIAL WORK IN A FORENSIC SETTING

The core social work tasks within a forensic mental health setting can be divided chronologically into the following six stages.

1. Preadmission
2. Admission
3. Formulation of and participation in care plan
4. Mental Health Review Tribunals/Mental Health Act managers review of detention
5. Liaison with outside agencies
6. Management of transfer and discharge

Clearly this is not a strict chronology as some tasks are recurring or ongoing and can occur at various stages of a patient's stay. Nevertheless, the sequence represents a progression through the treatment process, based on assessment and intervention, leading towards the rehabilitative options of care and support in conditions of lesser security or in the community.

The appropriateness of this chronological approach to core tasks is endorsed within the Review of Social Work Service in the High Security Hospitals (DoH 1999b) which recommends: 'whilst the role of the social workers should not be prescribed too rigidly, their primary function should be to provide a social care and liaison service at (a) pre-admission, (b) admission, (c) reviews including Mental Health Review Tribunal hearings, (d) planning and preparation for discharge (section 117) and (e) the point of discharge, including the arrangements for ongoing support and care planning'.

Preadmission

Under most circumstances, assessment by an Approved Social Worker is not a statutory requirement when a patient is admitted to a high security or medium secure forensic facility. Patients detained under part II of the Mental Health Act 1983 are usually being transferred from a setting of lesser security where an application for detention has already been made by an Approved Social Worker. Where a patient is detained under part III of the Mental Health Act 1983 the authorization for the patient's detention rests with the court or Home Secretary. Nevertheless, principles of good practice would indicate that it is desirable, where practicable, for the preadmission assessment process to include an autonomous social work assessment, which leads

to an independent social work report. The social work assessment has a particular importance in locating the prospective admission in its wider social context.

The social work assessment should be based on the following.

◆ Information gathered from outside agencies, including social services departments, probation service, prisons and the police.

◆ Consideration, where appropriate, of depositions and previous conviction documentation.

◆ Interview with the patient. The importance of this first contact in a secure environment cannot be overestimated.

◆ Interview with the patient's family or friends where appropriate. This is a key, lengthy but worthwhile process. The taking of a social history should remain of paramount importance in social work practice in secure settings.

The resultant social work report should refer to:

◆ possible alternatives to admission, including resource implications
◆ the social implications of admission for the patient and others
◆ the views on admission of the patient, the patient's family and significant others
◆ the patient's treatability, including likely outcomes of treatment
◆ significant cultural issues
◆ the patient's dangerousness, including the context of the index offence and of other offending or violent behaviour (actual or potential dangerousness in relation to children is of crucial significance)
◆ the patient's social history.

The preadmission social work report should be made available to those who have decision-making responsibility for the patient's admission. In the case of proposed admissions to high security hospitals, this will be the members of the hospital admissions panel. Criteria for considering admissions include: the presence or absence of a recognizable mental disorder; whether the individual presents a grave and immediate danger to the public; and whether that person will be amenable to treatment.

Admission

Admission to a secure forensic psychiatric facility can be a traumatic, frightening and distressing experience, for both the person admitted and the family. The social worker's task at the point of admission is to facilitate a two-way information-sharing process in respect of the patient's social care needs.

As soon as practicable after admission, the social worker should interview the patient, to reinforce their rights under the Mental Health Act 1983, which have been previously given by the Mental Health Act Manager from medical records, to offer transitional support in respect of any immediate problems precipitated by the admission and to discuss any appeal process against sentence or detention. There needs to be some flexibility in the timing of this process to take into account the patient's mental state and the impact this might have on their ability to understand. The social worker needs to be sensitive to the patient's cultural needs and their preferred language. An interpreter should be used whenever appropriate.

The social worker should contact the patient's nearest relative, offering appropriate information and advice in respect of the admission. It is essential that relatives are given information about visiting arrangements at the earliest opportunity. It is particularly important to ascertain whether there are any children, in whose interests it might be to visit the patient, so that the necessary preparation for this can be made.

The issue of contact between patients detained in forensic facilities and children is an important area of decision making which must be proactively addressed. Detailed guidance on assessment procedures and arrangements for children to visit patients in high security services is given within a document on visits by children to Ashworth, Broadmoor and Rampton hospitals (DoH 1999c). Arrangements for visits by children in other adult mental health settings, including regional secure units, are governed by the Mental Health Act 1983 code of practice: guidance on the visiting of psychiatric patients by children (DoH 1999d). Reference to these directions is incorporated into a document on working together to safeguard children (DoH et al 2000). In all cases the decision as to whether contact should be allowed should be based on assessment of the best interests of the child, and all contacts must take place under supervision and in a safe child-friendly environment.

It is essential at the time of admission for the social worker to undertake a full social history/assessment of the patient, leading to a detailed written report which will be incorporated into the patient's record. This report will draw on a variety of sources of information and might include:

◆ depositions
◆ medical files
◆ Social Services reports
◆ probation reports
◆ information from the voluntary sector
◆ information from family and significant others
◆ information from the patient
◆ education and employment history.

Wherever practicable, attempts should be made to corroborate information obtained from the patient, the family and other agencies. All sources of information should be identified and the distinction should be made between fact and opinion. Good practice should dictate the sharing of the completed social history/assessment with the patient, giving due regard to confidentiality and the protection of third-party information. This will create a platform for building trust in a difficult environment.

The social history/assessment report can usefully be structured under the following headings.

◆ *Header information.* To include patient's name, date of birth, date of admission, nationality, ethnic group, religion, first language, marital status, occupation, Mental Health Act 1983 section, legal classification, schedule one status (schedule one status refers to a person who has committed an offence against a child as defined in the Children's and Young Persons Act 1993).

◆ *Introduction.* The introduction will list sources of information, written and verbal. Interviews with individuals will contain statements of reliability.

◆ *Family history*. To include family structure, family psychiatric and forensic history, ethnic and cultural issues.

◆ *Childhood and adolescent developmental history*. Including perinatal history, account of birth and development problems, details of carers and upbringing, patient's home circumstances during childhood, relationships within the family and family dynamics, health, significant life events and education.

◆ *Relationships and sexuality*. Including psychosexual development and orientation, adolescent and adult relationships.

◆ *Patient's lifestyle*. To include occupation history, leisure activities and hobbies, addictive behaviour and substance use and patient's home circumstances before admission.

◆ *Psychiatric history*. History of previous admissions, behaviour problems and premorbid and morbid personality.

◆ *Offending history*. Offending behaviour and analysis of any patterns of offending and possible relationship to index offence.

◆ *Index offence*. Description and analysis.

◆ *Patient since admission*. Observed behaviour, attitudes and beliefs.

◆ *Conclusion*. Summary, needs assessment and risk assessment.

Formulation of and participation in care plan

To ensure that a patient's social care needs are fully addressed within the care plan, it is essential that the social worker participates as a full member of the multidisciplinary team. Within this multidisciplinary context, the unidisciplinary contribution of the social worker should be focused on the following areas.

◆ Engagement with the patient in order to: establish a supportive professional working relationship; monitor and develop social relationships and networks; assist in problem solving; and advocate as appropriate on behalf of the patient.

◆ Engagement with the patient's family and/or significant others.

◆ Needs and risk assessment including the security needs of other patients and the wider hospital environment in which the patient functions.

◆ Representation at case conferences in respect of social care issues.

◆ Any ongoing contact arrangements between the patient and children should be recorded in the care plan and monitored and reviewed on a regular basis.

Mental Health Review Tribunals

The Mental Health Review Tribunal hearing is arguably the most crucial event which takes place during a patient's period of detention in a forensic setting. The recommendations of the Mental Health Review Tribunal can have far-reaching consequences for the patient and their family and for the future management of the patient's treatment and care.

The Mental Health Review Tribunal rules give little indication as to the appropriate level of social work involvement in the tribunal process. Indeed, the only prescribed requirement in respect of the patient's social care needs is for the responsible authority to provide an up-to-date social circumstances report prepared for the tribunal, including reports on the following (HMSO 1983):

◆ the patient's home and family circumstances, including the attitude of the patient's nearest relative or the person so acting
◆ the opportunities for employment or occupation and the housing facilities which would be available to the patient if discharged
◆ the availability of community support and relevant medical facilities
◆ the financial circumstances of the patient.

However, these four headings do not address all the areas of social care which are likely to be key issues for patients detained in a forensic mental health setting. In particular, to make a meaningful contribution to the tribunal's decision-making process, the social circumstances report must also contain an assessment of the risks involved if the patient were to be discharged or transferred. This should also include a summary of the patient's needs and how these needs could be met in the community. This risk assessment should consider the patient's dangerousness in context, with reference to danger to self and others (including children and staff).

Consideration should be given to who is best placed to compile the social circumstances report, particularly in the case of patients detained in supraregional facilities such as high security hospitals. Whilst the hospital-based social worker will usually be the appropriate person to provide a current social work assessment, the local authority social worker is likely to have better knowledge of the local availability of community support. Liaison has to occur between the social workers in both settings to determine the authorship and contents of the report. Joint authorship or the submission of two reports are perfectly acceptable options.

The responsibilities of local authorities in relation to the tribunal process are highlighted within 'After-care under the Mental Health Act 1983 section 117: after-care services' (DoH 2000) which states: 'guidance in the revised Mental Health Act Code of Practice makes clear that where section 117 applies and there is to be a hearing of the Mental Health Review Tribunal, the "responsible authorities" should prepare an after-care plan under section 117 and submit this to the Tribunal to assist it in reaching its decisions.'

The social circumstances report should be compiled in accordance with principles of antidiscriminatory practice, giving due regard to issues of culture, race, gender and sexual orientation. Good practice indicates that the report should conclude with a recommendation by the social worker which reflects the information and assessment outlined within its contents.

The Mental Health Review Tribunal Rules (HMSO 1983) do not give any indication of the appropriate degree of social work participation in respect of the hearing itself. However, principles of good practice would again suggest that it is appropriate for the social worker to be actively involved prior to, during and after the tribunal hearing. In preparation for the Mental Health Review Tribunal, the social worker, where practicable, establishes a process of communication in order to:

◆ advise the patient on eligibility to apply for a Mental Health Review Tribunal hearing
◆ inform the patient of entitlement to legal representation and legal aid
◆ brief the patient about the purpose of the Mental Health Review Tribunal
◆ prepare the patient for the hearing itself and explain the role of all relevant participants
◆ facilitate the attendance of family members as appropriate.

In respect of the actual hearing, expectations concerning the participation of the social worker vary greatly and are largely determined by the outlook of the individual tribunal chairman. It is difficult, therefore, to be prescriptive about the nature and extent of the social work contribution. Attendance by the social worker at the hearing is desirable but this can be extremely time consuming and is of questionable value in respect of those hearings at which the social worker is not invited to participate. Best practice would indicate that the social worker always attends the tribunal hearing under the following circumstances.

◆ When the patient care team considers it likely that the patient will be conditionally discharged, transferred or absolutely discharged.
◆ When there is professional disagreement within the patient care team concerning the recommendations to the Mental Health Review Tribunal.
◆ When the patient requests the social worker to be present.

Following the tribunal hearing, the social worker continues the communication process in order to:

◆ assist the patient to come to terms with the outcome of the mental health review tribunal
◆ explain to the patient the meaning and implications of the decisions/ recommendations of the Mental Health Review Tribunal, e.g. conditional discharge, deferred discharge, aftercare under supervision, etc.

◆ advise the patient of rights in respect of future applications to the Mental Health Review Tribunal
◆ inform relatives of the outcome, where appropriate.

Liaison with outside agencies

Continuity of involvement by local authority Social Services departments in planning the delivery of social care to forensic patients on discharge is an essential component in the process of rehabilitation in the community. In accordance with the principles underlying the NHS and Community Care Act 1990, enabling patients to live independently in the community with appropriate support, and with the necessary safeguards to protect both the patient and the public, remains the fundamental rehabilitative goal.

The social care needs of forensic patients are invariably complex and they require full and detailed assessment which will often indicate the need for the commissioning of specialized resources. Consequently, it is essential that forensic patients are given adequate access to the care management process to ensure that resources are identified appropriate to their needs.

Initially, liaison needs to establish that the local authority accepts the patient is normally resident within its locality (DoH 1993). It is essential that local authorities and health authorities are contacted on the patient's admission to determine who will be responsible for commissioning the patient's care on discharge. Thereafter, there needs to be ongoing liaison at practitioner level to ensure the local authority social worker retains an active involvement.

However, in the high security hospitals, the distance from the local authority Social Services often militates against this. Sending an annual update of the patient's progress may be appropriate in these circumstances. This process is especially important for patients detained in supraregional facilities, such as high security hospitals. In the absence of a sustained commitment to joint working, these patients can become totally isolated from the social care services in their normal area of residence. Some patients may not return to their original place of residence, possibly because of victim proximity and the patient's desire to make a fresh start, and this causes additional problems of who pays for the care.

Since 1994 the liaison process between social workers in high security hospitals and local authorities has been underpinned by the Protocol for Work between High Security Hospital Social Work Services and Social Services departments. The protocol, which is included below, was ratified by the Association of Directors of Social Services in September 1997 and whilst its focus is on liaison with high security hospitals, it could equally be used as a model of good practice for liaison with other forensic mental health facilities.

Protocol for work between high security hospital social work services and Social Services departments

Admission High security hospital social work staff will:

1. inform the relevant local authority Social Services department that the patient has been admitted to the hospital and request acknowledgement of responsibility
2. request Social Services department to identify named responsible social worker who will be recipient of future case conference minutes
3. invite relevant Social Services department, and other relevant agencies, to initial care programme meeting
4. feed back to Social Services department staff relevant details of initial hospital assessment.

Social Services department social work staff will:

1. acknowledge responsibility or otherwise for the patient as soon as this has been determined
2. provide any relevant information about patient on request
3. attend or make representation to initial care programme approach meeting
4. liaise with other relevant agencies as appropriate.

Regular review High security hospital social work staff will:

1. invite Social Services department staff and other relevant agencies to regular care programme reviews and furnish minutes to named worker
2. request Social Services department to undertake the needs assessment
3. feed back to named social worker on patient's progress when appropriate.

Social Services department social work staff will:

1. undertake a patient's needs assessment leading to consequential care management and resource planning
2. cooperate in work with families and communities where appropriate
3. communicate with relevant agencies as appropriate.

Mental Health Review Tribunals High security hospital social work staff will:

1. inform the Social Services department of a patient's proposed application
2. negotiate with the Social Services department which agency is the most appropriately placed to prepare the social circumstances report
3. attend Mental Health Review Tribunals wherever possible
4. feed back tribunal decisions.

Social Services department social work staff will:

1. where agreed, prepare social circumstances report with special reference to resource implications and needs assessment
2. attend Mental Health Review Tribunals, where appropriate and possible
3. communicate outcome to purchasers and providers as appropriate.

Rehabilitation and preparation for departure High security hospital social work staff will:

1. ensure that the Social Services department social worker is invited to the section 117 conference

2. contact the Director of Social Services and Chief Probation Officer whenever a social supervisor has to be appointed
3. provide detailed transfer summary including an analysis of the index offence and reason for admission.

Social Services department social work staff will:

1. attend the section 117 conference and undertake subsequent planning and provision of resources
2. liaise with other relevant agencies as appropriate.

Additionally, the social worker will also need to liaise with the relevant local authority Child Protection Services on specific issues related to the patient's contact with children and any other child protection concerns. It is particularly important that liaison occurs about the movement of schedule one offenders. Guidance to prison governors on liaison with Social Services departments in respect of the movement of prisoners convicted of an offence within schedule one of the Children and Young Persons Act 1933 is contained within 'release of prisoners convicted of offences against children or young persons under the age of 18' (HM Prison Service 1994). Good practice indicates that these guidelines should also be followed for the movement of a patient detained under the Mental Health Act 1983 when the patient is also a schedule one offender. The social work team should also establish links with the area Child Protection Committee that has responsibility for the locality within which the forensic facility is based. The area Child Protection Committee can offer professional advice and access to local child protection training initiatives and can function as a focal point in the communication process.

Management of transfer and discharge

At the point of a patient's transfer or discharge from the forensic mental health facility, it is essential that the social work component of the aftercare plan has been fully prepared in accordance with the patient's future social care needs. Effective liaison with the social work services who will be taking over responsibility for the patient is crucial at this stage.

Essentially, there are three routes by which a patient detained in a forensic mental health facility is likely to move on: discharge into the community, transfer to conditions of greater or lesser security in another hospital or transfer to prison.

Discharge into the community

Discharge into the community presents the highest potential risk, requiring meticulous planning. All necessary components of a full social support network must be established in advance of discharge. Typically, this will include:

◆ accommodation with an appropriate level of support
◆ help with personal finances
◆ access to medical and day-care facilities
◆ contingency plans for an emergency or crisis.

The focus for this planning process will be the section 117 aftercare meeting. This needs to be a multidisciplinary and multiagency forum with representation from all interested parties. The specific role of the forensic social worker in preparation for this meeting is to liaise with the relevant local authority Social Services departments and other relevant agencies in order to achieve the following.

◆ To ensure that both the funding and receiving local authority Social Services departments are informed in writing of the proposed discharge and are invited to attend the section 117 meeting.
◆ To provide the appropriate Social Services department with relevant information including: (i) social history/assessment report; (ii) most recent social circumstances report to a Mental Health Review Tribunal; (iii) most recent care programme review documentation.
◆ To request a care management assessment from the funding Social Services department.

◆ To agree how patients' records will be transferred and to whom these will be made available.
◆ To establish who contacts whom if anything starts to cause concern.

For patients detained under part III of the Mental Health Act 1983, planning for the social aftercare should take into account the category of discharge, i.e. conditional discharge or absolute discharge. For a conditionally discharged patient the social worker has to write to the relevant Director of Social Services and, where appropriate, the Chief Probation Officer, specifying the conditions imposed and outlining the current care plan. An attempt must also be made to ensure that the patient understands the nature of the conditions and the potential consequences of failure to comply with these. For an absolutely discharged patient, the social worker liaises with the patient's Responsible Medical Officer to ensure that full consideration is given to making an application for guardianship under the Mental Health Act 1983 or supervised discharge under the Mental Health (Patients in the Community) Act 1995. Liaison also takes place with the receiving Social Services department to ensure the allocation, where possible, of an Approved Social Worker, to give full consideration to making a recommendation for supervised discharge.

In any event, when the patient is a schedule one offender within the Children and Young Persons Act 1933, the relevant details must be communicated to the receiving local authority. When the patient has been convicted of an offence under the Sex Offenders Act 1997, as well as taking steps to ensure that the patient is aware of responsibilities to register, consideration should be given to informing the appropriate police authority prior to the discharge (see DoH 1997).

Transfer to conditions of greater or lesser security in another hospital

The principal social work objective is to ensure continuity in the patient's social care, through a planned handover of casework involvement between the social workers in both settings. When the transfer is to conditions of greater security, for example from a regional secure unit to a high security hospital, often there will be a high level of urgency, in which case the social work handover needs to occur after the transfer has taken place. However, transfers to conditions of lesser security can generally be thoroughly planned over a period of time.

Key documentation which should be shared with the receiving social work team will include:

◆ the patient's social history
◆ a full social work assessment
◆ minutes of recent case conferences, CPA reviews
◆ the most recent social circumstances report to a Mental Health Review Tribunal.

The more difficult and sensitive task is the handover of any therapeutic relationship that has developed between the social worker and the patient. Wherever practicable, to facilitate this transition, a pretransfer meeting should take place between the existing and receiving social workers and the patient to clarify expectations of the new social worker's role. Ideally, this should be followed up after the transfer by another meeting in the new location. Both social workers need to liaise as appropriate with the patient's family to assist them through the transitional period.

The nature of all social work involvement should always be recorded within the section 117 documentation. Indeed, good practice indicates that a section 117 meeting should take place prior to transfer in the same way as for discharge. This should occur with the same degree of participation from those responsible for future social care provision.

Transfer to prison

When a patient detained in a forensic mental health setting is transferred back to prison to serve the remainder of a custodial sentence, there is a real danger that awareness of the patient's social care and mental health needs will be lost at the eventual time of release into the community. To avoid this, it is essential that communication takes place between the prison and the patient's responsible local and health authorities. The through-care

probation officer will often be the appropriate person to facilitate the process.

The social worker in the forensic mental health setting can assist by providing the prison with the relevant information pertaining to the patient's mental health and related social care needs at the time of transfer. Typically this will include:

◆ the patient's social history and social work assessment
◆ an account of any therapeutic work currently being undertaken with the patient
◆ the name and address of the patient's nearest relative and any other relevant community contacts
◆ details of the patient's through-care probation officer
◆ details of the patient's responsible local and health authorities.

COMPLEMENTARY ACTIVITIES

A wide range of activities can be compatible with the core forensic social work tasks detailed above. Some of these will involve direct work with patients and others will be focused more on developmental issues. Essentially, the patient-centred tasks can include any form of therapeutic input which assists the patient's social functioning. Clearly, there is an overlap here with the work of other professionals, such as clinical psychologists, occupational therapists, doctors and nurses, and agreement within the multidisciplinary team about specific therapeutic roles is vital. Tasks with a developmental focus will include participation in the fields of forensic social care research and social work education and training. The management structure of the forensic facility should include social work representation at all levels of service development, to ensure that policies and procedures give sufficient emphasis to social care issues. A few examples of appropriate complementary activities are listed below.

Individual psychotherapy and counselling

For social workers with the appropriate training in counselling or psychotherapy, the role of therapist can be compatible with that of caseworker. It is essential, however, that a distinction is made between the two roles and that psychotherapeutic involvement is not at the expense of the core social work tasks. Any individual counselling or psychotherapy must be planned with the multidisciplinary team and must be fully integrated into the patient's care plan.

Facilitation of group work

Within the restricted confines of a forensic mental health setting, group work can provide a valuable opportunity to improve a patient's social functioning, by working in a hands-on capacity with their personal interactions with others. A structured group work programme which is planned, recorded and reviewed can be a vital contribution to the patient's social assessment.

Research

For forensic social workers to achieve standards of excellence, their practice must be underpinned by a sound evidence base. This evidence base must be continually strengthened by an ongoing programme of research into issues pertaining to the social context of forensic mental health. Social workers in forensic mental health settings have access to a wealth of evidential social care data and the management of any forensic social work service should include a strategy for contributing to the forensic mental health research agenda.

Education and training

It is vital that social workers in forensic mental health settings participate actively in the broader arena of mental health social work training. This should be a reciprocal process: forensic social workers can offer specialized training opportunities, both prequalifying through Diploma of Social Work practice placements and postqualifying in relation to Approved Social Work and Advanced Award training. Likewise, forensic social workers need to be given access to wider social services training initiatives in order to ensure that they

keep abreast of mainstream practice, particularly in respect of community mental health services, care management and child protection. The training needs of each social worker should be assessed individually and monitored through the process of professional supervision.

The General Social Care Council will replace the Central Council for Education and Training in Social Work in regulating the training of social workers, setting conduct and practice standards for all social services staff, registering those in the most sensitive areas and developing new training strategy centred around a new national training organization for social care staff (DoH 1998).

CONCLUSION

The aim of all social work activity is to achieve improved social care outcomes for the client and others within the client system. Within forensic mental health practice, the client system needs to be seen in broad terms, and social care outcomes must accommodate not only the needs of the patient, but also the needs and the safety of the patient's family and others in his/her social network, actual and potential victims and the public at large.

The forensic social worker operates within a complex and continually evolving framework of social care legislation pertaining to those individuals who occupy the uncertain territory which exists at the interface of the criminal justice system and mental health services. It is the social worker who identifies the social context of psychopathology and behaviours which is an essential dimension of the patient's overall care, treatment and rehabilitation.

Forensic social work must be practised as a precisely described professional function within a clearly defined framework of accountability. The identification of core social work tasks within the chronology of the patient's pathway through care and treatment provides the foundation for the social worker to perform an essential unidisciplinary professional role within a comprehensive multidisciplinary and multiagency approach to forensic mental health care provision.

REFERENCES

Central Council for Education and Training in Social Work 1995 Forensic social work competence and workforce data. Black Bear Press, Cambridge

Department of Health 1993 Ordinary residence. LAC (93)7 DH. Department of Health, London

Department of Health 1997 Guidance to hospital managers and local authorities social services departments on the Sex Offenders Act 1997. Department of Health, London

Department of Health 1998 Modernising social services: promoting independence, promoting protection, raising standards. Stationery Office, London

Department of Health 1999a The Stephen Lawrence inquiry. Report of an inquiry by Sir William Macpherson of Cluny. Stationery Office, London

Department of Health 1999b Review of social work in the high security hospitals. Stationery Office, London

Department of Health 1999c Visits by children to Ashworth, Broadmoor and Rampton hospitals, HSC 1999/160. Department of Health, London

Department of Health 1999d Mental Health Act 1983 code of practice: guidance on the visiting of psychiatric patients by children, HSC 1999/222:LAC (99)32. Department of Health, London

Department of Health 2000 After-care under the Mental Health Act 1983 section 117: after-care services, HSC 2000/003:LAC (2000)3. Department of Health, London

Department of Health, Home Office, Department for Education and Employment 2000 Working together to safeguard children: a guide to interagency working to safeguard and promote the welfare of children. Stationery Office, London

Department of Health, Home Office, Welsh Office 1997 Notes for the guidance of social supervisors – Mental Health Act 1983. Supervision and after care of conditionally discharged patients. Stationery Office, London

Department of Health, Welsh Office 1999 Mental Health Act 1983: code of practice. Stationery Office, London

HM Prison Service 1994 Guidance notes: instructions to governors. HM Prison Service, London

HMSO 1983 Mental Health Review Tribunal rules (SI 1983 No. 942). HMSO, London

Mental Health Act Commission 2000 National visits 2: a visit by the Mental Health Act Commission to 104 mental health and learning disability units in England and Wales. Sainsbury Centre for Mental Health, London

Special Hospitals Social Work Service 1994 Beyond care? Social work in the special hospitals. Special Hospital Authority, London

FURTHER READING

Bean A, Mounser P 1993 Discharged from mental hospitals. Macmillan, London

Central Council for Education and Training in Social Work 1995 Achieving competence in forensic social work. Chameleon Press, Wandsworth

Munro A, McCulloch W 1969 Psychiatry for social workers. Pergamon, Oxford

Murphy E 1991 After the asylums. Community care for people with mental illness. Faber and Faber, London

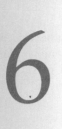

Chapter Six

Clinical governance: a framework for quality in forensic mental health care

David Duffy

INTRODUCTION

In recent years the British public has become increasingly concerned about the quality of care provided by the National Health Service in general, and mental health services in particular, demonstrated by the plethora of inquiries into these services. A long series of inquiry reports following homicides, suicides and other serious incidents involving mental health patients has placed the spotlight repeatedly on the mental health field and recently the Fallon Inquiry (DoH 1999a) into Ashworth Hospital has been the subject of intense media interest.

Unsurprisingly, therefore, the present government saw quality, alongside efficiency and fairness, as a central issue in its first major programme for change in the National Health Service, *The new NHS: modern, dependable* (DoH 1997). This White Paper was closely followed by another, *A first class service: quality in the new NHS* (DoH 1998a), which reinforced and elaborated on the quality theme through its threefold approach of setting, delivering and monitoring quality standards. It was in this document that the government formally set out its plans for introducing clinical governance.

Clinical governance must now be pursued at national, regional and local levels over the next 10 years, hopefully in a systematic, developmental and prioritized way. This new agenda places clinicians at the forefront of change. Clinical staff in forensic mental health services, required to suddenly divert a large amount of time and effort into what may seem a new set of priorities, are likely to pose some very probing questions. Clinical governance – what is it? What are our responsibilities as clinicians? Will there be a degree of local freedom or will clinicians have to simply comply with directives?

What will be the eventual outcome of clinical governance?

Such questions, whilst apparently easy to answer on one level, do raise some complex issues for clinicians working in forensic mental health services. The aim of this chapter is to provide an overview of clinical governance and to offer clinicians and others some suggestions on how they can engage in clinical governance activities to best effect for their patients. Before examining what clinical governance is and what it will mean for clinicians working on wards and in the community, it may be useful to look a little more closely at the broader policy context and background of clinical governance.

BACKGROUND AND POLICY CONTEXT

To begin with, it is important to recognize that efforts to improve quality of care were made for many years before the advent of clinical governance. Examples of such approaches to quality include:

◆ quality assurance
◆ clinical audit
◆ clinical risk management.

Quality assurance

Quality assurance, based on models developed in industry, was probably the first initiative and one that has not been embraced warmly by all clinicians. Although some quality assurance approaches base themselves firmly on 'bottom-up' ownership by those on the 'shop floor', the history of quality assurance in the National Health Service, exemplified by the 'top-down', government-initiated Patient's Charter (DoH 1992), has done little to promote ownership of assuring quality and as a result its original purpose seems to have been lost.

Clinical audit

Clinical audit emerged as a multidisciplinary expansion of medical audit a decade ago. Excellent examples of clinical audit have been seen and in some cases there has been genuine 'bottom-up' ownership, but it has tended to suffer from unsatisfactory links to organizational priorities and service demands.

Clinical risk management

Clinical risk management, involving the systematic monitoring and reviewing of adverse events in order to promote ways of reducing their recurrence, became an important priority for mental health services in reaction to the flood of mental health inquiries. However, many staff may feel that risk management has tended to be utilized defensively instead of supporting quality improvement initiatives.

Most recently, the concepts of clinical effectiveness and evidence-based care have gained common currency throughout the health service. However, the response of mental health professionals remains cautious as it is said to be difficult to specify expected outcomes and long-term health gain in the mental health field.

CLINICAL GOVERNANCE

Clinical governance is the present government's answer to the need to address inequalities in clinical practice and unacceptable levels of poor-quality care. The Department of Health has defined clinical governance as:

> *a framework through which healthcare organizations are accountable for continuously improving the quality of their services and safeguarding high standards of care by creating an environment in which excellence in clinical care will flourish. (DoH 1998a: 33)*

Clinical governance therefore requires organizations to ensure the quality of clinical care by making individual clinical staff, at all levels, accountable for setting, maintaining and monitoring standards of performance. The Health Act 1999 (DoH 1999b) outlines the new duty of quality which applies to NHS trusts, primary care trusts and health authorities. The Act requires arrangements to be implemented and maintained for monitoring and improving the quality of the health care provided.

Where chief executives were formerly accountable for the financial performance of their organization, they are now accountable for the overall clinical performance too. All quality and risk management activities are brought together as part of an integrated framework. This renewed focus on quality differs from previous central initiatives in that it seeks to marry individual clinical judgement with clear national and local standards. A specific example of clear national standards in the mental health context are those embodied in the National Service Framework for mental health (DoH 1999c).

To take forward clinical governance at a national level, the Commission for Health Improvement (CHI), a new statutory body, has been created as part of the government's NHS modernization reforms. Its purpose is to help the NHS assure, monitor and improve the quality of clinical care. The CHI has an important role in working to reduce unacceptable variations in services through its systematic review of clinical governance, National Service Framework adherence and monitoring the implementation of National Institute for Clinical Excellence (NICE) guidance. The legislative basis for the CHI is the Health Act 1999 (DoH 1999b) and it will work in a collaborative way with the Royal Colleges, professional organizations and regulatory bodies. The CHI will independently scrutinize local clinical governance arrangements every 4 years to ensure effective arrangements are in place to continuously improve the clinical quality of patient care. It is envisaged that the CHI will enquire into service failures by overseeing and assisting with NHS incident inquiries in England and Wales.

The government's reforms on modernizing the NHS show clinical governance working in the context set by the NICE and the CHI, supported by professional self-regulation and life-long learning. When considering the wider policy context of clinical governance, one must also take into account the programme *Modernising mental health services: safe, sound and supportive* (DoH 1998b); the National Service Framework for mental health (DoH 1999c); *Saving lives: our healthier nation,*

(DoH 1999d), together with other associated new national policy initiatives: *Making a difference*, the nursing, midwifery and health visiting nursing strategy (DoH 1999e); the new human resources strategy *Working together* (DoH 1998c); and the national information strategy (DoH 1998d), to name but a few.

What is this fertile ground in which clinical governance will grow and thrive? The answer lies in health-care organizations demonstrating features such as:

◆ an open culture in which education, research and the sharing of good practice are valued and expected
◆ a commitment to quality at all levels and by all professional groups, supported by clearly identified local resources
◆ an ethos of working closely with patients, carers and families and the public
◆ a 'top-down' *and* 'bottom-up' commitment to quality, demonstrated by regular discussion on key 'care' issues
◆ an ethos of multidisciplinary teamworking at all levels in the organization.

If clinical governance is to achieve its aims it must find ways of making a real difference in the practice setting, and the principles of clinical governance can best be illustrated through practical examples. The management of clinical risk is a crucial issue for forensic services and some varying approaches to the problem of suicide and suicide prevention will now be considered in order to bring out the key features of clinical governance.

Suicide is only one, particularly graphic, example of such clinical experience but it is of course very relevant to forensic care. The National Service Framework for mental health (DoH 1999c) has chosen suicide prevention as the subject of one of its seven standards and makes reference to *Safer services* (DoH 1999f), the recent report of the Confidential Inquiry into Suicide and Homicide by People with Mental Illness. This report states that:

◆ one in four of those who subsequently took their lives, around 1000 people each year, were found to have been in contact with

CASE STUDY

Lucy was a very disturbed Afro-Caribbean woman, troubled by a psychotic illness which often led her to behave violently towards herself and others and present significant challenges to the staff on the adult forensic unit. One morning, the nurse who entered Lucy's room to wake her found her lying dead on her bed, having apparently strangled herself with a ligature tied to the window but hidden by the bedclothes. Although staff had looked in on Lucy at intervals throughout the night, they had avoided going into the room, partly because she seemed to be sleeping in her usual posture and partly in order to avoid waking her with the noise of the door opening. According to the postmortem, she could have been dead for several hours whilst the staff had gone on observing her.

What was the trust's response to this incident? It is easy to imagine what might have happened not so long ago. An investigation would have been carried out as quickly as possible within the trust. The investigators would have met in private, a report would have been prepared and discipline would have been apportioned, singling out a few individuals, possibly those lowest in the organizational hierarchy but with most direct patient contact. Within a few weeks the incident would have been all but forgotten and the report would have been gathering dust on a shelf.

Under clinical governance, a very different approach should have been seen. The trust's response would have been characterized by a commitment to openness and fairness and the involvement of patients as well as staff at all levels. The aim would have been to discover the full explanation for this tragic incident rather than to find someone to blame. If there had been unprofessional behaviour by staff this of course would have been appropriately addressed, but the emphasis would have been on the organizational system within which the staff and the unit

functioned. For example, if it was possible for staff to carry out the observation procedure to the letter with a patient who had died, what did this say about the adequacy of the procedure? If the policy needed to be reviewed, how could the actual staff members responsible for carrying it out contribute, not to mention the patients who were the subjects of observation? Were the staff who carried out observation being appropriately supported, for example through clinical supervision? Perhaps they had tended to avoid waking Lucy less out of concern for her than out of fear of her aggressive behaviour. If there was some truth in this, was it not more important to consider the adequacy of their training with regard to aggression and the appropriateness of the staffing levels than merely to criticize them?

Most important of all, why had Lucy killed herself? Clearly, there could be all kinds of reasons, perhaps related to her psychotic experiences or to hopelessness about her future. Under clinical governance, the response would not restrict itself to such matters as the adequacy of risk assessments but would view the incident within the widest possible organizational framework: did the whole multidisciplinary team maintain a positive and proactive approach to Lucy's needs, taking into account vital concerns such as her ethnicity or her gender, and had the environment within the unit been appropriate in these respects? Had staff tried to develop a therapeutic relationship with her so that she could have communicated her distress before resorting to suicide? Even if they had, was further training and support indicated to promote relationship skills and if there were resource issues, how could these be addressed? These are just some examples of the kind of 'joined-up' thinking which should characterize clinical governance and which should ensure that real lessons are learned, and applied, from clinical experience.

specialist mental health services in the year before their death
◆ of these, 16% were inpatients at the time of their death

◆ 24% had been discharged from hospital in the previous 6 months
◆ many were not fully compliant with treatment when discharged

- in most case staff perceived the immediate risk of suicide to be low
- around half the suicides were committed by people with a history of self-harm and either substance abuse or previous admission to hospital.

Yet there is a long history of high-profile incident inquiries in mental health, often lengthy and expensive to carry out, whose recommendations have failed to make sufficient impact on practice, as underlined by the recurrence of incidents and the repetitiveness of many of the findings and recommendations of the different inquiries. If clinical governance is to achieve its aims, it must find ways of making a real difference to issues such as suicide prevention.

As an example of a systematic approach, Mental Health Services of Salford, a specialist mental health trust with a large forensic service, made a response to *Safer services* an early priority of its clinical governance agenda. The report was carefully analysed to identify the issues of most relevance to the organization and 10 standards were formulated, each with a practical action plan which was subject to continuous monitoring. Examples of standards with particular relevance to forensic care include the following.

Communication

Trust services have systems for adequately recording risk of self-harm and suicide and for communicating it to all those responsible for the care and treatment of people at risk.

Care planning

Allocation of patients to high-level care programme approach (CPA) encompasses the majority of patients at risk of self-harm or suicide.

- CPA plans take into account the heightened risk of suicide in the first 3 months after discharge and make specific reference to the first week.
- CPA documentation forms part of casenotes and is not maintained separately.

Compliance/engagement

All discharge care plans demonstrate explicit procedures for preventing non-compliance, encompassing interventions such as motivational interviewing, use of appropriate medication, involvement of families and carers and use of psychological interventions as an alternative or adjunct to pharmacological interventions.

Dual diagnosis

- All direct care staff are trained in the clinical management of patients with dual diagnosis, i.e. those with mental health problems who also engage in alcohol and/or substance abuse.
- Information on numbers of dual diagnosis patients is collected by the trust and used to inform decision making on resource allocation.

Family/carer involvement

- Families/carers of patients in the community are allocated an identified person and a clear mechanism for making contact with clinical teams at all times.
- Families/carers are given information regarding policies on non-compliance.
- Families/carers are routinely given appropriate information following a suicide.

Inpatient suicide prevention

- All wards are audited at least annually to identify and minimize opportunities for hanging.
- Environmental difficulties in observing patients are made explicit and remedial action taken as far as possible.

Preventing overdose

Patients at risk of suicide, including all patients with a recent history of self-harm, who are treated with psychotropic drugs receive modern, less toxic drugs and/or supplies lasting no more than 2 weeks.

Training

All direct care staff receive training in the recognition, assessment and management of risk of suicide/self-harm at intervals of no more than 3 years. The content of this training is approved by the trust board and reflects indicators of risk, high-risk periods, managing non-compliance and loss of contact, communication and the Mental Health Act. The quality and effectiveness of the training are continuously evaluated.

Aftermath of suicide

◆ All suicides are reviewed in a multidisciplinary forum, including as far as possible all staff involved in the care of the patient, in line with the trust's policy for serious incidents.
◆ All staff and patients affected by a suicide have the opportunity to receive appropriate and effective support as soon as they need it.

These standards demonstrate many of the features of the clinical governance ethos:

◆ they are based on sound evidence, in this case the major research programme behind the National Confidential Inquiry
◆ although 'top down', they involve staff at every level, since all direct care staff, qualified or unqualified, come into contact with mental health service users, who are at a much greater risk of suicide than people without mental health problems
◆ they are achievable
◆ they can be audited
◆ they bring together all relevant stakeholders in the organization, managers, trainers, quality assurance staff, clinicians of all disciplines, not to mention users and families/carers, in a corporate endeavour to continuously improve quality, linking leadership at all levels with accountability and seeking to promote best practice.

CONCLUSION

Clinical governance will evolve, change and improve, it will challenge organizational behaviour and professional practice, it will impact on professional and service boundaries and will create status and power shifts. There will be problems with transparency and openness due to perceived threats of exposure and challenges to competence. There is much for services to embrace if clinical governance is to bring about the expected changes in clinical practice and to sustain the improvements in clinical care delivery in the forensic mental health setting. Nonetheless, if it succeeds, clinical governance may come to be seen as a major landmark in the history of the NHS and of the sometimes turbulent but always challenging and exciting field of forensic mental health care.

REFERENCES

Department of Health 1992 The patient's charter. HMSO, London

Department of Health 1997 The new NHS: modern, dependable. Cm 3807. HMSO, London

Department of Health 1998a A first class service: quality in the new NHS. HMSO, London

Department of Health 1998b Modernising mental health services: safe, sound and supportive. HMSO, London

Department of Health 1998c Working together: securing a quality workforce for the NHS. HSC 1998/162. HMSO, London

Department of Health 1998d The national IM & T strategy: an information strategy for the modern NHS. HMSO, London

Department of Health 1999a The Report of the Committee of Inquiry into the Personality Disorder Unit, Ashworth Special Hospital. Stationery Office, London

Department of Health 1999b The Health Act. Stationery Office, London

Department of Health 1999c Mental health national service framework: modern standards and service models. Stationery Office, London

Department of Health 1999d Saving lives: our healthier nation. Stationery Office, London

Department of Health 1999e Making a difference: strengthening the nursing, midwifery and health visiting contribution to health and health care. Stationery Office, London

Department of Health 1999f Safer services: the National Confidential Inquiry into Suicide and Homicide by People with Mental Illness. Stationery Office, London

FURTHER READING

Crinson I 1999 Clinical governance: the new NHS, new responsibilities? British Journal of Nursing 8(7): 449–453

Isherwood J 1999 Clinical governance in mental health services: a view from the shop floor. Psychiatric Bulletin 23(12): 718–720

McSherry R 1999 Evidence-based healthcare: its place within clinical governance. British Journal of Nursing 8(2): 113–120

Oyebode F 1999 Clinical governance: application to psychiatry. Psychiatric Bulletin 23(1): 7–10

Williams R, Cohen J 2000 Substance use and misuse in psychiatric wards. A model task for clinical governance? Psychiatric Bulletin 24(2): 43–46

Chapter Seven

7

Evidence-based practice and clinical monitoring

Maggie Clifton   Ros Harvey

INTRODUCTION

Research and development (R&D), clinical effectiveness and evidence-based practice are all key components of clinical governance, the policy for improving the quality of services and care for all patients of the NHS. This chapter sets out an overview of these policies, provides some examples of how they have been implemented in forensic mental health services and identifies some of the issues in implementation specific to forensic mental health services.

The key distinction is between *doing* and *using* research: the NHS R&D strategy and funding mechanism is concentrated on doing R&D whereas clinical effectiveness and evidence-based practice are concerned with using the products of R&D. There is a blurring of boundaries at the point of raising the R&D profile in an organization, where training and education in research might be intended to increase the level of general research awareness and research implementation in an organization (using research) or to develop specialist academic research skills (doing research).

The first section of this chapter examines doing R&D, NHS policy, sources of information and issues for forensic mental health whilst the second looks at using research, in particular evidence-based practice and clinical effectiveness.

DOING RESEARCH AND DEVELOPMENT

Research and development – what is it?

NHS R&D is defined as activity designed to generate new, potentially generalizable knowledge which will be disseminated and subject to public scrutiny, generally through publication (DoH 1994).

A simple 'rule of thumb' is that R&D is carried out by or under the supervision of academic staff, often with close links (through joint appointments and honorary contracts) with the NHS. The quality system of peer review which applies to academic work should also apply to NHS-funded R&D, whether located in higher education or not. These functions of R&D, and the connection with academic activity and quality, distinguish R&D from similar activities such as clinical audit, professional development and management information.

NHS R&D is concerned with clinical interventions, the organization and delivery of services. NHS R&D funding supports basic research carried out by partner agencies such as the Medical Research Council, universities and charities carrying out non-commercial R&D within the NHS, as well as funding academic and management infrastructure, projects and programmes of research.

What is the NHS R&D strategy trying to achieve?

The first comprehensive NHS R&D strategy was introduced in 1991 (DoH 1991), followed in 1994 (DoH 1994) by recommendations for organizational structures and funding systems to implement the strategy. At the time of writing, both strategy and funding mechanisms are under review.

The key principle behind the strategy is that the NHS puts significant resources into R&D, not as an end in itself but as a means to an end, which is continuous improvement of services for patients. NHS R&D produces knowledge for health and social care. The primary aim of the strategy is to 'improve the health of the nation by promoting a knowledge-based health service in which clinical, managerial and policy decisions are informed by sound information about R&D findings and scientific developments' (DoH 1998: 1).

The NHS R&D strategy aims to:

◆ shift the imbalance of resources away from acute medical specialities and towards community and primary care services and nursing and professions allied to medicine
◆ improve transparency in accounting for resources put into R&D and value for money
◆ promote quality standards relating to scientific and ethical standards and ensuring R&D has relevance to, importance for and potential to impact on health services and clinical care.

How is R&D supported in the NHS

At the time of writing the details of the funding mechanisms are under review, but the broad approach remains. Resources allocated for R&D are taken from health authority budgets and then returned to NHS services and research providers for the sole purpose of supporting or doing R&D. Because this funding (or levy) is taken from the resources available for patient care, it is crucial that research is focused not only on improving patient care and service delivery, but also on meeting the same priorities and needs which are the province of service provision.

Funding is made available to NHS trusts and other service providers to support R&D: in mental health, this might include costs of clinical staff time as research subjects or to provide patient related or other information for research purposes, to fund academic posts and to provide management and administrative support. Additionally, regional programmes provide funds for developing research capability (particularly amongst nursing and professions allied to medicine, in general practice and in community services), for commissioning research projects and units to provide academic support to researchers from within the NHS. A number of national programmes are also funded.

How do I find out what's going on in R&D?

The most relevant of the standard databases of published research are PsychLIT and CINHAL. In addition, there are a number of sources of information about R&D in the NHS, including:

◆ Department of Health R&D website: http://www.doh.gov.uk/research/index.htm
◆ National Research Register (NRR): http://www.doh.gov.uk/research/nrr.htm
◆ the proposed Research Findings Electronic Register (ReFER)
◆ National Forensic Mental Health R&D Programme: http://www.open.gov.uk/doh/fmhrd.htm

The above sources have the benefit of providing information about research in progress and research findings prior to publication in academic journals. The R&D information pack (DoH 1998) includes details of the NHS R&D strategy, its associated structure, contact details and publications, as well as information about centrally funded research programmes. This includes the mental health programme (which funded 33 projects) and associated Medical Research Council (MRC) priorities, and the policy research programme, which includes work on mental health policy and social care for people with mental health problems.

Basic information about all research projects funded by the NHS should be submitted to the NRR which is the most comprehensive register of current research. It enables unpublished research to be identified, helps avoid unnecessary duplication in research and facilitates contact between researchers (and practitioners) with particular research and practice interests. The current NRR projects database includes 53 972 items, of which only 127 are accessed by a search using the keyword 'forensic'; 26 are accessed by a search using the keywords 'mentally disordered offenders'; 92 are accessed by 'severe mental illness'; and

115 by 'personality disorder'. Relevant topics include:

◆ pathways out of medium security
◆ ethnic differences amongst adolescents who attempt suicide
◆ behavioural disturbance and borderline personality disorder
◆ staff stress in forensic settings
◆ medication amongst discharged mentally disordered offenders.

ReFER is still in the development stage but is intended to provide information about the findings of completed R&D projects which have been supported by the NHS prior to publication in the academic press, thus facilitating speedier access to relevant research.

Of specific relevance is the National Programme on Forensic Mental Health Research & Development (NPFMHRD). Its main aims are to develop a research programme which:

◆ encourages academic units to become involved in forensic mental health research
◆ broadens opportunities for individuals to undertake research and strengthen their skills
◆ involves all disciplines and agencies relevant to providing services for mentally disordered offenders
◆ develops people and networks
◆ strengthens the forensic mental health research community.

The ultimate aim of this activity is to improve forensic mental health services for those who use them.

The NPFMHRD website contains details of the projects, fellowships and bursaries which have been funded, conference reports and details of relevant events. A wide range of topics has been funded by the programme. Some examples are:

◆ the therapeutic environment in secure mental hospitals
◆ personality disorder in primary care
◆ risk assessment and management in relation to sex and violent offending
◆ professional roles in secure settings

◆ randomized controlled trials relevant to the management of offenders
◆ deliberate self-harm in a maximum secure setting
◆ care, custody and control in high secure settings
◆ prevalence of personality disorders and their comorbidity with other psychiatric disorders
◆ review of sex offender treatment programmes.

Overall, this site provides a mine of information about research and other activities relevant to improving services for mentally disordered offenders. One of the main initiatives has been the creation of the Virtual Institute for Severe Personality Disorder (VISPED). This brings together 11 academic units with established and new researchers with the express aim of contributing to the evidence base and supporting clinical governance. Its objectives are to:

◆ bring together and generate networks of people in the field
◆ facilitate an interdisciplinary research agenda
◆ develop researchers
◆ carry out research
◆ produce discussion papers.

Further information can be found on its website at: http://www.visped.org/

What are the challenges and opportunities for forensic mental health R&D?

The challenges and opportunities for forensic mental health R&D are similar to those for other non-acute, non-medical services and disciplines. There is a scarcity of high-calibre specialist researchers in all disciplines and therefore a need to develop capacity, particularly at doctorate and postdoctorate levels.

In addition to research capacity, the development of a high-quality R&D evidence base requires input from a range of agencies and disciplines. For forensic R&D, this involves not only the health, social care, housing and educational services that many client groups require but also those from criminal justice agencies (probation,

police, prisons and courts). This adds to the multiplicity of structures, perspectives and values which need to be brought together, coordinated and integrated, some of which may have conflicting priorities such as the tension between public safety and client-focused therapy, much debated in relation to high security hospital provision and to mental health services in general.

One approach to addressing these issues, and making a start in bringing together the relevant individuals and agencies, has been a project to develop a multidisciplinary and multiagency North West R&D network relating to mentally disordered offenders (led by Dr Tom Mason, Senior Research Fellow, Caswell Clinic, Cardiff University and supported by funds from the NHSE North West R&D Directorate). This involved a large steering group representing the range of NHS forensic mental health service providers, academics, psychiatry, psychology, nursing, social work, managers and criminal justice liaison schemes. A smaller management group representing academic and national health service interests oversaw the development of the project.

The first phase involved the collection of contact details from as many relevant agencies and institutions as could be identified in the North West, followed by a stakeholder conference in January 2000. Over 100 participants from the range of interest groups, including service users, heard about the practical and theoretical importance of collaborative working in research, current research evidence of effectiveness and contributed to workshops on developing a collaborative R&D strategy for forensic mental health in the region, identifying research priorities, developing research contributions, overcoming barriers to research and research dissemination and use. This conference is intended to form the foundation for collaborative groups of researchers and practitioners to develop and implement a research agenda for meeting the needs of mentally disordered offenders.

Experience of the project to date confirms that:

◆ collaboration approaches to R&D in this field are crucial: without involving the whole range of stakeholders, at least in the overall approach to developing a strategy and priorities, the effort and energy expended will only have partial relevance to meeting the needs of the various services, disciplines and ultimately service users

◆ collaboration on this scale requires a degree of coordinating, negotiating and support to bring the disparate interests together in a fruitful collaborative endeavour.

USING RESEARCH AND DEVELOPMENT

A vast amount of research findings are published. Over 2 million articles are published each year in the biomedical literature, there are over 20 000 biomedical journals and over 400 nursing journals. Managing this amount of data, identifying that which is relevant, appraising and interpreting it all and putting it into practice is clearly an impossible task for busy practitioners and service managers.

There are a number of approaches to using research-based evidence in practice, two of which are discussed here: clinical effectiveness and evidence-based practice. Evidence-based practice is the process whereby clinicians, practitioners (and managers, although it has primarily been focused on health-care practitioners) put research into practice in meeting individual patient or client needs whereas clinical effectiveness is an organizational approach to improving the effectiveness of clinical managerial practice.

Standards of research evidence are relevant here. The consensus of opinion is that the highest level of evidence of effectiveness of interventions is the randomized controlled trial (RCT). Other experimental models, observational studies and expert opinion have lesser validity and should only be used when good-quality RCT evidence is not available. Elliot et al (1995) provide a readable account of the scientific method and the characteristics and assumptions which distinguish evidence from experience or opinion. They also indicate the limits to evidence-based practice,

specifically in relation to psychiatry, and the need for sound clinical judgement to complement scientific evidence. A search of both PsychLIT and CINHAL from 1994 to 1999 using the terms 'randomized controlled trial' with 'forensic' and 'mentally disordered offenders' produced no results.

A particular source of evidence relevant to forensic mental health services comes from the inquiries into homicide and other serious incidents. Despite the limitations of the inquiry method for generating evidence, recommendations can contribute to improvements in clinical and managerial decision making and practice. Inquiry reports recommend what should be done but not how it should be done (Clifton & Duffy in press). Implementation of these recommendations must, however, be tempered by a recognition of the potential for inconsistencies and even contradictions between reports. The UKCC & University of Central Lancashire (1999) note that the Fallon Report (DoH 1999) into Ashworth Hospital was critical of the political response to the Blom-Cooper report (DoH 1992) and of the way in which its recommendations had been implemented, which had led to the problems which triggered the Fallon Inquiry.

Clinical effectiveness

Clinical effectiveness is based on the principle that:

> the overall purpose of the NHS is to secure through the resources available the greatest possible improvements in the physical and mental health of the people of England. (DoH 1996)

This will be achieved by ensuring that 'decisions about clinical services are increasingly driven by evidence of clinical effectiveness and cost effectiveness, coupled with systematic assessment of health outcomes to secure the greatest health gain from the available resources' (DoH 1996).

Clinical effectiveness is a general term incorporating a range of activities which ensure and demonstrate that the best possible care is given.

The following stages have been identified in this process:

◆ identifying a current practice or issue to be examined
◆ finding evidence/information on effective practice
◆ acting on the information, e.g. recommendations or guidelines
◆ monitoring and evaluating practice.

Clinical leadership and multidisciplinary collaboration are key to driving this initiative at a local level, thus leading to a cultural shift which may require significant structural changes to the organization. More importantly, it requires the pooling of expertise and experiences of all staff to maximize its potential for success. Such coordination of effort emphasizes that clinical effectiveness is everyone's business and that awareness, collaboration, good evidence, communication, dissemination, enthusiasm and persistence are integral to its success.

Whilst it must be acknowledged that changes to organizational structure do not provide an easy or complete solution, the underpinning notion is that these activities cannot be done in isolation from each other. If the process of information, change and monitoring is to be successful, it requires a structure which incorporates the relevant experts into a group of activity and draws upon expert advice as necessary, thus reducing duplication and maximizing use of time.

Levers for change include: professional education to suit local purposes, clinical audit, R&D, support systems, empowered/ educated patients, contracts/finance and staff trained in evidence-based practice. Additionally, it requires investment in training and education to get the clinical effectiveness message across and the integration of medical and non-medical workforce planning, with a special emphasis on multidisciplinary education. Finally, information systems need to be integral to the delivery of care and provision of data.

These levers for change are usually under the control of disparate groups, so successful clinical effectiveness will require effective and sustained collaborative working.

A structure for improving clinical effectiveness

This proposed structure attempts to address these multifarious issues and also connect systems with mechanisms for effective work across organizational structures and professional boundaries. The proposed structure includes a core group, whose membership should consist of representatives from clinical and operational management, education and training, quality, R&D and clinical audit. The primary responsibility of this autonomous core group is to process suggestions and prioritize projects relating to clinical issues. It is a clearing house for activity, with staff collaborating with other bodies as necessary, which ensures that all projects comply with the strategic direction of the organization.

Once a project has been agreed, a project leader, project team and time scales should be identified to progress the work. Project teams should be small but comprise the necessary expertise and commitment to examine an issue. They need to be flexible, so expertise can be brought into the team at any stage of the process if required.

The project teams focus their activity on the key elements of the clinical effectiveness process.

◆ *Inform*. Collating information via clinical audit, evidence-based research, local practice and clinical expertise. From this information they will offer recommendations and guidelines relating to best practice.
◆ *Change*. Implement the changes recommended by the project teams; this is a difficult part of the process which requires effective support from all staff.
◆ *Monitor*. After a specified period a clinical audit tool will be developed to monitor the success of the change process.

The process requires the identification of clinical issue(s) and obtaining the best evidence to answer these questions from clinical research, published literature and other sources. Evidence-based practice requires that key players should be skilled in both critically appraising the evidence and then applying the results of this appraisal to clinical practice. If agreed, the changes to practice should be implemented with the support of rigorous monitoring systems. There will then be a feedback loop, whereby the monitoring feedback is communicated to the core group, who will direct the project team if further work or research is required.

The proposed structure is intended to encourage effective and focused collaboration, reduce time spent attending meetings and help involve all staff in the clinical effectiveness process. It is also suggested that a review of the effectiveness of this structure should take place after 12 months.

What is evidence-based practice?

Evidence-based practice is an approach to decision making which draws explicitly on four types of information:

◆ research evidence
◆ clinical judgement
◆ patient preferences
◆ available resources.

In forensic mental health services, decision making will additionally be constrained by decisions of the criminal justice system (the courts' sentencing policy and practice), Home Secretary's decisions (restricted patients) or mental health tribunal (civil sections). The UKCC & University of Central Lancashire (1999) report highlights the politicized context of secure services and the lack of public and media support which intrude upon the pursuit of a research evidence-based service.

According to Geddes (1996) the process of evidence-based practice consists of:

◆ converting a clinical or service issue or problem into an answerable question
◆ finding the best evidence to answer the question
◆ critically appraising the evidence for validity and usefulness
◆ combining the research evidence with clinical judgement, patient preferences and the available resources
◆ applying the results in practice

◆ evaluating performance against evidence-based standards.

A study of nursing in secure environments (UKCC & University of Central Lancashire 1999) found that provision of library facilities and journals was good and that nurses claimed to use evidence to inform their work. In practice this evidence tended to be anecdotal and experiential rather than research based.

Where do I find research information to improve clinical effectiveness and support evidence-based practice?

The most relevant of the standard databases of published research are PsychLIT and CINHAL. Both these should be accessible from local NHS and university health libraries and librarians will be able to assist in searching these sources of published information. The primary sources of information about research-based evidence designed to be more 'user friendly' to practitioners are:

◆ Cochrane Library
◆ Bandolier
◆ *Effective Health Care* bulletins
◆ NHS learning zone
◆ ImpAct.

The first three focus on the 'gold standard' of evidence of effectiveness, the RCT, whereas the others contain expert opinion and examples of service developments.

Cochrane library

The Cochrane Library is the output of the Cochrane Collaboration, an international network of individuals (researchers, practitioners, consumers) who work together to prepare, maintain and disseminate systematic reviews of the effects of health-care interventions. About 50 review groups prepare and maintain reviews, identifying up-to-date and reliable evidence about particular health-care problems.

The main output of the Cochrane Collaboration is found on the Cochrane Library which contains five databases. It is updated quarterly and is available by subscription basis on disk, CD-ROM and the Internet. The relevant databases are:

◆ systematic reviews – reviews produced by Cochrane Collaboration groups
◆ reviews of effectiveness – reviews published elsewhere
◆ controlled trials register – information (not quality assured) about tens of thousands of controlled trials.

Systematic reviews are produced to exacting quality standards which are applied to all reviews, regardless of topic area. Because they are rigorously quality assured they will include all relevant evidence, using an agreed hierarchy of types of evidence, and extensive and comprehensive search strategies. They produce better evidence than individuals working alone, because the methodology and the peer review of decisions on what to include and exclude reduce bias. In keeping with best scientific practice, the Cochrane Collaboration targets RCTs as the best evidence of effectiveness.

There are four Cochrane Review Groups with relevance to forensic mental health services: schizophrenia group; development, psychosocial and learning problems group; drugs and alcohol group; and effective practices and organization of care group. Each group includes researchers and reviewers: membership and contact details are available on the Library database.

Further information about the Library and how to subscribe to it can be accessed from Update Software Ltd, Summertown Pavilion, Middle Way, Oxford OX2 LG, UK, tel: 01865–513902, e-mail info@update.co.uk. The Cochrane Library's website is: http://www.cochrane.co.uk

Bandolier

Bandolier is published monthly and contains information about evidence of effectiveness of a whole range of interventions (conventional and complementary medicine), as well as information on how to convert research findings into useable information. This includes numbers needed to treat (NNT) and numbers needed to harm (NNH), both relatively straightforward techniques for translating statistical concepts into more meaningful information. The former indicates how many patients need to be treated with a particular intervention to achieve one 'successful outcome' (so that a low number means that the intervention is more effective) and the latter gives the number needed to receive an intervention before harm is caused (so that a high number means that the intervention is less harmful).

Examining the issues of Bandolier published in 1997 and 1998 indicates that very little of the content is relevant to mental health in general, let alone forensic mental health services. The publication can be viewed at: http://www.j+2.ox.ac.uk/bandolier/

Effective Health Care bulletins

These publications are intended to make research findings relevant to the needs of health-care practitioners and service providers and are usually based on a systematic review of the literature on specific interventions or types of intervention for specific health-care problems and in specific settings. Those specifically relevant to mental health cover drug treatments in schizophrenia (NHS Centre for Reviews and Dissemination 1999a) and deliberate self-harm (NHS Centre for Reviews and Dissemination 1998). The bulletins follow the format of identifying the particular clinical problem under consideration, reviewing the evidence of effectiveness of interventions, identifying implications for practice and implications for further research. Both these reviews note the limitations in the research evidence but make recommendations about practice on the basis of the best available information. Both recommend further research.

NHS learning zone

This recent website produces a different type of evidence, namely examples of good practice which are published to enable others to learn. This resource contains the Database of Service Delivery Practice, which is in pilot form. The objective is to enable staff to access and enter information in a preset format to disseminate ideas for good practice throughout the NHS. Contributions relevant to forensic mental health services include: information about local forensic services for people with learning disabilities in Teeside; assertive outreach in Wandsworth; and a comprehensive multidisciplinary service for mentally disordered offenders in Leeds. Service providers are encouraged to contribute information about their own innovative developments. Further details are at: http://www.doh.gov.uk/learningzone/index.htm

ImpAct

A second publication which supports transfer of examples of good practice and innovation in service delivery is ImpAct, published bimonthly as an insert to Bandolier. It aims to cover, amongst other things:

◆ clinical governance and clinical quality
◆ integration of services across institutional boundaries
◆ involving patients and the public
◆ developments in human resources including staffing and skill mix.

An initiative will be reported if there is evidence that it works, is transferable and affordable within normal budgets. Since the first issue was published in June 1999, there have been no reports of service developments specific to forensic or general mental health services, although there may be some transferable key points arising from service developments in other fields of health care. The September 1999 issue of ImpAct has nothing specifically about mental health but articles about introducing innovation in other areas (cardiac care, sexual health, career paths for junior doctors) seem to have transferable lessons. For example:

◆ services that are outward looking and care about how they are perceived are more likely to succeed: influence is born of good relationships, not internal structures and systems
◆ make sure you know what needs to change before making detailed plans; don't rely on anecdotes; make sensible use of questionnaires.

How can I make best use of available information?

Regardless of the type of information produced, it will still require critical appraisal to ensure its relevance to the clinical or service problem in question. This applies whether one is using the organizational model of clinical effectiveness, the model of evidence-based practice or, preferably, both.

Critical appraisal is key to clinical effectiveness; it assists in identifying the validity, value, rigour and applicability of the evidence to support the process. Organizations should draw upon the expertise of the critical appraisal skills programme (CASP) schemes to ensure that their staff are sufficiently skilled in appraising the literature.

It must be remembered that searching the published literature will reveal:

◆ evidence that may be unsuitable for that particular research project
◆ evidence that is rigorous enough to inform the research project
◆ that evidence may be absent in that particular field, a finding that will help to drive a relevant research agenda.

If a search of the literature via databases and the Internet locates relevant reviews, CASP (1996) determines that there are three broad issues which need to be considered when appraising research reviews:

1. screening questions – are the results of the review valid?
2. detailed questions – what are the results?
3. will the results help locally?

Screening questions – are the results of the review valid?

It will need to be determined that the review article was clearly focused in relation to interventions and outcomes. In addition, it is essential that the authors of the review accessed appropriate research studies and consequently produced an appropriate design. This will require a detailed examination of the search strategy, quality and quantity of bibliographic databases used.

Importantly, questions need to be asked in relation to access to unpublished works and non-English language research and the author's personal contact with the experts. It should be remembered that clinical information is a combined approach from two sources, the patient information and the research, both of which will inform the care of the patient. As such, it is vital that the appraiser assesses the quality and rigour of the study. Careful attention should be given to metaanalysis within combined studies to ensure that the results were similar and clearly displayed and that the rationale for variations is presented within the study.

Detailed questions – what are the results?

The study should clearly display the results numerically, using ratios if applicable. Precision is also essential in ascertaining the validity of the study; this will be expressed by confidence limits.

Will the results help locally?

The suitability of the study's application to the local population should be considered; for example, if the patients examined in the review are vastly different from those in your specific area it will negate the relevance of the research. In addition, it will be necessary both to check the outcomes and to undertake an economic appraisal of the results, given that there could be cost implications to changes in practice and treatment.

Overall, critical appraisal assists practitioners by increasing their confidence and ability in using evidence to inform decision making. It allows them to be more discriminating about the validity and results of the available research and thus facilitates more rigorous contributions to the clinical effectiveness process.

What are the barriers to evidence-based practice?

An *Effective Health Care* bulletin (NHS Centre for Reviews and Dissemination 1999b) focused specifically on getting evidence into practice, although it did not draw on evidence related specifically to forensic mental health settings. The bulletin acknowledged the need for routine mechanisms for enabling individual and organizational change. It concluded that:

◆ an analysis of factors likely to influence change should be carried out
◆ dissemination and implementation strategies should be selected in the light of that analysis along with relevant research evidence
◆ a range of interventions targeting different barriers to change are more likely to be effective than single interventions
◆ adequate resources and skilled people are required
◆ successful management of change requires plans to monitor, evaluate and maintain change.

Although the research base for forensic mental health services is growing, limited research evidence is still a barrier to implementing evidence-based practice. There is a momentum towards generating more research relevant to forensic mental health services but it is in the nature of good scientific evidence that this will take time. Other barriers have been identified (UKCC & University of Central Lancashire 1999).

◆ Time (or rather the lack of it) is a significant problem facing all practitioners in all forensic services.
◆ Staff may not have the necessary skills or interest to appraise and use research evidence.
◆ The organizational culture may not facilitate its implementation in practice.

Literature suggests that nursing as a profession does not yet have a 'culture' of research interest or research utilization; that organizations do not provide adequate support for nurses to develop research awareness and utilization skills; and that the culture of closed institutions does not necessarily promote changes in practice to take on board research evidence (UKCC & University of Central Lancashire 1999). Lack of easy access to research findings has also been identified in studies of nursing in other settings (Carroll et al 1997).

One approach to facilitating access to research evidence is the provision of literature databases (CINHAL and PsychLIT) on a hospital network (Bradshaw & Dale 1999). Starting from evidence that nurses in general hospitals tended to use literature that was close to hand (i.e. on the ward) and that CD-ROM services in libraries were of limited value to ward-based staff, Bradshaw & Dale argue the potential value of making these databases available at ward level and providing the necessary training and support for staff.

CONCLUSION

This chapter has described the national health service R&D strategy, sources of information about the national research programmes and some of the forensic mental health research projects currently under way. It has been noted that there is a paucity of published research which meets the highest standard of evidence of effectiveness, in relation to mental health in general and forensic services in particular. The importance of, and particular complexities associated with, collaborative approaches to R&D in this field were highlighted.

Two approaches to using research evidence have been discussed. The policy for improving clinical effectiveness was described and a proposed structure for implementing that policy in forensic mental health services was indicated. This structure would bring the relevant disciplines and activities to bear on the process of inform, change and monitor. The process of evidence-based practice was also described, noting the need to balance high-quality research evidence with clinical experience and judgement. Again, the limited amount of research evidence made available through the main dissemination routes was noted. The CASP approach to evaluating research evidence was described and a brief overview of barriers to research utilization was provided.

Using research evidence to improve clinical effectiveness and as a basis for evidence-based practice in forensic mental health services is an area of growing importance with the introduction of the National Institute for Clinical Excellence and the Commission for Health Improvement but the challenge lies in moving from a weak to a strong evidence base and overcoming the individual and organizational barriers to research utilization in services which attract a high level of political and media interest.

REFERENCES

Bradshaw C, Dale C 1999 Informed choice. Nursing Management 6(3): 8–12

Carroll DL, Greenwood R, Lynch KE, Sullivan JK, Ready CH, Fitzmaurice JB 1997 Barriers and facilitators to the utilization of nursing research. Clinical Nurse Specialist 11(5): 207–212

CASP 1996 Critically appraising research evidence: making sense of the evidence about clinical effectiveness. Anglia and Oxford Regional Health Authority

Clifton M, Duffy D (In press) Mental health inquiries. In: Cotterill L, Barr W (eds) Targeting in mental health services: a multi-disciplinary challenge. Ashgate, Aldershot

Department of Health 1991 Research for health. Department of Health, London

Department of Health 1992 Report of the Committee of Inquiry into complaints about Ashworth Hospital. HMSO, London

Department of Health 1994 Supporting research and development in the NHS (The Culyer Report). HMSO, London

Department of Health 1996 Promoting clinical effectiveness: a framework for action in and through the NHS. Department of Health, London

Department of Health 1998 Research and development information pack. Department of Health, London

Department of Health 1999 The Report of the Committee of Inquiry into the Personality Disorder Unit, Ashworth Special Hospital. Stationery Office, London

Elliot M, Goldner MD, Blisker D 1995 Evidence-based psychiatry. Canadian Journal of Psychiatry 40: 97–101

Geddes J 1996 On the need for evidence-based psychiatry. Evidence-Based Medicine 1(7): 199–200

NHS Centre for Reviews and Dissemination 1998 Deliberate self-harm. Effective Health Care Bulletin 4(6). FT Healthcare, Harlow

NHS Centre for Reviews and Dissemination 1999a Drug treatments for schizophrenia. Effective Health Care Bulletin 5(6). Royal Society of Medicine Press, London

NHS Centre for Reviews and Dissemination 1999b
Getting evidence into practice. Effective Health Care
Bulletin 5(1). Royal Society of Medicine Press, London

United Kingdom Central Council for Nursing, Midwifery
and Health Visiting, University of Central Lancashire
1999 Nursing in secure environments. UKCC, London

FURTHER READING

Department of Health 1996 Clinical effectiveness
reference pack. Department of Health, London

Dunning M, Abi-Aad G, Gilbert D, Hutton H, Brown C
1999 Experience, evidence and everyday practice:
creating systems for delivering effective health care.
King's Fund, London

Kyle C 1993 Evaluating provider effectiveness. Health
Services Management 89(6): 10–12

Murphy M, Dunning M 1997 Implementing clinical
effectiveness: is it time for a change of gear? British
Journal of Health Care Management 3(1): 23–26

Summerton N 1995 The burden of proof. Health Service
Journal 105(5481): 33

Chapter Eight

Education and training developments in the context of clinical governance

Tony Thompson   Fran Aiken   Ros Harvey

INTRODUCTION

This chapter explores some of the policy changes in education and training which can be linked to clinical governance and which are intended to reshape the way in which interprofessional care is provided throughout the health services and associated agencies.

It has long been recognized that the quality of most public services and the efficiency with which they are delivered are extremely difficult to measure. In a recent statement Le Grand, Richard Titmuss Professor of Social Policy at the London School of Economics and Political Science, reinforced the fact that there may be a public service ethos, or a reservoir of public spiritedness, on which policy makers can draw to ensure that the proper implementation of their policies is carried out (Steel 1999).

The claim has been made that if managers are imbued with an ethos of public service then they can be trusted to try their best to do what that ethos actually implies. In other words, those who work within services such as the health and custodial services serve the public. If they fail in various ways in that task, if they produce low-quality services or if they are inefficient and therefore waste resources that could have gone into providing more services, then it is not because of malice or lack of goodwill; rather, it is more likely to be because of ignorance of what they are supposed to be doing or of best practice or perhaps simply a lack of the necessary skills. Le Grand elaborates by stating that the appropriate management response is therefore to provide employees with the knowledge concerning the aims to be achieved, with information concerning good practice and with suitable training and then leave them to get on with their job.

Forensic mental health services, and organizations with similar goals, depend upon the people who constitute the workforce to make the organization actually function. The importance of the motivation and job satisfaction of staff is recognized by managers throughout the services. However, this is not an easy task; motivation is complex and is not easily triggered in areas where the pathology of the patient can provoke public outrage. Further, it requires a great deal of attention and support, if individuals working at all levels are to function effectively together to help the organization achieve its aims. To remain motivated within forensic mental health services over time demands that the visions and strategies be communicated on a continuous basis, not just occasionally. The concept of professional development has to go beyond just informing; it needs to excite people by connecting to their personal values.

Considerable progress has been made in the past 2 years within the health services around a framework for continuing professional development. This development is considered absolutely necessary to support the delivery of a high standard of patient care, together with the assurances offered by the concept of clinical governance. For a number of years, personnel working within forensic mental health services have been conscious of the need to fulfil their potential and to recognize their own capacity and capability, as a means of delivering effective outcomes with regard to the mental health priorities of the health service.

The new emphasis on clinical governance and the basis of the National Service Framework for mental health (DoH 1999) strongly reinforce the principle that lifelong learning should be designed to meet organizational needs, as well as the individual expectations and aspirations of contributing professionals. The development of a locally managed approach to continuing professional development and the associated personal development plans required for all the staff working within services cannot be achieved overnight. It is a long-term arrangement but the local initiatives being applied to forensic services are an important milestone towards building a learning environment within these services which supports necessary change and lifelong learning for its personnel.

The National Health Service Executive (1998a) identified a number of proposals which were intended to support the delivery of a consistent and better quality service to patients. These were classified in the following way.

◆ The setting of clear national quality standards through the National Service Frameworks and the National Institute for Clinical Excellence.
◆ Effective local delivery of quality clinical services. This was to be channelled through the concept of clinical governance, reinforced by a new statutory duty supported by programmes of lifelong learning and local delivery of professional self-regulation.
◆ Accurate and effective monitoring of the delivery of standards. This is to be carried out by a new statutory Commission for Health Improvement superimposed on an NHS performance assessment framework.

Innovations and novel ideas in relation to continuing professional development are being seen in a number of areas within forensic mental health services. The long-term history of attempting to improve recruitment and retention within the services has made this an essential component of organizational management and it is also highlighted as a necessary remedy by numerous critical inquiries and reports. Whatever the style of introduction, those charged with the responsibility for initiating professional development and clinical governance are tending to focus on the following criteria.

◆ Development should be participative and the focus should be on involving the practitioner.
◆ It should be targeted towards direct patient care.
◆ It should be aimed at meeting an identified educational need.
◆ It should be based on accurate evidence which is educationally effective.
◆ It should be lodged within the wider organizational strategic and development plans.
◆ It should transfer across professional and service delivery boundaries.
◆ It should reflect previous knowledge and experience of practice.

The fundamental aspects of programmes of continuing professional development revolve around the requirement that it should meet the professional needs of the person, together with their individual aspirations, but these have to be integrated with the needs of the service. It follows, then, that the best way to target professional development within the forensic mental health service is to organize and manage the programmes on a local basis. The local education consortia can play a most useful supportive role, as can postgraduate deans, as they are able to work in partnership with higher education providers, professional associations, regulatory bodies and staff associations.

A good example of locally based educational initiatives and programmes which are accessible and at the same time validated by external bodies is that seen within the Ashworth Centre at the Ashworth Hospital Authority. The comprehensive programmes designed within the centre can be delivered on or off site but they are rooted within the need for work-based learning and clinical identification of need.

The forensic mental health services have in common with other aspects of the health service the need to develop a locally managed, systematic approach to continuing professional development during the year 2000. The plans to design relevant locally supported programmes have to be linked with the strategic plans for implementing clinical governance. Such demands and initiatives are serious and require a high level of resource investment; this can be seen in the way in which the services as employment authorities have to take stock of their current patterns of professional development investment.

The health service circular *Agenda for change* (NHSE 1999a) identified the government's aims for a modern pay system for the health service. A key component of these reforms will be the greater flexibility of roles which are underpinned by the concept of lifelong learning. Parallel debate is taking place between government departments on the need to invest in lifelong learning and professional development, alongside other key personnel issues which include security of tenure of employment and the development of family-friendly policies.

In the government's circular *Working together* (NHSE 1998b), there was a reiteration of the intention, set out in *A first class service* (DoH 1998), that all NHS employers should have in place training and development plans for the majority of health professional staff. It is also the aim that the notion of personal development planning will be extended to all staff groups throughout the health service. The forensic mental health services in particular are urged to capture the essence of previous adverse inquiries and reports and reflect these in plans for local professional development. These concepts are in keeping with the government's strategy for lifelong learning which is set out in the publication called *The learning age* (Department of Education and Employment 1998).

There is nothing unique in the implications of the above initiatives for the forensic mental health services and the pressure in the forthcoming years will be to ensure that the practical aspects of introducing these changes are in place. These will include:

◆ the capacity of new technology and distance learning to maximize learning opportunities
◆ identifying how the expertise of professional and statutory bodies can best support local professional development within the context of clinical governance
◆ the role of monitoring, peer review and appraisal in determining the structure of continuing professional development programmes
◆ the need within every health organization to have an educational infrastructure designed to identify, analyse and meet the needs of its professional staff.

The push for work-based learning is a welcome development within forensic mental health services and tends to focus on finding solutions to practical problems. Some of these are unique to services that often have to work within a high-risk environment and are likely to include:

◆ the design of learning sets
◆ work-based projects
◆ job rotation

- job shadowing
- mentoring
- coaching
- accurate clinical supervision.

The critical element of work-based development is the ability to reflect on and learn from the knowledge and experience of practice. This includes identifying 'near misses', service failure and subsequent public concerns. This is a sensitive process and one where forensic mental health services sometimes become locked in defending a situation rather than turning the consequences to the advantage of future planning. In common with their colleagues, forensic mental health professionals will be looking to the guidelines produced by the National Institute for Clinical Effectiveness (NICE) as a focus for professional development activities. These are likely to be interlinked with more far-reaching and sophisticated audit activities linked to clinical guidelines and national standards.

ORGANIZING CONTINUING PROFESSIONAL DEVELOPMENT PROGRAMMES

The way in which professional development is integrated with clinical governance is often dependent upon the way in which it is financed. This would include local training and development budgets, access to charitable and educational trusts and professional body sponsorship.

Many health personnel share the financial responsibility for their professional development. One of the problems of introducing consistent systems is that there is sometimes inequity between the professions with regard to how much money is available for individual professional development. It is the government's aim for employers to align their existing training funds with local service objectives and clinical governance plans and throughout these plans, there should be a clear strategy to introduce work-based learning. Clinical governance demands the creation of more appropriate and better quality

learning environments within each locality. It is considered that to meet this demand robust leadership at board level will be required and that board members should be local champions of professional development and lifelong learning (DoH 1998).

The whole process of continuing professional development, which is required to support clinical governance, has to be based upon local identification of need and represented at board level. Its status is such that board members will wish to include regional education and development groups, postgraduate deans and the education consortia in meeting their strategic aims.

The government guidance on continuing professional development and quality in the new NHS (NHSE 1999b) advises on robust criteria in order to establish systematic approaches to professional development, which should:

- be closely linked to local clinical governance plans
- have a clear infrastructure with explicit lines of accountability
- include a multidisciplinary remit
- provide local mechanisms for ensuring that all staff have a personal development plan
- set out the local approach to appraisal for all staff
- incorporate effective processes for identifying the education and developmental needs of individuals and service teams
- focus on local service objectives and priorities within the health improvement programme
- promote the understanding and use of up-to-date knowledge by linking together continuing professional development, clinical audit and research and development activities
- be open and transparent in their working and reporting arrangements
- actively promote equality of opportunity, regardless of professional background, level of seniority and current achievement; this includes part-time staff
- ensure that the continuing professional development programmes meet professional and educational standards which are flexible

enough to accommodate different styles of learning

◆ be appropriately integrated and compatible with the requirements of Royal Colleges and the regulatory bodies for the professions
◆ be supportive of those tasked with leading continuing professional development and address their own specific development needs.

The way in which the forensic mental health services integrate and inform the wider mental health services is becoming increasingly important. Those who work within these services have to be tuned in to political developments and strategic activities which are reconfiguring the nature of the workforce available to people with a mental health problem. The end product of many of these forces is likely to be focused on the need to create a mental health-care delivery system which can meet the needs of service users in a competent manner, that it is available in the required numbers and mix of skill and embedded in a framework of qualifications linked to national occupational standards and that the total workforce is committed to lifelong learning.

These developments will tie into and rely heavily upon the training strategies which are being developed by Health Work UK National Training Organization. This organization, alongside the training organization for the Personnel Social Services, will definitely impact upon the training demands to be placed upon the forensic mental health services.

Whilst both the organizations share concerns about the workforce, Health Work UK is taking the lead on mental health issues, specifically relating to the development of national occupational standards. Its work will cover the whole mental health service, so that mental health roles and functions and the competence of the workforce can be matched to the needs of service users and associated carers. Naturally, the National Service Frameworks in mental health will impact heavily on the development of occupational standards within the mental health field.

PERFORMANCE MANAGEMENT PROCESS

The planned cycle of clinical governance which is designed to improve the quality of service delivery requires organizations to have the following:

◆ an appraisal system
◆ monitoring arrangement to identify training and development needs
◆ leadership programmes to develop clinical teams
◆ strategy for workforce planning, including lifelong learning.

Continuous improvement and a culture which encourages and supports organizational (lifelong) learning are key to organizational success. All of this will require the total integration of training and development, on all levels, to meet the standards and contracts with purchasers and at a corporate level by meeting the professional and individual development needs.

Implicit within a plan for organizational success is the requirement for a capable and motivated workforce. It is also acknowledged that improving the performance of employees against specified corporate aims will simultaneously improve individual ability and organizational performance. It is widely accepted that there are recruitment and retention concerns in nursing generally and more specifically within the field of mental health services. As such, it is imperative that organizations provide both current and prospective employees with a framework for managing performance through personal development plans and thus ensure the effective delivery of suitable education and training programmes which impact upon practice.

Organizations need to clearly identify training needs, prioritize and communicate these needs and finally identify the physical and financial resources to support these needs. This performance management process will need to be strategically led and managed and become an integral part of the organization's culture and philosophy to be truly effective. Additionally, proper feedback and evaluation must take place to ensure that spending on training becomes an investment.

The offer of self-development and good training is clearly motivational and will assist in the primary goal of keeping skilled employees. Recruitment is also essential to the growing success of organizations so they will have to demonstrate that they take individual development and training seriously.

To be effective and successful, performance management processes should be led and supported at a senior level within the organization. Guidelines should outline a commitment by the organization to providing the opportunity for all staff to discuss their role, job function and performance on a regular basis. The main objective is to help all staff to perform their current job to the best of their abilities and to enable the identification and development of skills which ensure that staff can reach their potential, both for personal growth within job role and function to meet the organizational goals.

Importantly, this should be a corporate process which embraces all staff. It should offer a consistent approach to review on an annual basis (incorporating updating meetings). It is vital that the process is seen as developmental and not punitive in the production of a developmental plan which includes clear objectives.

Staff review is a two-way process where, prior to the interview, both the manager and employee complete review preparation forms. A staff review interview form is completed during the interview process which offers a statement of the discussion and agreements reached.

The following factors may contribute to a failure to successfully implement the process.

◆ It is not corporately driven – needs to be supported strategically and operationally.
◆ There is a lack of ownership resulting in fragmented implementation.
◆ It is not integrated into the business planning cycle.
◆ Unworkable documentation.
◆ Non-existent or inappropriate training for managers.

Non-compliance within the performance management process will prevent the effective identification and evaluation of training and developmental requirements. Organizations need to support and lead the review process to ensure total compliance. This will ultimately provide essential information for the organization to improve the way it operates in the following areas of people management.

◆ Human resource planning.
◆ Training and development – to assist in undertaking a training needs analysis, linking this to the business planning objectives and bidding constructively for funding.
◆ Internal job market and the identification of potential within the organization.
◆ Recruitment and retention of staff.

The entire process is essential to the business planning cycle in that it captures much of the information required for human resource planning, ultimately ensuring that there are sufficient numbers of people with the right skills and experience to meet future requirements.

LIFELONG LEARNING

Professional development for staff as outlined by the Department of Health (1997) will be pivotal in achieving the objectives of clinical excellence and quality improvement in health organizations. Practice professional development plans are required as a keystone of clinical governance and will help staff and organizations to recognize education and training needs, to budget for these needs and to measure outcomes.

Professional development or lifelong learning is now a favourite theme not just in institutional policy but also in political directives (DoH 1998, European Commission 1995) and professional standard setting (English National Board 1995). These policy makers see lifelong learning as continuous professional development and essential for health practitioners to respond quickly to service needs and to enable purchasers and providers to achieve their objectives (English National Board 1995). Communities and patients will benefit from professionals whose skills and knowledge are keeping pace with change: 'a continuing process of updating and maintaining expertise will support the delivery of high-quality, modern, effective healthcare in a fast-changing world' (DoH 1998).

The policy makers have also identified the need to prepare for the disappearance of geographical boundaries (Affara 1997) and to update knowledge to overcome obsolescence of preregistration courses. Dissolution of the applicability of knowledge has meant that professional obsolescence can start from between 2 and 5 years after registration (Grant 1992). There is also the drive to update and develop new skills to respond to the changing nature of employment where rapid and global change is a constant and where technological progress and social change require workers to be more flexible. The deliberate strategy of career development through continuous learning (Hall & Mirvis 1995) is maybe as much a stimulation for individuals as organizational or professional requirements.

The prerequisites for lifelong learning

Psychological factors

Individuals need intrinsic motivation to develop, to be self-directed and to learn. They may find they enjoy learning for its own sake and plan their learning in advance; this type of learner, the 'self-directed' or proactive learner, is often overlooked by educationalists (Jarvis 1987). Nevertheless, most adults learn because they want to use the knowledge or skills, to cope with change in their lives such as moving to a new clinical area or working with a different client group. Other triggering events or transitional periods may be life events such as children leaving home. They will also be highly motivated to lifelong learning, recognize their needs and have a self-concept that is helpful to lifelong learning.

Lifelong learners need to be aware of their weaknesses and learning needs, be able to self-diagnose learning needs (Carpenito 1991) and evaluate how learning has altered or affected these needs and deficits (Hinchliff 1994): self-awareness and self-evaluation skills are therefore required. Learners also need a sense of control over what is learned and the pace of learning: if the locus of control is held by the learners, rather than enforced by an organization or institution, the learning achieved will be more significant and the learners will become more autonomous and avoid learned helplessness, becoming more proactive and taking more responsibility for their own learning, for example through using a learning log.

Competencies/skills

Lifelong learners must set realistic learning goals commensurate with life circumstances and individual needs. They must have good study skills and awareness of the learning style best suited to them, possess skills in using learning aids, such as open learning material, and knowledge of resources and the ability to access them. This may require additional resources and requirements beyond the individual. Self-managed learning is a requirement for lifelong learning but it requires personal commitment, devotion to goal setting and record keeping and openness to appraisal and support from others (Fair 1995).

Conditions

The individual cannot learn in a vacuum; there must be a culture of learning to support and augment the learning strategies and opportunities. A preregistration culture of emphasizing individuals' responsibility for learning strategies and development of inquiry skills rather than only focusing on gaining knowledge and psychomotor skills will encourage lifelong learning (Appel & Malcolm 1998).

Process-focused learning in the preregistration curriculum will develop the student's ability to question, challenge and learn independently (Carpenito 1991), skills necessary for lifelong learning. Course content of postregistration programmes must be adapted to allow the learner to use and interpret materials and information from different fields; this is particularly effective in interdisciplinary shared learning. The practitioner is then more likely to be ready for decision making in the real world where resources have to be shared, teamwork is the norm and different viewpoints taken on board (Maslin-Prothero 1997). An active learning approach in preregistration programmes has been suggested as an effective way of facilitating skills acquisition (McManus & Sieler 1998). Through utilizing resource-based learning such as skills laboratories, the programme is more likely to produce competent, confident and reflective practitioners who are also self-directed and motivated to continue their professional development.

The organization needs to value practice based on relevant research. The clinical learning environment will then allow practitioners to question practice and add to their own and colleagues' understanding (Maslin-Prothero 1997). The process of continuing professional development in a healthy, quality-driven organization has been identified in the document *A first class service: quality in the NHS* with assessment through training needs analysis and performance review which take the form of organizational and personal development plans taking into account individuals' learning styles, identifying opportunities for shared, interdisciplinary and practice-based learning (DoH 1998).

According to Carpenito (1991), Janhonen (1991) and Jarvis (1987), educationalists need to be aware that a preregistration education policy which will develop lifelong learners and promote lifelong learning should encourage:

◆ learners identifying their own needs and experiences required in the clinical setting
◆ directing the learner to other learning experiences
◆ allowance for individual learning styles and personality differences
◆ more effective study skills
◆ self-evaluation
◆ peer review
◆ sharing between lecturer and learner of development of learning objectives
◆ responsibility for own learning.

A strong continuing educational policy is a vital requirement for lifelong learning. When formal courses are planned, they must be based on organizational needs by incorporating problem identification in the curriculum that focuses on health care (Jarvis 1987), using flexible strategies with facilitation and experiences that will meet learning objectives.

Strategies for lifelong learning

An organizational training needs analysis is essential to formulate a robust training strategy that will provide professionals who are 'fit for purpose' at a cost that can be met within the available resources. However, individual learning needs assessment and action plans are also required for personal development plans that will meet the statutory body's needs for the minimum acceptable levels of continuous professional development.

Through systematic and regular assessment and planning of learning experiences (Box 8.1), professionals will develop a strategy for lifelong learning that is more meaningful to them, to the service and the client. The assessment can consist of objectives, assessment of time and resources, reflection of their own practice, analysis of current research, identification of other colleagues, research and development officers (Browne 1998) and educationalists as support or as a resource and an action plan with time scales and identification of costs (Pedder 1998). Reflection on learning can be enhanced through a learning diary in which individuals record key points learned, how those might be applied to their practice and issues or areas that need further work and then assesses how well they are using opportunities to learn in and outside work, to review whether they are getting the most out of their learning and then possibly involve other colleagues, mentors or supervisors on getting feedback on their development.

Evaluation of lifelong learning

Methods of evaluation can include self-report, record audit (independent review of patients' records) and direct observation by an independent professional (Grant 1992). A wider perspective of evaluative methods is required, however, to capture the changes, through professional development, in attitude and values, the impact on the

---

Box 8.1 A personal development plan

STAGE 1: ASSESSMENT
- ◆ What do I need to do?
- ◆ What do I want to learn?
- ◆ Do I want to fulfil a personal training objective?
- ◆ Do I want to carry out practice at a higher standard?
- ◆ How much time have I got?
- ◆ What resources have I got already or are available?
- ◆ What aspects of my current practice do I need to change?
- ◆ What quality research is there already that might help me?

STAGE 2: PLANNING
- ◆ What are my short-term goals and the time scales for these?

- ◆ What are my long-term goals and the time scales for these?
- ◆ What resources do I need to achieve these?

STAGE 3: REFLECTION
- ◆ What are the key points I have learned?
- ◆ How might these be applied to my practice?
- ◆ Are there issues or areas that need further work?
- ◆ How well am I using opportunities to learn in and outside work?
- ◆ Am I getting the most out of my learning?
- ◆ What feedback do my colleagues, mentor or supervisors give me on my development?

---

whole organization and the profession as well as a narrower focus on outcomes in a particular area of practice. Tripartite planning and evaluation of needs, function and outcomes may provide a more meaningful framework (Sunter 1993).

Issues and dilemmas of lifelong learning

Surveys have shown that nurses have had difficulty with presenting evidence of the learning process and linking learning with practice needed to compile the required personal professional profile (Redfern 1998), although in reality the nurses did set goals and action plans (Williams 1998).

Educationalists themselves need to be more committed to self-directed learning: Janhonen (1991) found that nurse instructors failed to practise self-directed learning despite supporting it in principle. Yet there is little research that proves the effectiveness of reflective learning (Grant 1992) and self-directed learning (Maslin-Prothero 1997) although these are central tenets in nurse

education today as part of a humanistic and liberal ideology.

Other constraints that need to be addressed by managers and educationalists are the individuals' ability and willingness to undertake proactive and self-directed learning:

- ◆ Perceived and disabling views about a lack of control over learning.
- ◆ Peer pressure leading to indifference or even antagonism to the learner from family or colleagues.
- ◆ Gatekeepers to learning placing obstacles in the way of learners, such as giving misleading information.
- ◆ Academic or professional language that distinguishes an experienced learner from an inexperienced learner (Candy 1991).

FUTURE TRENDS AND NEEDS

Flexibility in provision of continuing professional development programmes will be even more essential as local needs drive educational programmes. The long, developmental academic course will become a rarity as modular programmes become the norm; learners will demand strategies and resources that are accessible and equitable, such as distance learning, that might be increasingly used in local training and education centres. Technological teaching and learning methods are continually advancing. Innovations include the virtual university, where video and TV programmes, mail systems and video-conferencing are combined so that learners can participate in class discussions, communicate with peers and access tutorials or lectures, nationally and internationally (Davison & Rhodes 1996). Accessibility and flexibility are the obvious benefits. Issues such as a need for a shift from competition to common goals, rethinking to take full advantage of the potential of the new technology, copyright and ownership of knowledge, reliability of knowledge and problems related to openness of systems all need to be addressed. The philosophical debate around how electronic communication in education separates the speaking body from the listening body also needs to be explored (Cheek & Doskatch 1998).

Ensuring standards of education provision, strategic direction of education and training and coordination of service needs with continuing education delivery at a regional and national level will be the role of the regional education and development groups proposed in the White Paper *The new NHS* (DoH 1997). These groups will need to have real powers and resources as well as having a pragmatic perspective as there is a danger that they may become gatekeepers who can place obstacles or unrealistic specifications on continuing education delivery.

Priority areas for continuing professional development to achieve clinical governance will include training in mentoring for leads in clinical governance and training in informatics to support evidence-based practice, to use the evidence to help in change management and to monitor outcomes. Training in interdisciplinary and inter-agency working is vital, as will be training in audit. Learning in a multidisciplinary context will affect the lifelong learning of mental health professionals (Affara 1997), where constructive and effective team consolidation in the delivery of care must be taught and practised. Through more interprofessional education there will be more understanding and communication within teams (Skeil 1995).

Other future directions for continuing professional development include international links and exchanges, possibly between institutions or non-governmental organizations, for example nursing exchanges across professional organizations. Some of the educational activities for health professionals across international boundaries might be funded by multinational companies where scholarships or sponsorships could be utilized as long as these partnerships were in an ethical framework (Affara 1997). If international educational activities increase, there would be an accompanying need for accreditation to allow a mutual recognition of learning. The International Council of Nurses is currently looking at these issues.

CONCLUSION

Fundamental to any success in continuing professional development is the ability of the organization to raise the profile of the concept of lifelong learning. This poses a real challenge for those who lead the organization in these areas. Recent government guidance and the push for social inclusion mean that those who contribute to the service have to be prepared to harness all the appropriate ways to ensure that the professionalism of the service is underpinned by sound knowledge and experience of practice.

The forensic mental health service has many participants who are deeply committed to providing the best possible standards of treatment and care and the approaches mentioned above should help develop the proper climate to ensure that they can continue to extend their skills. If education and training strategy is well grounded, it will in turn ensure that those who hold roles within the forensic sector are fit for purpose and fit for practice.

REFERENCES

Affara F 1997 Why lifelong learning? International Nursing Review 44(6): 177–180

Appel A, Malcolm P 1998 Specialist education and practice in nursing: an Australian perspective. Nurse Education Today 18: 144–152

Browne A 1998 The role of the research and development officer. Nursing Standard 13(8): 41–42

Candy P 1991 Self-direction for lifelong learning. Jossey-Bass, California

Carpenito L 1991 A lifetime commitment. Nursing Times 87(48): 53–55

Cheek J, Doskatch I 1998 Information literacy: a resource for nurses as lifelong learners. Nurse Education Today 18: 243–250

Davison D, Rhodes D 1996 The virtual university. Nursing Standard 10(27): 21–22

Department of Education and Employment 1998 The learning age: a renaissance for a new Britain. Cm 3790. Stationery Office, London

Department of Health 1997 The new NHS. Stationery Office, London

Department of Health 1998 A first class service: quality in the NHS. Department of Health, London

Department of Health 1999 Mental health national service frameworks: modern standards and service models. Stationery Office, London

English National Board 1995 Creating lifelong learners: partnerships for care. ENB, London

European Commission 1995 European year of lifelong learning: guidelines. European Commission, Brussels

Fair N 1995 Set up and grow. Nursing Management 2(2): 24–26

Grant R 1992 Obsolescence or lifelong education: choices and challenges. Physiotherapy 78(3): 167–171

Hall D, Mirvis P 1995 Careers as lifelong learning. In: Howard A (ed) The changing nature of work. Jossey-Bass, California

Hinchliff S 1994 Learning for life. Nursing Standard 8(48): 20–21

Janhonen S 1991 Andragogy as a didactic perspective in the attitudes of nurse instructors in Finland. Nurse Education Today 11: 278–283

Jarvis P 1987 Lifelong education and its relevance to nursing. Nurse Education Today 7: 49–55

Maslin-Prothero S 1997 A perspective on lifelong learning and its implications for nurses. Nurse Education Today 17: 431–436

McManus E, Sieler P 1998 Freedom to enjoy learning in the 21st century: developing an active learning culture in nursing. Nurse Education Today 18: 322–328

National Health Service Executive 1998a A first class service: consultation document on quality in the new NHS. HSC 1998/113. Department of Health, London

National Health Service Executive 1998b Working together – securing a quality workforce for the NHS: a framework for managing human resources in the NHS. HSC 1998/162. Department of Health, London

National Health Service Executive 1999a Agenda for change – modernising the NHS pay system. HSC 1999/035. Department of Health, London

National Health Service Executive 1999b Continuing professional development: quality in the new NHS. Department of Health, London

Pedder L 1998 Training-needs analysis. Nursing Standard 11(6): 50–53

Redfern L 1998 Time to ban the certificate culture. Nursing Times Learning Curve 2(10): 2

Skeil D 1995 Individual and staff professional development in a multidisciplinary team: some needs and solutions. Clinical Rehabilitation 9: 28–33

Steel J 1999 Wasted values – harnessing the commitment of public managers. Public Management Foundation, London

Sunter S 1993 The effectiveness of continuing education. Nursing Standard 8(6): 37–39

Williams M 1998 Surveys reveal nurses getting the message about PREP. Nursing Times Learning Curve 2(10): 2–3

FURTHER READING

National Health Service Executive 1998 Working together – securing a quality workforce for the NHS: a framework for managing human resources in the NHS. HSC 1998/162. Department of Health, London

National Health Service Executive 1999 Continuing professional development: quality in the new NHS. Department of Health, London

UKCC 1999 Fitness for practice: a report of the Commission of Education. UKCC, London

9

Chapter Nine

Risk assessment and management

Phil Woods

Chapter Contents

INTRODUCTION

This chapter explores some key issues of risk assessment and management within forensic mental health care, first, from the individual patient perspective and second, from the organizational perspective. However, before this the issue of dangerousness is explored briefly, so as to place this within the context of risk. Some indicators of good practice will be discussed in terms of risk assessment and management. This chapter is aimed predominantly at the practising clinician so emphasis will be placed on clinical risk assessment and management, although actuarial assessment will be placed within the clinical context.

DANGEROUSNESS

Dangerousness is an emotive word which has gradually been replaced by issues of risk assessment and management. However, for anyone tasked with risk assessment and management, there is a need to understand this concept which is entangled within the risk assessment process and how this relates to it.

Dangerousness is the potential ability to cause serious physical and psychological harm to others. It also includes those fear-inducing, impulsive and destructive behaviours that are displayed or have been known to be displayed. Chin (1998) questions the whole usage of dangerousness as a concept in mental health practice, advocating that the risk concept should be used instead. Indeed, Duggan (1997) informs us that there has been a critical shift by theoreticians from assessing dangerousness to assessing and managing risk. This is perhaps not surprising since extreme burden is placed upon mental health providers to protect the public by identifying dangerous persons and taking the proper professional action.

RISK ASSESSMENT

Risk may, generally, be defined as the probability of a bad consequence or as the likelihood that a particular adverse event will recur (Prins 1996). It involves such issues as outcome and probability.

Risk assessment can exist in many contexts: for instance, the safe storage of medicines or when parents allow their child to return home from school by themselves. Within forensic mental health care risk assessment is mainly concerned with three highly interrelated components: the risk posed in the past, now and in the future. Moreover, the most important points at issue are: will reoffending occur and what is the potential for change?

Risk assessment and its related management are the guiding force for clinicians working in forensic care and this is the central component in the assessment process (Woods 1996). However, it is no magical process (Scott 1997) but a complex issue determined to a large degree by who defines the risk and how it is defined (McClelland 1995). Pollock & Webster (1990) and Monahan & Steadman (1994) highlight that assessments need to be systematic and based on the population undergoing assessment, with identified risk factors required to be broken down into more manageable components, further assessed through effective treatment planning and outcomes evaluated through recovery status.

Forensic mental health professionals are expected to be able to assess risk adequately (Bingley 1997). However, as this is a key skill and one which relies heavily on clinical judgement since 'no other measurement device is available' (Chiswick 1995), the difficult question arises as to how we prepare ourselves for this task.

The expert literature reveals that three foci for the future of risk assessment research have been suggested. First, there should be an actuarial focus (a statistical approach to assessment based on predetermined, often historical variables, which have been shown to be predictive of risk). This should be inclusive of clinical information presented in statistical tables, to assist in clinical judgements. Second, there are the situational variables, such as characteristics of the family, the work and peer group environment. Third, attention should be on varied populations upon which predictions are made (Monahan 1984).

Borum (1996) makes three recommendations to improve clinical practice in risk assessment:

1. improve assessment technology
2. develop clinical practice guidelines
3. develop training programmes and curricula.

Therefore, these expert researchers are giving clinicians some pointers for developing their practice towards improving risk assessment and management.

Although these indications appear to be straightforward, it needs to be borne in mind that even the most careful risk assessment is complicated by the assessor's inability to control for future physical and social circumstances. For example, the patient may do something completely out of the blue, something which could never have been predicted. Clinicians want to achieve the best possible grasp of the likely behaviour of an individual and to elicit detail sufficient for risk factors to be minimized and appropriately managed (Vinestock 1996). Furthermore, the Royal College of Nursing (1998) suggest that the aims of risk assessment are to:

1. identify the hazards
2. identify who is at risk
3. evaluate the risks
4. make a record of the findings
5. review and revise the assessment.

Approaches to risk assessment

As in any behavioural analysis, to assist in risk assessment there are two main approaches. First is the *actuarial* or *statistical*, which has been briefly mentioned above. This approach seeks to assess the individual on predetermined, often historical variables, which have been shown to be predictive of risk. It is based on the assumption that an individual coming from a population within which a certain type of behaviour is common is more likely to display this form of behaviour (Pollock & Webster 1990).

Second, in contrast, there is the *clinical* approach, which is based upon professional opinion concerning a patient's self-presentation and on consideration of situational or clinical variables. This approach looks for explanation of specific violent behaviour and is concerned with how individuals behave; how they react in various situations; how they have been known to behave; how willingly they accept treatment; and how much insight they have into their condition.

So which approach is 'better' or more valid? Some leading researchers in the field of risk assessment are opposed to the clinical approach on the grounds that it may be contaminated by 'assessor bias' and that it is only as good as its theoretical base. Indeed, some empirical studies indicate that on occasion, predictions from clinicians are no better than chance (Monahan 1988).

Testing the predictive ability

There are many ways of testing the predictive ability of risk assessments, to evaluate if outcomes have been successful or not. Although many of these tests are statistically complex a useful way for clinicians to do this is through the use of two-by-two contingency tables to display results (see Fig. 9.1). This enables correct predictions and error rates to be examined.

If violence is used as an example, two possibilities exist in this design: either the violence did occur or it did not. Typically, this is reported as a *true negative* (the patient was predicted as not violent and was not violent); a *true positive* (the patient was predicted to be violent and was violent); a *false negative* (the patient was predicted to be not violent and was violent); and a *false positive* (the patient was predicted to be violent and was not violent).

Webster et al (1995) rightly point out that in their endeavour to produce 'safe' conclusions,

clinicians tend to vastly overrate the likelihood of future violence, thus making 'false-positive' errors, where an individual is predicted as potentially violent but in fact does not turn out to be so. The first study to clearly show this was 'Baxstrom', where clinicians and administrators were found to be assuming that patients were more dangerous than they actually proved to be (Steadman & Cocozza 1974). It has been suggested that these errors should not be viewed entirely as poor clinical practice but may be part of the risk itself, with the social pressure of false-positive errors being better than false negatives (Shah 1978). This is not surprising, since what is being asked is, will an individual be violent in the future? This is rather like crystal ball gazing, as violent behaviours stem from a complex array of causal factors including personality, developmental influences and environmental effects.

Good practice in risk assessment

Over the past few decades researchers have looked at virtually all aspects of the risk assessment process. However, they have shown little appreciation of the clinical complexities and practical impediments in making risk assessments (Webster et al 1995) and little effort has been made to develop frameworks for clinical usage (Borum 1996). Although predictions made in relation to dangerous behaviour are poor, factors can be identified that predispose an individual to behave dangerously (McClelland 1995, Pollock & Webster 1990). Thus, 'any criticism of the professionals' lack of ability to predict risk should not detract from the search for answers' (McClelland 1995).

Within the findings of research studies many similarities can be found and these should serve as indicators for good practice in risk assessment. Pollock & Webster (1990) introduced an assessment model which included many predictive factors. Included were: established patterns of violence; negative social history; antisocial value systems; underlying hostility; nature of the current offence and surrounding circumstances; sadistic orientation; drug and alcohol abuse; history of mental ill health; suspicion; irritability; potential

Prediction	Outcome	
	Risky	Not risky
Risky	True positive	False positive
Not risky	False negative	True negative

Figure 9.1 An example of a two-by-two contingency table.

for change; current attitudes; current mental health status; motivation; socially acceptable values and goals; and attitudes to the self.

Currently, there is strong consensus that actuarial factors should serve as an anchor for more dynamic clinical risk assessment. Commonly recognized, but generally static, variables are:

◆ previous history of violence
◆ age under 30
◆ male gender
◆ concurrent drug/alcohol abuse
◆ active psychotic symptoms.

The important point to stress here is that these actuarial risk markers only provide a guide for risk management planning and any assessment must be individualized to the particular person. It has been previously highlighted that clinical experience informs that risky incidents are situation specific. That is, they may only occur when certain circumstances precede the risky behaviour. For instance, a patient may only be verbally or physically threatening following a family visit or at the anniversary of their index offence. Therefore, risk assessment needs to include both actuarial and individual risk factors; for instance, history of behaviour(s) and how recent and severe they are, their frequency and the pattern with which these have occurred. There needs to be an indication of the effect that identified risk factors have on any planned intent on the part of the patient, which may be apparent.

Current assessment instruments available

There are currently a number of instruments available to assist in the risk assessment and management process. Some which are undergoing research evaluation will be discussed. However, this is only a handful of those which are available and the reader is directed to the literature for others. Ryan (1999) particularly is a good source of information on related measures.

HCR-20

The HCR-20 risk assessment scheme (Webster et al 1997) consists of a mixture of static historical variables and dynamic clinical and risk management variables (see Box 9.1). Each of the 20 items is measured on a three-point scale, with a lower score indicating less risk than a higher score. The former historical variables are given the same

---

Box 9.1 HCR-20 variables

Historical
◆ Previous violence
◆ Young age at first violent incident
◆ Relationship instability
◆ Employment problems
◆ Substance use problems
◆ Major mental illness
◆ Psychopathy
◆ Early maladjustment
◆ Personality disorder
◆ Prior supervision failure attempts

Clinical
◆ Lack of insight
◆ Negative attitudes
◆ Active symptoms of major mental illness
◆ Impulsivity
◆ Unresponsive to treatment

Risk
◆ Plans lack feasibility
◆ Exposure to destabilizers
◆ Lack of personal support
◆ Non-compliance with remediation
◆ Stress

Box 9.2 VRAG variables
◆ PCL-R score
◆ Elementary school maladjustment
◆ Personality disorder
◆ Age at index offence (negatively related)
◆ Separated from parents under age 16
◆ Failure on prior conditional release
◆ Non-violent offence history
◆ Never married
◆ Schizophrenia (negatively related)
◆ Victim injury in index offence (negatively related)
◆ Alcohol abuse
◆ Female victim index offence (negatively related)

Box 9.3 ASSESS-list variables
◆ Antecedent history
◆ Self-presentation
◆ Social and psychosocial adjustment
◆ Expectations and plans
◆ Symptoms
◆ Supervision
◆ Life factors
◆ Institutional management
◆ Sexual adjustment
◆ Treatment progress

weight as both the clinical and risk management variables combined. Extensive research has focused on the instrument's predictive ability and although the researchers say that the results are only preliminary, the HCR-20's predictive ability looks promising. For a full discussion of the HCR-20 the reader is directed to its manual (Webster et al 1997).

Violence Prediction Scheme

The Violence Prediction Scheme (Webster et al 1994) combines both an actuarial and a clinical component. The actuarial component (see Box 9.2) is the Risk Assessment Guide or the RAG (Harris et al 1993) which has been renamed the Violence Risk Appraisal Guide or the VRAG (Rice & Harris 1995). This instrument is receiving considerable attention in the UK at present and is one of the preferred instruments being evaluated as part of the proposed research on the assessment of severe personality disorder (Home Office & DoH 1999). Again, results of the research on this instrument indicate promising predictive ability.

Although it has been suggested that scoring of the predictor variables which form the VRAG is not

overly complex, this should not be undertaken by anyone without suitable training and experience. Furthermore, scores given to each variable carry certain weights within the overall predictive score.

The second clinical component of the scheme is a mnemonic, the ASSESS-list (see Box 9.3), and it was suggested that this should be undertaken as part of the above actuarial VRAG component. Here, scores are given, as either favourable or unfavourable, for each item.

For a full description of the Violence Prediction Scheme the reader is directed to its manual (Webster et al 1994).

Behavioural Status Index

The Behavioural Status Index (BSI) was developed by the author of this chapter and others (Robinson et al 1996, Woods et al 1999) to assist in the clinical assessment of social risk. The structural properties of the BSI make it a suitable instrument for investigation of a particularly intriguing problem. Clinical logic suggests that there may exist certain patterns, or behavioural diatheses, which predispose to (that is, increase the risk of) occurrence of offending behaviour. Such diatheses may consist of behavioural elements or skills repertoire, thus allowing for assessment of baselines, appropriate interventions designed to ameliorate specific deficits or promote insightful adjustment and

---

Box 9.4   BSI risk subscale items

- Family support
- Serious violence to others without apparent trigger event
- Serious violence to others following trigger event
- Minor violence to others without apparent trigger event
- Minor violence to others following trigger event
- Serious self-harm
- Superficial self-harm
- Verbal aggression without apparent trigger event
- Verbal aggression following trigger event
- Attacks on objects without apparent trigger event
- Attacks on objects following trigger event
- Breaches of security
- Disruptive episodes
- Imitative disruption
- Inappropriate sexual behaviours
- Sadomasochistic behaviours
- Macho gear and adornment
- Obsessive-compulsive behaviours
- Substance abuse
- Psychiatric disturbance

---

social learning and evaluation of remeasurement data (Woods et al 1999). In this way it is postulated that the BSI could meet the needs of professionals seeking an appropriately operationalized version of constructs commonly used in the multidisciplinary planning of individualized treatment in forensic care (Robinson et al 1996). The current version of the BSI consists of three related subscales. These include behaviours which are associated with risk in a forensic context; the degree of insight into causality and current status shown by an individual; and assessment of current communication and social skills. Each item is carefully described and measured on a five-point ordinal scale, using a stepwise method of worst case to best case scenario.

The risk subscale measures such constructs as violence to others; violence inwardly directed; verbally directed aggression; violence directed towards property or objects; generally disruptive or antisocial behaviours; supportive family links; and psychiatric disturbance (see Box 9.4).

The insight subscale examines an individual's cognitive constructs of reality. Items are theoretically grouped into tension-orientated and anger-related items; strategies for reducing tension; features of personal and shared situations; treatment and problem solving; antecedent events leading to treatment; and ascription of responsibility (see Box 9.5).

Finally the communication and social skills subscale principally examines social skills or adaptive social behaviour. Items are theoretically grouped into habitual facial expression; various aspects of proxemics; paralinguistic features; aspects of conversational interaction; potential conflict; self-presentation and interpersonal skills (see Box 9.6).

A case study has been provided as an example of how the BSI can be used to assist social risk assessment (Woods 2000). By focusing thought around other areas of individual functioning, such as insight and communication and social skills, for an individual displaying risky behaviours, there is the possibility of working therapeutically to reduce the risky behaviours. This is the central thrust of the BSI: to search for logical links between items which are specific to the individual, in order to construct meaningful and measurable intervention strategies.

RISK MANAGEMENT

As has been discussed it is vitally important that once a risk assessment has occurred, a risk

Box 9.5 BSI insight subscale items

- Awareness of tension
- Description of tension
- Tension-reducing strategies
- Recognition of negative or angry feelings
- Tension-producing thoughts
- Tension-producing events
- Personal strategy for reducing tension
- Identifying relaxing thoughts
- Identifying relaxing activities
- Attributes disliked in others
- Attributes liked in others
- Events producing insecurity
- Events producing security
- Antecedent events leading to treatment
- Ascription of responsibility
- Self-appraisal
- Prioritization of problems
- Goal planning
- Compliance with therapy
- Expectations

Box 9.6 BSI communication and social skills subscale items

- Facial expression
- Eye contact
- Orientation to others
- Body posture
- Expressive gestures
- Social distance
- Tone of voice
- Voice modulation
- Verbal delivery
- Conversational initiative
- Amount of speech
- Fluency
- Turn taking
- Listening skills
- Response to questions
- Conversational topics
- Egocentric conversation
- Frankness
- Expressing opinions
- Disagreement
- Arguments
- Making requests
- Assertiveness
- Self-presentation
- Social activities
- Emotional control
- Relationship with others
- Ease of communication
- Sociability and support
- Deferring to others

management plan focuses on the likelihood of the probability or outcome occurring. Vinestock (1996) describes this as a method of balancing probable consequences of decisions which assists in formalizing the decision-making process in relation to the risk of harm to self or others. In essence, it is the link between risk assessment information and the known or potential interventions.

The risk management plan should state precisely the nature or level of the risk. However, this needs to be very specific. The situational context of the risk should be stated and the relationships between the risky behaviours presented. Next, for the plan to be effectively evaluated, it must be continuously reviewed. These reviews need to be time bound, and above all, the plan and evaluations need to be communicated to all relevant people involved in the care process.

Doyle (1999: 49) indicates seven key questions which assist in estimating the level of risk and offer good practice guidelines.

1. What is the likelihood of harm occurring?
2. How often is this likely to occur?
3. What possible outcomes may there be?
4. Who is at risk?
5. What is the immediacy of the risk?
6. What is the time scale for assessment?
7. What are the circumstances which are likely to increase or decrease the risk?

However, in order for risk management to be effective clear statements of anticipated risk and how these can be avoided need to be made; thus the impact of any risk is minimized.

In effect, therefore, if one has a detailed knowledge of the individual's personal, mental health, forensic histories, etc., then the early warning signs of any risk can be anticipated. In turn, the risk management plan can focus specifically on the responses required to deal with these potential or anticipated risks, and effectively and clearly monitor the effects of the risks and any progress made through the implementation of the plan. In essence, this is dynamic risk assessment.

Good practice should dictate which responses are made when crisis happens (i.e. the risk occurs). This may range from physical restraint or isolation from others on the unit to allowing the individual to ventilate their feelings on a one-to-one basis. The crucial task is that the individual is informed of the risk(s) which have been identified, what will happen if they occur and why. In practice, this may involve the individual being given the opportunity to select from a range of alternative management strategies. For instance, some very powerful men are petrified of being injected with a major tranquillizer and therefore other forms of medication in crisis may be more beneficial. Women who have been sexually abused may be terrified of being physically restrained whilst on their back, as this was the position they were held in when being abused, and it may be more appropriate to only restrain whilst on their front.

If this is to occur therapeutically to allow the individual to develop and hopefully learn from risky situations, thus reducing potential risk, creative thinking which promotes positive risk taking is necessary.

Further questions that need to be asked are:

◆ Do we have the personal and professional experience and resources to manage the risk?
◆ Is our working environment conducive to managing the risk (for example, physical layout, potential weapons)?
◆ Particularly within the community, are the carers, friends or neighbours likely to hinder the risk management plan?

An organizational risk management strategy

So far this chapter has been concerned with individual patient risk assessment and management. However, just as important is the organizational risk management strategy in forensic mental health care. The strategy proposed below provides a framework which recognizes that risks are managed every day, but that this often occurs on an ad hoc basis and in an uncoordinated way. Thus, the strategy aims to create a more coordinated, systematic and focused approach to the management of risks. The strategy has been previously described in relation to a community nursing service (Dale & Woods 2000).

Based around a six-point action programme, the strategy embraces organizational, cultural, clinical, employee, environmental and incident reporting issues, all of which are developed around a risk management policy statement. This statement must:

◆ describe the role of the forensic service, to provide the highest standard of care and treatment, encompassing its duty of care to identify potential individual patient risks

- highlight that all managers and clinicians own and accept that the identification and management of risks is a fundamental duty
- indicate that honesty and openness are vital, with mistakes or untoward accidents treated positively and responsively
- highlight that the ultimate aim of risk management is to achieve optimum balance between good-quality care, treatment and rehabilitation, through improved prevention, control and containment of risks.

Organizational issues

Line management responsibility Line management responsibility has to be accepted as a fundamental tenet of the strategy; all managers, at all levels, must believe in the approach. They must own the process and take action, both proactively and retrospectively, to identify, assess and tackle any risk issues affecting their areas of responsibility. One of their primary roles must be to stimulate the inclination of their staff to spot and report risks.

Risk management team Coordination of risk management activity throughout a service should be undertaken by a multidisciplinary risk management team. This team should be led by a project manager, who is personally responsible for ensuring that the strategy action points are implemented. Other managers and clinicians with specific knowledge and skills should be coopted when needed. This helps to provide a more systematic and focused approach; support to the line managers on the risk profile of the service; changing trends in risks; and the priorities for action.

Risk awareness Staff need to recognize and appreciate the importance of their own responsibilities in identifying and reporting hazardous and risk situations. It is vital that feedback is given on all reports which they make.

Identifying, assessing, controlling and monitoring of risks No risk can be managed until one has been identified so this fundamental process is vital if a service's risk management process is to succeed. Identifying risk should embrace both proactive and retrospective approaches. A retrospective review gives an opportunity to learn lessons about why an adverse incident occurred but more importantly, appropriate action can be taken to avoid a recurrence. However, this should not detract from the proactive approach, predicting where an incident may occur and taking appropriate steps to avoid it.

Once a service has identified a risk, analysis has to take place to assess: the likelihood of it recurring; how often it is likely to occur; and the likely impact should it occur, in terms of damage or loss to patients, staff, the public and the assets of the service. Following on from risk identification and assessment, the options on how to deal with the risk should be considered. Although a risk cannot always be eliminated entirely, it should be possible to control the frequency and severity of it, individually or in combination with other control measures. Finally, the control measure(s) must be monitored at all times, thus enabling assessment of the effectiveness of the systems and changes that have been put in place.

Cultural issues

Organizational attitudes An attitude of openness and honesty within a service, which takes all the necessary steps to avoid cover-ups of adverse incidents and mistakes, can help to reduce risk. The overall approach within a service should be to help and support each other, rather than recrimination and blame. Indeed, what appear at times to be overwhelming difficulties should be seen as manageable challenges.

All managers should ensure a quick and decisive response to any report of an adverse incident or complaint, with quick feedback on any action taken, or not, and a clear indication of how the particular risk situation has been reduced or eliminated. Therefore, staff and patients will be encouraged to report similar incidents more readily in the future.

Communications One of the greatest risk factors in an organization is inadequate communication. Indeed, it can lead to misunderstanding between care professionals, a failure to pass on vital patient information or the wrong information being cascaded to staff. The fundamental and key feature is that risk-free communications is a two-way process. It should be easy for staff to raise issues of concern to them with their manager(s); for staff to be consulted on proposed organizational or other changes; for managers to keep staff informed of progress on issues; for patients, their relatives and advocates to identify points of concern or worry; and for the media to be kept advised of developments in the service.

Clinical issues

Policies, procedures, protocols and guidelines The importance of easily understood clinical policies, procedures, guidelines, treatment protocols and agreed standards, which are up to date, cannot be over emphasized in relation to risk reduction. A major cause of risk can be that members of staff are uncertain of what is expected of them, particularly in emergency situations. This can be compounded when other members of the same team have different understandings.

Policies and procedures should be issued to those who need to use them, read, understood and put into action by those people. Furthermore, regular audit should be undertaken. Medical and nursing procedures should be based on the best available evidence and procedure manuals and documents should include a reference section. Service-wide policies and procedures should be sufficiently flexible to be of practical use in different situations, yet at the same time avoid inconsistency in interpretation. Accordingly, all new policies should make it clear what must be strictly followed and what is open to discretion.

Patient treatment plans Every individual patient should have an individual treatment plan, which is based on a multidisciplinary assessment and patient and family involvement. Review should occur on a regular basis, so all members of the patient's clinical team are fully aware of its current content. Without such up-to-date plans, there will be considerable risk of patients' care being compromised. To ensure that all patient treatment plans are valid, there should be regular audits of a random selection of plans, under the auspices of the risk management team.

Professional staffing and competencies Formal assessment should be undertaken to analyse relative risks of the adequacy of the staffing levels; patient needs analysis; the utilization and skill mix of staff; and the ongoing competencies of professional staff. This should be underpinned by a system of formal audit of effectiveness.

Infection control The risk management team should regularly review and control for actual, or potential, crossinfection leading to severe risk to patients and staff. This should be operated within an agreed infection control policy.

Employee issues

A charter for staff Wide recognition exists that staff who feel more valued will be more efficient and effective in their work. A useful approach to assist in this is to produce a charter for staff which includes: development and education needs; provision of a safe and pleasant working environment; offer of help, support and counselling when required; provision of satisfactory occupational health services; and training in lifting and handling, together with appropriate health and safety obligations.

Induction and exit issues In order to minimize risk, all new staff must undergo a satisfactory induction programme, if not before commencing employment then as soon as possible after this. This should apply to all locum, agency or bank staff, however short their length of duty. Equally important is the provision of an exit interview for staff before they leave. This not only can obtain their views about various aspects of the service, but may also be an opportunity to collect items owned by the organization. Moreover, a particular emphasis should be given to a series of prepared questions on various aspects of risk.

Employee responsibility for risk management and health and safety Through the Health and Safety at Work Act 1974, all employees are obliged to accept some responsibility for maintaining a safe workplace environment. It is vital that all staff are informed of this and also that they should highlight their concerns about any health and safety issue, either directly to their manager or through their appointed health and safety representative.

Environmental issues

Security Services are often open to the risk of theft, both from their service premises and when visiting patients' homes. It is necessary for security to have a direct link with clinical care and that procedures are minimally intrusive and respect the rights and dignity of all those which they may affect. Furthermore, not only is greater awareness of security issues necessary, but also specialist training for staff to deal with patients in confrontational situations.

Health and safety The introduction of the Health and Safety at Work Act 1974 lead to a steady growth in the codification of health and safety legislation which sets detailed standards of compliance. On 1 January 1993, a whole body of new regulations universally known as 'the Six Pack' became law. These were: Display Screen Equipment Regulations (HMSO 1992a); Management of Health and Safety at Work Regulations (HMSO 1992b); Manual Handling Operations at Work Regulations (HMSO 1992c); Personal Protective Equipment at Work Regulations (HMSO 1992d); Provision and Use of Work Equipment Regulations (HMSO 1992e); and the Workplace (Health, Safety & Welfare) Regulations (HMSO 1992f).

All these regulations are underpinned by good risk assessment, control and monitoring. Moreover, they impose criminal, not civil law sanctions and if they are breached, the service's senior officers, or individuals deemed responsible, may be fined or imprisoned. Therefore, health and safety improvements should be an integral part of a risk management strategy, with the service's health and safety officer a key member of the risk management team.

Incident reporting

Reporting systems Reporting of risk situations, including adverse incidents, near misses, accidents to staff, staff mistakes and complaints from patients, is a vital part of effectively managing and controlling risk. Chapter 10 provides details of a number of incident reporting systems but any system used should be monitored by the project manager and the risk management team. Moreover, this should entail ensuring that staff know what to report; how they should report; which form they should complete; where they can obtain the form; who should complete and countersign the form; and to whom they should send it.

Data collection, analysis and feedback The importance of centralized data collection cannot be overemphasized, in order that it can be analysed, thus allowing the provision of meaningful and useful information on data trends of incidents occurring.

Desire to report Fundamental to any reporting system is the desire of staff to report those incidents, mistakes and accidents they have been asked to report. Underreporting of incidents occurs for a number of reasons: for instance, staff are too frightened to report because of possible recriminations or disciplinary actions; they are too lazy; they do not think it is important; they are not sure what to report; they are ambivalent; or because they have reported so many times before without any apparent notice being taken of it. Therefore, any reporting system should aim to overcome underreporting issues.

Complaints and claims Data and information should be brought together on: adverse patient incidents; staff accidents; medical and clinical audit results; quality assurance initiatives; patient complaints; and legal claims from both patients and staff. Aggregate information should be supplied to the risk management team to allow them to effectively examine trends, initiate corrective actions and monitor the success of these.

CONCLUSION

Within this chapter it has been impossible to discuss all aspects of risk assessment and management but it has highlighted the fundamental aspects of risk assessment and management, both from the individual patient perspective and the forensic service perspective. The author has also tried to indicate good practice issues.

From the individual patient perspective, some of the instruments which are currently available have been discussed and the way has been pointed towards others. It has been highlighted throughout that any risk assessment and its related management needs to be systematic and based on the population being assessed. Furthermore, it is necessary to effectively and systematically monitor the whole process. From the wider forensic service perspective, the fundamental underpinning issue to any risk management strategy must be a coherent and manageable communication and evaluative process, that encompasses all relevant legislation. Thus, the chance of harm or litigation when things inevitably go wrong is minimized. Moreover, there are some key points which need to be borne in mind when considering risk assessment and management.

◆ In an increasingly litigious environment and with the heightened likelihood of an inquiry or major investigation, the existence of a systematic and considered approach to risk is a good defence for the practitioner who may find themselves called to task about their practices. Although this may be deemed a defensive reaction, it is in fact a reality.

◆ Following discharge from forensic settings, mentally disordered offenders do not necessarily offend quickly. Evidence suggests that on average reoffending occurs some 3 years after discharge. Consequently, there is a critical need for vigilance with regard to changes in circumstances. For example, a new relationship or a breakdown in an existing one, a bereavement and loss of a support system, a job loss, recommencing drinking, etc. can all be the triggers for increased risk of offending.

◆ Serious consideration needs to be given to how often to reassess and what may trigger a reassessment.

◆ Assessments need to remain as objective as possible. A supervisor who is not directly involved in the care team, who is emotionally detached, can assist in identifying flaws in the assessment and management processes.

Finally, the whole process of risk assessment and management was perhaps summed up over two decades ago by Scott (1977):

It is patience, thoroughness and persistence in the process rather than any diagnostic brilliance that produces results. In this sense the telephone, the written requests for past records and the checking of information against other informants are the important diagnostic devices.

REFERENCES

Bingley W 1997 Assessing dangerousness: protecting the interests of patients. British Journal of Psychiatry 170(32): 28–29

Borum R 1996 Improving the clinical practice of violence risk assessment. American Psychologist 51(9): 945–956

Chin CJ 1998 Dangerousness: myth or clinical reality? Psychiatric Care 5(2): 66–71

Chiswick D 1995 Dangerousness. In: Chiswick D, Cope R (eds) Seminars in practical forensic psychiatry. Gaskell, London, pp 210–242

Dale C, Woods P 2000 Safe as houses: a risk management strategy for community nursing. British Journal of Community Nursing 5(6): 286–291

Doyle M 1999 Organizational responses to crisis and risk: issues and implications for mental health nurses. In: Ryan T (ed) Managing crisis and risk in mental health nursing. Stanley Thornes, Cheltenham, Ch 4, pp 40–56

Duggan C 1997 Assessing risk in the mentally disordered. Introduction. British Journal of Psychiatry 170(32): 1–3

Harris GT, Rice ME, Quinsey VL 1993 Violent recidivism of mentally disordered offenders: the development of a statistical prediction instrument. Criminal Justice and Behavior 20: 315–335

HMSO 1992a Display Screen Equipment Regulations. HMSO, London

HMSO 1992b Management of Health and Safety at Work Regulations. HMSO, London

HMSO 1992c Manual Handling Operations at Work Regulations. HMSO, London

HMSO 1992d Personal Protective Equipment at Work Regulations. HMSO, London

HMSO 1992e Provision and Use of Work Equipment Regulations. HMSO, London

HMSO 1992f Workplace (Health, Safety & Welfare) Regulations. HMSO, London

Home Office, Department of Health 1999 Managing dangerous people with severe personality disorder: proposals for policy development. Home Office and Department of Health, London

McClelland N 1995 The assessment of dangerousness: a procedure for predicting potentially dangerous behaviour. Psychiatric Care 2: 17–19

Monahan J 1984 The prediction of violent behaviour: toward a second generation of theory and policy. American Journal of Psychiatry 141: 10–15

Monahan J 1988 Risk assessment of violence among the mentally disordered: generating useful knowledge. International Journal of Law and Psychiatry 11: 249–257

Monahan J, Steadman HJ (eds) 1994 Violence and mental disorder: developments in risk assessment. University of Chicago Press, Chicago

Pollock N, Webster C 1990 The clinical assessment of dangerousness. In: Bluglass R, Bowden P (eds) Principles and practice of forensic psychiatry. Churchill Livingstone, Edinburgh, pp 489–497

Prins H 1996 Risk assessment and management in criminal justice and psychiatry. Journal of Forensic Psychiatry 7(1): 42–62

Rice ME, Harris GT 1995 Violent recidivism: assessing predictive validity. Journal of Consulting and Clinical Psychology 63(5): 737–748

Robinson D, Reed V, Lange A 1996 Developing risk assessment scales in psychiatric care. Psychiatric Care 3(4): 146–152

Royal College of Nursing 1998 Dealing with violence against nursing staff: an RCN guide for nurses and managers. Royal College of Nursing, London

Ryan T (ed) 1999 Managing crisis and risk in mental health nursing. Stanley Thornes, Cheltenham

Scott PD 1977 Assessing dangerousness in criminals. British Journal of Psychiatry 131: 127–142

Shah S 1978 Dangerousness: a paradigm for exploring some issues in law and psychology. American Psychologist 33: 224–238

Steadman HJ, Cocozza JJ 1974 Careers of the criminally insane: excessive social control of deviance. Lexington Books, Lexington MA

Vinestock M 1996 Risk assessment: 'a word to the wise'? Advances in Psychiatric Treatment 2: 3–10

Webster CD, Harris GT, Rice ME, Cormier C, Quinsey VL 1994 The Violence Prediction Scheme: assessing dangerousness in high risk men. Centre of Criminology, University of Toronto, Toronto

Webster CD, Eaves D, Douglas K, Wintrup A 1995 The HCR-20 scheme: the assessment of dangerousness and risk, version 1. Simon Fraser University and Forensic Psychiatric Services Commission of British Columbia, Vancouver, Canada

Webster CD, Douglas KS, Eaves D, Hart SD 1997 HCR-20: assessing risk for violence, version 2. Mental Health Law and Policy Institute, Simon Fraser University, Vancouver, Canada

Woods P 1996 How nurses make assessments of patient dangerousness. Mental Health Nursing 16(4): 20–22

Woods P 2000 Social assessment of risk: the Behavioural Status Index. In: Mercer D, Mason T, McKeown M, McCann G (eds) Forensic mental health care: a case study approach. Churchill Livingstone, Edinburgh, pp 333–339

Woods P, Reed V, Robinson D 1999 The Behavioural Status Index: therapeutic assessment of risk, insight, communication and social skills. Journal of Psychiatric and Mental Health Nursing 6(2): 79–90

FURTHER READING

Duggan C (ed) 1997 Assessing risk in the mentally disordered. British Journal of Psychiatry 170 (Suppl 32): 1–39

Monahan J, Steadman HJ (eds) 1994 Violence and mental disorder: developments in risk assessment. University of Chicago Press, Chicago

Morgan S 1998 Assessing and managing risk: a practitioner's handbook. Pavillion Publishing, Brighton

National Health Service Executive 1993 Risk management in the NHS. NHSE, London

Ryan T (ed) 1999 Managing crisis and risk in mental health nursing. Stanley Thornes, Cheltenham

Chapter Ten

10

Incidents: reporting and management

Phil Woods

INTRODUCTION

Introduced within this chapter is the violent incident, one of those untoward incidents which occur in forensic mental health settings. The literature and the time that the media dedicate to violence in the workplace indicate that it is a real problem. This applies not only to forensic mental health professionals who are dealing with known violent individuals but also to those in accident and emergency departments; psychiatric inpatient facilities; nursing homes; day centres; and of course the community. Brakel (1998) discusses how workplace violence is an ongoing concern, with an alarming total number of incidents. The Royal College of Nursing (1998) asks if the problem is getting worse and concludes that the available evidence suggests that it is. A recent survey by the National Audit Office (1996) found that the third most common staff accident in National Health Service acute hospital trusts in England was physical assault.

Incidents are important factors when considering the risk an individual poses, not only in the short term but also in the long term. They are also fundamental components of evaluating a hospital's risk assessment and management strategies. It is not surprising that Berg et al (1994) report how injuries, stress, anxiety and psychosomatic illness have resulted from the exposure to violence. More recently, Gournay & Carson (2000), reporting preliminary findings from a survey in two English high security hospitals, suggest how being assaulted clearly has an effect on staff, with those assaulted being significantly younger, having lower job satisfaction and having more than twice the amount of sickness in the last 12 months.

It is vitally important that incident monitoring is maintained on a regular basis and placed within the context of key situational, environmental and demographic variables. Indeed, the National Audit Office (1996) highlights in its survey that reporting systems were either inadequate or unreliable. The Royal College of Nursing (1998) states that reporting systems must be accessible and straightforward and that employers need to know what is happening, to whom, by whom and where, why and when. Further, health service guidelines indicate that systems should:

◆ be simple to use (ideally based on a standard form for all incidents which can be used by all staff – one form should be used in all situations)
◆ be based on a standard definition of incidents to ensure comparability across the organization
◆ allow for the timely collation of data and investigation of incidents (near misses) and accidents
◆ be able to record the people involved (e.g. names, ages or training), the cause(s) of both the accident and the injury (e.g. falls or chemicals), the location and time of the incident, treatment given, any resulting staff absence and most importantly, action taken by management to prevent a recurrence. (NHSE 1997)

Further, it states that it is:

the line manager's responsibility to ensure that the system works. Staff involved in completing incident report forms should receive training in the purpose for which the forms will be used and in how to fill them in. Written guidelines may be useful. (NHSE 1997)

Over the past three decades extensive research has been undertaken in relation to all aspects of violent incidents, with a view to developing our understanding of how and why these occur. This has occurred from the forensic perspective (Carton & Larkin 1991, Coldwell & Naismith 1989, Dooley 1986, Kelsall et al 1995, Larkin et al 1988) and general mental health care (James et al 1990, Noble & Rodger 1989, Pearson et al 1986, Walker & Seifert 1994). However, it is extremely difficult to generalize from the literature considering the differing definitions and measurements of violence used.

INCIDENTS

The first and perhaps the most important issue to be considered when developing any incident-reporting system is what exactly is meant by an incident. At face value this would appear to be an easy task, especially for forensic mental health professionals. However, if the literature is studied many conceptual ambiguities will be found. Definitions range from the vague, such as 'untoward events that adversely affect the well being of patients' (Drinkwater & Gudjonsson 1989, Haller & Deluty 1988), to the more complete which include passive aggression, verbal abuse, threatened aggression and actual aggression (Way et al 1992) or physical violence against the person, categorized by seriousness of the injury (Coldwell & Naismith 1989, Fottrell 1980, Noble & Rodger 1989, Walker & Seifert 1994). Kelsall et al (1995) offer a definition which is perhaps the most useful: 'any behaviour which could physically damage the individual, another individual or property'. However, this only goes part of the way because any definition should also include psychological damage. Thus, a suitable definition may well be: 'any behaviour which could be physically or psychologically damaging to the individual, another individual or property'.

The next important issue is what factors are considered, or need to be reported on, when an incident has occurred? Ideally, one should be as inclusive as possible but not at the risk of monitoring meaningless numbers of variables. If one again looks at the literature for assistance, there is considerable agreement that high priority should be given to a number of factors which are related to violence:

◆ predisposing factors
◆ environmental factors
◆ the nature of the incident.

Factors predisposing to violence

The *Concise Oxford Dictionary* definition of *predispose* is to influence favourably in advance. Therefore, factors predisposing to violence could be understood to simply mean the things which make someone more likely to be violent. Generally, the literature suggests that these factors form the actuarial base of any risk assessment and management strategy and are the anchor for clinical opinion.

Within the literature many predisposing factors have been examined as being important such as: the individual characteristics of age; gender;

ethnicity; diagnosis; length of stay; and previous history of violence. Indeed, some of these have been shown to be reliable indicators of future violence: see Chapter 9 for a discussion of these. Moreover, for the localized incident reporting and management system, monitoring of these variables following an incident not only allows the individual patient groups to be monitored but also encourages comparisons to be made with the vast research base existing in relation to these variables. Thus, underpinning the local reporting system within a research and development programme provides vital information which can feed into the larger national and international perspective.

The evidence base for each of the predisposing factors identified above will now be briefly discussed.

Age

The general trend reported within the literature is that younger patients tend to be involved in more violent incidents.

Gender

Inconsistencies exist within the literature as to whether men or women are involved in more violent incidents. Many have commented on high levels of violence in women patients (Carton & Larkin 1991, Cooper & Mendonca 1991, Fottrell 1980, Hodgkinson et al 1984, Larkin et al 1988). Within one high security forensic mental health setting, it was reported that women accounted for 75% of all violent incidents but for only 25% of the hospital population (Larkin et al 1988). Others note that the majority of their assaultive sample were men; however, stratifying by age, it was found that the majority of assaultive patients under 25 years of age were women (Tardiff & Sweillam 1979).

Ethnicity

This has received the least research attention over the years. Although the general population's perception is that mentally disordered blacks are more violent than mentally disordered whites, what few studies there have been provide contradictory evidence. For instance, no evidence of racial difference has been found by some (Gray 1989, Tanke & Yesavage 1985), whilst a small number report that Afro-Caribbean patients showed a disproportionately high level of assaultive behaviour (Noble & Rodger 1989, Walker & Seifert 1994).

Diagnosis

This has one of the most controversial associations with violence. Evidence can be found to support no link (Gray 1989, James et al 1990, Tanke & Yesavage 1985) or that schizophrenia is the most commonly represented diagnosis in violent patients (Coldwell & Naismith 1989, Fottrell 1980, Hunter & Carmel 1989, Kennedy 1993, Noble & Rodger 1989, Tam et al 1996). Others have reported personality disorder to be more linked to violent incident than mental illness (Dooley 1986). However, one of the diagnostic categories most frequently associated with violent incidents is substance abuse (Davis 1991, Palmstierna & Wistedt 1989, Steadman et al 1998, Walker & Seifert 1994).

Length of stay

Associations have been shown between length of stay in hospital and violent incidents. For instance, the more violent patients have been inpatients for a longer period of time (Dooley 1986, Krakowski & Czobor 1994, Miller et al 1993). More importantly, findings have revealed that the majority of aggressive incidents occur within the first 2 months following admission, with a marked decrease thereafter (Barnard et al 1984).

Previous history of violence

There is little doubt that previous violence is linked to future violent incidents and is generally thought to be the best predictor (Davis 1991, Fottrell et al 1978, Morrison 1994, Noble & Rodger 1989). Morrison (1994) found links between previous violence and length of stay.

The strongest evidence is that a small proportion of patients is responsible for the majority of violent incidents (Depp 1983, Fottrell 1980, Kelsall et al 1995, Larkin et al 1988, Pearson et al 1986). For instance, one study reported that 50% of assaults were committed by 20% of the patients (Hodgkinson et al 1984) and another in a regional secure unit found that two patients were responsible for 189 of the 389 incidents (Rix & Seymour 1988). Similarly, high security hospital studies have found that, in special care wards, 19% of the patients were responsible for 62% of the incidents (Coldwell & Naismith 1989) and one patient was responsible for 40% of the incidents (Carton & Larkin 1991).

Environmental factors

The importance of environmental factors is often overlooked. The type of ward the incident occurred on: was it an admission ward or a high, medium or low dependency one? What was the location of the incident? Did it occur on the ward or in an off-ward area such as the work area or education department; at the social activities; in the hospital grounds; on a patient movement; in the medical centre; or external to the hospital setting? If it occurred on the ward, where was the sublocation of the incident? Did it occur in the day area, bedroom, night station, dining room, corridor, television lounge, staff area, library/quiet room, seclusion room, kitchen, toilets, garden area, bathroom or somewhere else? Did the fact that many patients were congregated together in one area have any bearing on the incident? What time of day, week or month did it occur? Was it during shift change, medication time or meal time? Are there seasonal variations and was it affected by staffing levels? These are all important questions that can assist in monitoring the occurrence of violent incidents. The evidence for these environmental factors will now be examined.

Type of ward

Although violent incidents occur on all types of ward there appears to be considerable agreement within the literature that admission, intensive care and locked wards, within general psychiatric hospitals, have the most incidents (Coldwell & Naismith 1989, Fottrell 1980, Hodgkinson et al 1984, Powell et al 1994). Importantly, studies have shown that wards which care for alcohol and drug abusers have higher levels of violence (Krakowski et al 1989, Palmstierna & Wistedt 1989, Powell et al 1994). Perhaps not surprisingly, secure and forensic settings have been shown to have more violent incidents than in general psychiatry (Dietz & Rada 1982, Kelsall et al 1995, Larkin et al 1988, Rix & Seymour 1988).

Location of incident

Generally it has been shown that the majority of incidents occur within ward areas (Coldwell & Naismith 1989, Fottrell 1980, Hodgkinson et al 1984, Kelsall et al 1995). Moreover, more violent incidents occur in communal ward areas (Hunter & Love 1996, Larkin et al 1988). Some studies have demonstrated that ward sleeping areas accounted for a small but significant proportion of the incidents (Coldwell & Naismith 1989, Hodgkinson et al 1984, Kelsall et al 1995).

Patient density

Although Drinkwater & Gudjonsson (1989) argue that there is little support for associating patient density with aggression, there is extensive research which indicates a link (Brooks et al 1994, Coldwell & Naismith 1989, Dietz & Rada 1982, Harris & Varney 1986).

Time of day

Considerable evidence is available in relation to the time of the day when most incidents occur. Some report peak times are in the morning (Ekblom 1970, Fottrell 1980, Hodgkinson et al 1984), whereas others report the evening (Ekblom 1970). Others have indicated the afternoon (Coldwell & Naismith 1989, Lanza et al 1994).

Less specifically, some have just reported day time for most violent incidents (Ghaziuddin & Ghaziuddin 1992, Noble & Rodger 1989, Tam et al 1996, Walker & Seifert 1994). Walker & Seifert (1994) reported that most incidents occurred at medication times.

Day of the week and seasonal variation

The evidence here is conflicting and all indications are that this is related to patient density.

Nature of the incident

The importance of recording the nature of the incident cannot be overestimated. For instance, who were the victim(s)? Were they staff, patients or others? What was the severity of the incident? Was it serious, moderate or minor? Evidence will now be examined in relation to each of these.

Victim

Staff appear to take the brunt of most violent incidents (Carton & Larkin 1991, Fottrell 1980, James et al 1990, Larkin et al 1988, Noble & Rodger 1989, Whittington & Patterson 1996). Moreover, Carmel & Hunter (1993) indicated that attacks on male nursing staff were 50% higher than on female nursing staff. However, it has to be borne in mind that nursing staff are involved in direct patient care and therefore are more likely to be available for attack. Conversely, Dooley (1986) found that patients were more likely to be assaulted than nursing staff.

Severity of incident

There is considerable evidence to suggest that the majority of incidents are minor in nature (Fottrell 1980, Kelsall et al 1995, Noble & Rodger 1989, Rix & Seymour 1988). However, within high security care, it has been suggested that they are more serious in nature (Carton & Larkin 1991, Larkin et al 1988).

REPORTING

Many variables have been examined in relation to violent incidents. Although conflicting evidence can be found to support or refute their usefulness in the process of monitoring violent incidents, there is little doubt that they serve as reliable measures to include in any system which may be developed. A few authors have published incident-reporting systems which have been empirically examined in order to determine their usefulness. The best known of these is the Staff Observation Aggression Scale (SOAS) (Palmstierna & Wistedt 1987), with a recently revised version (SOAS-R) presented by Nijman et al (1999). The main variables measured are as follows.

1. *Provocation*. Subdivided into: (1) no understandable provocation; (2) provoked by other patient(s), help with ADL, patient being denied something, staff requiring patient to take medication or other provocations.
2. *Means used by the patient*. Subdivided into: (1) verbal aggression; (2) ordinary objects, chair(s), glass(ware) or other; (3) parts of the body, hand (hitting, punching, etc.), foot (kicking), teeth (biting) or other; (4) dangerous objects or methods, knife, strangulation or other.
3. *Target of aggression*. Subdivided into: (1) nothing/nobody; (2) object(s); (3) other patient(s); (4) self; (5) staff member(s); (6) other person(s).
4. *Consequence(s) for victim(s)*. Subdivided into: (1) no; (2) objects, damaged but not replaced or damaged and replaced; (3) persons, felt threatened, pain for less than 10 minutes, pain for over 10 minutes, visible injury, need for treatment by a physician.
5. *Measure(s) to stop aggression*. Subdivided into: (1) none; (2) talk to patient; (3) calmly brought away; (4) peroral medication; (5) parenteral medication; (6) held with force; (7) seclusion/isolation (locked door); (8) physical restraints; (9) other measures.

The form is completed when aggressive behaviour occurs. Aggression here is defined as any verbal, non-verbal or physical behaviour that was threatening (to self, others or property) or physical behaviour that actually did harm (to self, others or property) (Morrison 1990). This is widely used within many European countries and has been the standard instrument used in Norwegian psychiatric hospitals for nearly a decade. Indeed, it is given here as an example of good practice for staff in-service training.

Others have used the SOAS in conjunction with the Brøset Violence Checklist (Almvik & Woods 1998, 1999), to measure violence in the first 3 days following admission. The Brøset Violence Checklist assesses confusion, irritability, boisterousness, verbal threats, physical threats and attacks on objects as either present or absent. It is hypothesized that an individual displaying two or more of these behaviours is more likely to be violent in the next 24-hour period. All variables have been shown to be predictive of violence occurring.

A comprehensive computerized incident-monitoring system was discussed by Dale et al (1999). This system was introduced into a high security setting following an inquiry recommendation but it serves as a good example of a comprehensive system which could be used in any forensic setting. The aims of the incident-reporting system were:

◆ to provide an accurate record of all relevant information appertaining to incidents
◆ to produce a system of incident reporting which is accessible and versatile and would assist in reviewing the patient's care
◆ that the system should be viewed positively by those involved, including patients, and should underpin good practice and help improve standards of care and treatment (Ashworth Hospital, internal document, 1994: 1).

The system functions from the operational definition of 'any event, untoward or unusual, which is counter to the therapeutic activity or smooth running of the ward or department, which involves patients and/or staff and/or visitors, and which may adversely affect their safety and welfare, then or later' (Ashworth Hospital, internal document, 1994: 1). Incidents are categorized through the system into four groups, which are in descending order of seriousness.

◆ Category A – which includes any unexpected death.
◆ Category B – which includes life-threatening activity (e.g. attempted suicide); severe assault with a weapon or attempted strangulation; escape; hostage taking; serious fire.
◆ Category C – which includes serious assault; significant destruction of property; drug/alcohol abuse; security breaches (e.g. escape plot).
◆ Category D – which includes others within the definition of incidents above: minor assaults; verbal altercation between patients; verbal abuse against staff.

The list was not intended to be exhaustive and staff were expected to exercise judgement regarding this.

MANAGEMENT

In order for such an incident-reporting system to feed into the management of incidents from the organizational perspective, it is necessary for information to be reported or collated from all the variables which have been discussed. First, the predisposing factors: age; gender; ethnicity; diagnosis; length of stay; and previous history of violence. It may not always be necessary for staff involved in the incident to report these when using a computerized system, as information can be linked to existing patient information systems.

Second, the environmental factors: type of ward (admission, high, medium or low dependency); location of incident; if on the ward, what was the sub-location of the incident (day area, bedroom, night station, dining room, corridor, television lounge, staff area, library/quiet room, seclusion room, kitchen, toilets, garden area, bathroom, or somewhere else) or if off the ward (the work area, education department, at the social activities, in the hospital grounds, on a patient movement, in the medical centre or external to the hospital setting); did the fact that many patients were congregated together in one area have any bearing on the incident; what was the time of day and date; was it during shift change, medication time or meal time?

Third, the nature of the incident: the victim or victims (staff, patients or others); and the severity (serious, moderate or minor).

If all this information is collected it allows analysis of the incidents which occur, according to all the variables or multiples of these; for instance, differences between men and women, seasonal variations, time variations or whether staffing levels or congregation of patients are affecting the level of incidents. These are all important questions that can assist in monitoring the occurrence of violent incidents. In the system described above, monthly printouts are sent to clinical areas and the hospital-wide picture is discussed at hospital board meetings. The information is readily available for clinical teams to look at individual patients in the light of the overall hospital picture.

UNDERREPORTING ISSUES

We cannot leave this chapter without mentioning the all too troubling underreporting of incidents. A number of researchers have reported on the level of this (Braff et al 1986, Convit et al 1988) whilst some have been more specific and reported that up to five times as many assaults occurred as were actually reported. They offered some possible explanations, such as:

◆ the frequency of minor assaults is so high that staff become inured to them and therefore do not report all incidents
◆ staff consider it too troublesome to fill out reports, especially when they see no change forthcoming as a result of reporting
◆ staff fear accusations of negligence and inadequate performance when assaults occur (Lion et al 1981: 498).

It has been reported that with an observer-based instrument such as the SOAS (Palmstierna & Wistedt 1987), the level of actual incident reporting is between 87% and 98%, whereas using a rating method based on charts and records alone, typically levels are between 27% and 53% (Silver & Yudofsky 1991). More specifically, Carton & Larkin (1991), who replicated an earlier study by Larkin et al (1988), reported that even with a prospective study, underreporting was high, with only 42% of incidents being reported. This was verified by crosschecking incident reports with ward day reports.

So, as can be seen, this is a real problem which has no easy answer. However, if all staff are trained in the use of a user-friendly computerized incident-reporting system this may perhaps go some way to providing a solution.

CONCLUSION

It is vitally important, within forensic mental health care, to have an effective system of monitoring violent incidents. Whether this is a computerized or paper system, it must be well managed and address issues of underreporting. It must also define what exactly is meant by an incident. Furthermore, it needs to be clear and precise in what is being monitored, in relation to predisposing and environmental factors, as well as the nature of the incident itself. All this helps to promote understanding of why and how the incident occurred and what, if any, measures can be taken to reduce the likelihood of recurrence.

REFERENCES

Almvik R, Woods P 1998 The Brøset Violence Checklist (BVC) and the prediction of in-patient violence: some preliminary results. Psychiatric Care 5(6): 208–211

Almvik R, Woods P 1999 Predicting in-patient violence using the Brøset Violence Checklist (BVC). International Journal of Psychiatric Nursing Research 4(3): 498–505

Barnard GW, Robbins L, Newman G, Carrera F 1984 A study of violence within a forensic treatment facility. Bulletin of the American Academy of Psychiatry and the Law 12: 339–348

Berg HM, Olsen DL, Sveipe EJ, Hoy BIØ 1994 Threats of violence – a psychological strain to staff personnel. Norwegian College of Nursing, Norway

Braff J, Way BB, Steadman HJ 1986 Incident reporting: evaluation of New York's pilot incident-logging system. Quality Review Bulletin 12: 90–98

Brakel SJ 1998 Legal liability and workplace violence. Journal of the American Academy of Psychiatry and the Law 26(4): 553–562

Brooks KL, Mulaik JS, Gilead MP, Daniels BS 1994 Patient overcrowding in psychiatric hospital units: effects on seclusion and restraint. Administration and Policy in Mental Health 22: 133–144

Carmel H, Hunter M 1993 Staff injuries from patient attack: five years data. Bulletin of the American Academy of Psychiatry and the Law 21(4): 485–493

Carton G, Larkin E 1991 Reducing violence in a special hospital. Nursing Standard 5: 29–31

Coldwell JB, Naismith LJ 1989 Violent incidents on special care wards in a special hospital. Medicine, Science and the Law 29: 116–123

Convit A, Jaeger J, Lin SP, Meisner M, Volavka J 1988 Predicting assaultiveness in psychiatric patients: a pilot study. Hospital and Community Psychiatry 39(4): 429–434

Cooper AJ, Mendonca JD 1991 A prospective study of patient assaults on nurses in a provincial psychiatric hospital in Canada. Acta Psychiatrica Scandinavica 84: 163–166

Dale C, Woods P, Allan G, Brennan W 1999 Violence in high secure hospital settings: measuring, assessing and responding. In: Kemshall H, Pritchard J (eds) Good practice in working with violence. Jessica Kingsley, London, Ch 11, pp 207–230

Davis S 1991 Violence by psychiatric in-patients: a review. Hospital and Community Psychiatry 42: 585–590

Depp FC 1983 Assault in a public mental hospital. In: Lion JR, Reid WH (eds) Assaults within psychiatric facilities. Grune and Stratton, New York

Dietz PE, Rada RT 1982 Battery incidents and batterers in a maximum security hospital. Archives of General Psychiatry 39: 31–34

Dooley E 1986 Aggressive incidents in a secure hospital. Medicine, Science and the Law 26: 125–130

Drinkwater J, Gudjonsson GH 1989 The nature of violence in psychiatric hospitals. In: Howells K, Hollin CR (eds) Clinical approaches to violence. Wiley, Chichester, pp 287–307

Ekblom B 1970 Acts of violence by patients in mental hospitals. Scandinavian University Books, Uppsala

Fottrell E 1980 A study of violent behaviour amongst patients in psychiatric hospitals. British Journal of Psychiatry 136: 216–221

Fottrell E, Bewley T, Squizzoni M 1978 A study of aggressive and violent behaviour among a group of psychiatric in-patients. Medicine, Science and the Law 18: 66–69

Ghaziuddin M, Ghaziuddin N 1992 Violence against staff by mentally retarded in-patients. Hospital and Community Psychiatry 43: 503–504

Gournay K, Carson J 2000 Staff stress, coping skills and job satisfaction in forensic nursing. In: Robinson D, Kettles A (eds) Forensic nursing and multidisciplinary care of the mentally disordered offender. Jessica Kingsley, London, Ch 12, pp 152–164

Gray GE 1989 Assaults by patients against psychiatric residents at a public psychiatric hospital. Academic Psychiatry 13: 81–86

Haller RM, Deluty RH 1988 Assaults on staff by psychiatric in-patients: a critical review. British Journal of Psychiatry 152: 174–179

Harris GT, Varney GW 1986 A ten year study of assaults and assaulters on a maximum security psychiatric unit. Journal of Interpersonal Violence 1: 173–191

Hodgkinson P, Hillis T, Russell D 1984 Aggression management: assaults on staff in a psychiatric hospital. Nursing Times 80(16): 44–46

Hunter M, Carmel H 1989 Staff injuries from in-patient violence. Hospital and Community Psychiatry 40: 41–46

Hunter ME, Love CC 1996 Total quality management and the reduction of in-patient violence and costs in a forensic psychiatric hospital. Psychiatric Services 47: 751–754

James DV, Fineberg NA, Shah AK, Priest RG 1990 An increase in violence on an acute psychiatric ward: a study of associated factors. British Journal of Psychiatry 156: 846–852

Kelsall M, Dolan M, Bailey S 1995 Violent incidents in an adolescent forensic unit. Medicine, Science and the Law 35: 150–158

Kennedy MG 1993 Relationship between psychiatric diagnosis and patient aggression. Issues in Mental Health Nursing 14: 263–273

Krakowski MI, Czobor P 1994 Clinical symptoms, neurological impairment, and prediction of violence in psychiatric in-patients. Hospital and Community Psychiatry 45: 700–705

Krakowski MI, Convit A, Jaeger J 1989 In-patient violence: trait and state. Journal of Psychiatric Research 23: 57–64

Lanza ML, Kayne HL, Hicks C, Milner J 1994 Environmental characteristics related to patient assault. Issues in Mental Health Nursing 15: 319–335

Larkin E, Murtagh S, Jones S 1988 A preliminary study of violent incidents in a special hospital (Rampton). British Journal of Psychiatry 153: 226–231

Lion JR, Snyder W, Merrill GL 1981 Underreporting of assaults on staff in a state hospital. Hospital and Community Psychiatry 32: 497–498

Miller RJ, Zadolinnyj K, Hafner RJ 1993 Profiles and predictors of assaultiveness for different psychiatric ward populations. American Journal of Psychiatry 150: 1368–1373

Morrison EF 1990 Violent psychiatric in-patients in a public hospital. Scholarly Inquiry for Nursing Practice 4(1): 65–82

Morrison EF 1994 The evolution of a concept: aggression and violence in psychiatric settings. Archives of Psychiatric Nursing 8: 245–253

National Audit Office 1996 Health and safety in NHS acute hospital trusts in England. National Audit Office, London

NHS Executive 1997 NHS health and safety issues. HSG(97)6. Department of Health, Wetherby

Nijman HLI, Muris P, Merckelbach HLGJ et al 1999 The staff observation aggression scale – revised (SOAS-R). Aggressive Behavior 25: 197–209

Noble P, Rodger S 1989 Violence by psychiatric in-patients. British Journal of Psychiatry 155: 384–390

Palmstierna T, Wistedt B 1989 Risk factors for aggressive behaviour are of limited value in predicting the violent behaviour of acute involuntarily admitted patients. Acta Psychiatrica Scandinavica 81: 152–155

Palmstierna T, Wistedt B 1987 Staff observation aggression scale, SOAS: presentation and evaluation. Acta Psychiatrica Scandinavica 76: 657–663

Pearson M, Wilmot E, Padi M 1986 A study of violent behaviour among in-patients in a psychiatric hospital. British Journal of Psychiatry 149: 232–235

Powell G, Caan W, Crowe M 1994 What events precede violent incidents in psychiatric hospitals? British Journal of Psychiatry 165: 107–112

Rix G, Seymour D 1988 Violent incidents on a regional secure unit. Journal of Advanced Nursing 13: 746–751

Royal College of Nursing 1998 Dealing with violence against nursing staff: an RCN guide for nurses and managers. Royal College of Nursing, London

Silver JM, Yudofsky SC 1991 The overt aggression scale: overview and guiding principles. Journal of Neuropsychiatry 3(2): 522–529

Steadman HJ, Mulvey EP, Monahan J et al 1998 Violence by people discharged from acute psychiatric in-patient facilities and by others in the same neighborhoods. Archives of General Psychiatry 55: 393–401

Tam E, Engelsmann F, Fugere R 1996 Patterns of violent incidents by patients in a general hospital psychiatric facility. Psychiatric Services 47: 86–88

Tanke ED, Yesavage JA 1985 Characteristics of assaultative patients who do and do not provide visible clues of potential violence. American Journal of Psychiatry 142(12): 1409–1413

Tardiff K, Sweillam A 1979 Age and assaultative behaviour in mental patients. Hospital and Community Psychiatry 30: 709–711

Walker Z, Seifert R 1994 Violent incidents in a psychiatric intensive care unit. British Journal of Psychiatry 164: 826–828

Way BB, Braff JL, Hafemeister TL, Banks SM 1992 The relationship between patient–staff ratio and reported patient incidents. Hospital and Community Psychiatry 43: 361–365

Whittington R, Patterson P 1996 Verbal and non-verbal behaviour immediately prior to aggression by mentally disordered people: enhancing the assessment of risk. Journal of Psychiatric and Mental Health Nursing 3: 47–54

FURTHER READING

Gray R, Thomas B 1998 Violent behaviour and locked wards: a review of the effects on patients. Mental Health Care 1(12): 410–411

Kemshall H, Pritchard J (eds) 1999 Good practice in working with violence. Jessica Kingsley, London

Kho K, Sensky T, Mortimer A, Corcos C 1998 Prospective study into factors associated with aggressive incidents in psychiatric acute admission wards. British Journal of Psychiatry 172: 38–43

Nijman HLI, Muris P, Merckelbach HLGJ et al 1999 The staff observation aggression scale – revised (SOAS-R). Aggressive Behavior 25: 197–209

Powell G, Caan W, Crowe M 1994 What events precede violent incidents in psychiatric hospitals? British Journal of Psychiatry 165: 107–112

Rasmussen K, Levander S 1996 Individual rather than situational characteristics predict violence in a maximum security hospital. Journal of Interpersonal Violence 11(3): 376–390

Royal College of Nursing 1998 Dealing with violence against nursing staff: an RCN guide for nurses and managers. Royal College of Nursing, London

Royal College of Psychiatrists 1998 Management of imminent violence: clinical practice guidelines to support mental health services. Royal College of Psychiatrists, London

Wykes T (ed) 1994 Violence and health care professions. Chapman and Hall, London

11

Involving services users

Nicola Lees   Jeff Withington

INTRODUCTION

The involvement of service users with serious mental illness in individualized care, as well as in planning and implementation of services, must be one of the most important issues of this edition. Without a successful range of methods to engage service users and their representative bodies, forensic mental health services cannot move forward effectively. It is not possible, however, for user involvement, patient advocacy and patient councils to exist in isolation; they are concepts that require thought, awareness and a rethink in attitude. The concepts should not be seen as a threat but embraced as a partner. User involvement is here to stay and is growing, in all areas of mental health, including forensic.

There already exists a substantial movement which, on behalf of users of mental health services, has achieved extraordinary success in empowering them in redressing the imbalance of power that has existed from the time mental health became a medical concern.

This chapter will put forward the issues of user involvement so that the reader can formulate their own opinions about the need for service user involvement, advocacy services and patient councils. Explanations as to why user involvement is necessary may either confirm your understanding of the concept of involvement and people's rights or at times seem controversial and argumentative. This chapter will also discuss and demonstrate by example the good practice that has been developed over many years, to bring about the changes that will eventually produce a reduction in the pervading stigma associated with mental health.

DISEMPOWERMENT OF

SERVICE USERS

Empowerment is a term frequently used within mental health-care settings today. It is applied to a wide variety of issues: the black power movement (Davis 1988, Minkler & Cox 1980); gay rights

(Minkler & Cox 1980); powerlessness and oppression in women (Edwards 1997); and empowerment of people with AIDS (Haney 1988, Kirp & Epstein 1989).

Within health-care settings managers appear to have satisfied themselves that empowerment is achieved by delegating decision making and involvement to those further down the hierarchy. The empowerment of users, however, appears to be perceived as a totally separate issue, which on the surface appears superficial. Issues of user involvement and empowerment are readily identified within information booklets, operational policies and service and resource plans, many believing that this seriously addresses the issue in a meaningful way. Many would be found guilty of this and whilst wishing to radically change our inclusion philosophies, few have truly succeeded.

There are no quick-fix solutions. It is a lengthy process of attitude and cultural change requiring personal reflection and a compulsion to reverse the balance of power. Few professionals are truly able to do this without feeling that their own professional standing would be compromised.

For John (see Box 11.1) and many like him, institutions have been their only home, compelled by society to reside there because it was felt to be in their best interests. Whilst the 1980s saw a shift in models of care from institution to community, those in secure conditions were left with the traditional power imbalance between patients and those described as their carers. Empowerment is better understood by its absence when individuals feel hopeless, oppressed, powerless or dependent (Hegar & Manzeker 1988); it is viewed as a continuum rather than in absolute terms. It is concerned with power and control and its effect upon people's lives (Webb & Tossell 1991).

Those who come into contact with forensic mental health services are particularly susceptible to the effects of disempowerment and vulnerability. The majority of individuals will have been in contact with the criminal justice system, often resulting in some type of conviction. Many will be placed on a section of the Mental Health Act 1983 and could be subject to a restriction order, the sex offender register or supervised discharge. The motivation behind many of these is purposefully to restrict, contain and deny an individual's liberty and in many instances deny involvement in care and treatment (see Box 11.2). Many are labelled by society as both 'mad' and 'bad'.

Madness carries far greater stigma than simple criminality; society fears people who are unpredictable or incomprehensible far more than those who are simply dishonest career villains. It is understandable that society should demand to be protected from the risk of recurrence of a violent or sexual offence but at present society's response to even modest degrees of risk tends to be overtly repressive and restrictive (Murphy 1991).

Box 11.1   Case study – John

John is 55 years old. He currently resides in a medium secure unit in the north of England. He has been receiving care and treatment there since his transfer from the high security services 6 years ago. John has spent much of his adult life in institutional care, after an unprovoked assault on his mother in the 1970s, which left her paralysed from the waist down. His family visit periodically. John describes his relationship with his family as predominantly unsupportive, his sister believing that he should remain in institutional care for the rest of his life. In truth, they still remain afraid of John. Whilst John's clinical team agree that the ideal model of care for him would be based around the concept of long-term medium security, nothing exists locally, or indeed nationally, which would fulfil his needs. John therefore remains in a care environment that neither meets his needs nor conforms to the principles of treating people in the lowest level of security possible. John sits and waits for the development of appropriate services, his only active advocate being his solicitor, who campaigns for him at the highest levels for appropriate service provision.

Box 11.2 Case study – Katie

Katie, 48 years old, was discharged from a medium secure unit on a Mental Health Act 1983 section 41 restriction order 12 months ago. The conditions of her restriction order are that she receives social supervision from her social worker, including weekly visits, and that she resides in a named hostel. Katie has recently met a man and would like to move into his flat with him. The community team responsible believe that this relationship is not in her best interests, because they both indulge in excessive bouts of alcohol intake. The team are unsupportive in Katie's regular pleas to be transferred from the hostel. Katie feels that this is contributing to her feelings of frustration and anger which culminate in regular verbal outbursts to others within the hostel. As a result Katie's boyfriend has been banned from visiting the hostel until Katie is better able to control her temper. The situation has escalated to the point where Katie is perceived by others to be a risk in relation to her angry outbursts and the clinical team are considering contacting the Home Office about the possibility of formally recalling her. Katie feels helpless and powerless to do anything in this situation, resulting in feelings of oppression and a sense of lack of purpose. In reality, whether the care team are justified or not in their plans, they have disempowered and disabled Katie's ability to have any influence and control over her own destiny. The balance of power is tipped truly in favour of the carers.

Traditionally, professionals have exerted dominance and power over those individuals within their care, creating the 'we know best' culture. The key task placed before professionals and clinical teams today is not only to empower individuals but to facilitate the empowerment of cultures and environments. Whilst this philosophy is nationally recognized and driven by organizations, many are unwittingly disempowering their staff and in turn inhibiting the empowerment of patients.

HISTORY OF THE USER MOVEMENT

The user movement began as early as 1620 with 'the petition of the poor distracted people in the house of Bedlam' and 'the Alleged Lunatics Friend Society' in the 1980s (Read & Wallcraft 1992).

The 1960s and 1970s saw the beginning of the anti-psychiatry movement, inspired by the work of people such as Ronald Laing and Thomas Szasz who criticized the concept of 'mental illness', suggesting its foundations were in moral and social judgements with no scientific validity (Read & Wallcraft 1992).

The move towards community care in the 1980s gave rise to the rundown of the traditional asylum concept and the closure of large psychiatric institutions began to accelerate. The planning and development of new services enabled health-care workers and service planners, for the first time, to consult in a limited but meaningful way those who would use the services. The mid 1980s saw the emergence of a plethora of user organizations, self-help groups and advocacy schemes. Organizations began to pay more than lip service to involving users in every sphere of health-care delivery. The imbalance of power began to be redressed.

In 1990, the United Kingdom Advocacy Network (UKAN) was established, whose purpose was to develop group self-advocacy, through patient councils, peer advocacy schemes and working directly with individuals and support groups. A number of these are currently involved in the planning, development, monitoring and running of mental health services. Funders of UKAN include the Sainsbury Centre for Mental Health Development and the Mental Health Foundation.

Hundreds of organizations exist today to represent and advise people from all ethnic backgrounds, genders, ages and sexual orientations.

Many organizations focus around the specific needs of service users; for example, the Afro-Caribbean mental health projects, Women In Secure Hospitals (WISH), National Schizophrenia Fellowship, MIND and Survivors Speak Out.

More recently, a number of citizens' advice bureaux (CAB) and community health councils have also taken on the role of advocate or provide management contracts for advocacy schemes. Users themselves have been facilitated to form self-help groups, peer advocacy schemes and schemes in institutional settings, such as patient councils.

As the user movement has evolved, the expectation placed upon professionals to include the contribution of users in the development and running of services has increased. The consumerism culture that has developed has been driven at governmental level, with the importance of considering the views of service users further reinforced within policy development (DoH 1991, 1994).

CONTROLLING BEHAVIOUR AND STIGMATIZATION

The need for service user involvement is clear and essential in all mental health services, from the shared community care of the care programme approach to the inherent restrictions that can be found in the forensic mental health services. The same philosophy can be used in every area; the greater the involvement, the greater the response and the better the outcome for the patient. Rae (1993) indicates 'There must be absolute commitment to patient–staff collaboration. Patients' voices must be heard, their opinions sought, their concerns and problems listened to…'.

History shows that mental health was seen as something to be controlled and, indeed, a hundred years ago control was one of the few interventions available. The need to control still exists today and this is dependent on the level of risk presented by the patient.

In expounding the theories of spatial organization, Prior (1988) explains how the early asylums were designed and that madness necessitated a special architecture. Prior developed the theory of the sociology of space which exists as a direct result of architectural design and suggested that present-day hospital buildings for psychiatry were inextricably linked with the birth of psychiatry and the involvement of the medical discipline in madness.

The study of alterations of elements of hospital and ward design can thus reveal changing objects of medical attention or disclose innumerable principles concerning the conceptualization of disease and illness. Prior (1988) outlines that space and sociology are inseparable and links this with institutional life and how space should be viewed as not just 'out there' but as a form of social interaction or discourse.

Drinkwater (1982) puts forward ideas about control by describing 'the social learning theory of aggression' and suggests that 'aggressive behaviour is similar to all other types of behaviour, and, therefore, can be environmentally controlled'. The literature therefore shows that buildings were designed with the specific purpose of controlling individuals with mental health problems. Control means a loss of autonomy for the individual. By exerting control from the moment someone enters a mental health building, the controlling effect puts the patient at a disadvantage; it reduces the notion of equal respect and the general recognition that the patient has the capacity to determine their own destiny (Beauchamp & Childress 1994).

One of the most disempowering issues that surrounds mental health is that once someone becomes a service user, they are different. That is, they have become outwardly different in some way. When someone has an outward difference which appears unusual or bad, society often stigmatizes them to explain the inferiority and account for the danger presented. Therefore, for a psychiatric patient, the illness or the treatment they receive may result in an outward difference and in them being stigmatized. Once stigmatized, they are often made to fit into one of a limited number of stereotypes and effectively sidelined by society (Byrne 1997).

It can be asked whether this is the fault of the service user or of those who recognize the difference and act unjustly towards them. Is this a form of social exclusion or unwitting prejudice? Maybe the individual begins to see themselves as different, a process of self-stigmatization (Gallo 1994), as they become isolated from society because of unemployment, media castigation or personal stressors.

In a survey undertaken by Read & Baker (1996) of 778 MINDLink members, it was reported that in relation to their mental illness, 47% had been abused or harassed in public. Of these, 14% had been subjected to physical assault, 34% had been sacked or forced to resign from employment and 26% had moved home because of harassment. It has been suggested that stigma or negative attitudes are a result of the general public's lack of knowledge and that the general public will have a significant bearing on the success of initiatives, such as care in the community (Wolff et al 1996). Indeed, the evidence is overwhelming that the general public maintains a state of fear about mental illness that results in social exclusion and that the need for control of the individual by hospitalization outweighs the possibilities of adopting a more tolerant attitude towards the mentally ill (Byrne 1997, Richards 1982, Sayce 1998, Taylor & Dear 1981, Wilcocks 1968, Wolff et al 1996).

How prevalent are negative attitudes towards the mentally ill in mental health workers? It could be argued that, if negative attitudes did not exist within professional groups, then there would be no need for advocacy, user involvement or patient councils. But as the previous passages have described, present-day mental health workers have inherited systems of social and environmental control and the negative attitudes associated with the labelling of people who show an outward difference.

A gap exists between patients and health professionals which stems from the validity ascribed by professionals to the views of patients, especially in the process of satisfaction with services. The problem is similar in general health care but even greater in mental health (Williams & Wilkinson 1995). It surrounds the assumption that those with mental disorder are less able to accurately evaluate the services they receive. This view is supported by Trivedi (1996) who

advocates working in partnerships with patients and not seeing them as adversaries. Effective partnership essentially involves changes in attitudes on both sides, as well as a change in cultural norms.

An example to highlight this can be taken from the issue of consent, in relation to how much information is supplied to patients to enable them to make valid choices about their medication (Withington & Renoden 1997). Studies show that improvements could be made in this area and that patients will become more active and responsible partners in treatment if they are provided with education and information about the drugs they take (Goldman & Quinn 1988). People don't feel it is their place to question or they are too frightened to ask about the medication they are taking or to question what is being put into their bodies by depot injection. Sometimes they don't question because of fear of the psychiatrist's response (Withington & Renoden 1997). Tempier (1996) points out the legal necessity for patients to have information about their medication, so that they are able to give informed consent. However, Gilbert (1995) notes that the vast array of information produced by statutory agencies and pharmaceutical companies includes very few examples of reliable or unbiased reports which summarize the current state of knowledge about risks and benefits of treatment options, to assist patients in making informed choices.

The Code of Practice for the Mental Health Act 1983 (DoH & Welsh Office 1999) offers guidance on how consent should be obtained from all patients, both informal or detained. It is unclear to what extent mental health workers uphold this right or provide information for patients on a range of issues that is easily read and understood (Withington & Renoden 1997).

The issue of control is not necessarily a deliberate exclusion of people with mental health needs. The vast majority of professionals have been unwitting contributors to stigma and although mental health services have gone through massive changes in the past 30 years, mental health workers are still subject to, and confronted by, disturbed behaviour and therefore reluctant to cast off the security given by their professional status. They are not truly engaging in partnerships with users, arguing that those with communication problems or in a state of distress are unsuitable for collaborative relationships.

There are lessons to be learnt from all walks of life and philosophies, which may explain the situation. The most recent analogy can be taken from the Macpherson Report into the death of Stephen Lawrence (DoH 1999a). Sir William Macpherson was extremely brave in his statements about the Metropolitan Police Service, when he referred to institutional racism. He suggested that:

Institutional racism consists of the collective failure of an organization to provide an appropriate and professional service to people because of their colour, culture or ethnic origin. It can be seen or detected in processes, attitudes and behaviour which amount to discrimination through unwitting prejudice, ignorance, thoughtlessness, and racist stereotyping which disadvantage minority ethnic people. (DoH 1999a: ch 6 para 6.34)

He further stated that 'It is incumbent upon every institution to examine their policies and practices to guard against disadvantaging any section of our communities' (DoH 1999a: ch 6, para 46.27).

These statements are offered as points of debate. If the words 'colour, culture and ethnic origin' were replaced by 'mental health', the issue would still be the same and extremely pertinent. The debate about unwitting prejudice, ignorance and thoughtlessness is one that should be ongoing within forensic mental health services.

Does unwitting prejudice exist within forensic mental health care? For example, a decision may be made by a forensic mental health worker not to supply a patient with a piece of information or to omit certain items from an explanation. Often the decision has been made, on the patient's behalf, that they do not need to know or are not capable of understanding. Surely, as well meaning as this action may be, this person has been discriminated against or singled out as different. Therefore, one might say that this person has been subject to unwitting prejudice. If a patient does not understand about their illness or their

medication, because a health worker has not ensured that they understand, surely this thoughtlessness, unwitting as it may be, has prejudiced this person's treatment?

Under part 4 of the Mental Health Act 1983, the law lays down the right of an individual to give consent to treatment; to go through a process where the treatment, its nature, effects, side effects and alternatives are explained and an opinion is supplied as to their ability to understand. The law also ensures, under section 132, that explanations should continue to be discussed in an endeavour to help the person understand. Indeed, statements have to be made on whether they do or do not understand. One wonders how much effort is made to ensure that an informally admitted patient or a patient in the community is afforded that same right.

Pugh & Eastwood (1997), in a study of attitudes to and knowledge about their depot injection, found that patients were unaware of their rights. Box 11.3 provides a case study to provoke thought in relation to this matter.

Box 11.3   Case study – Thomas

Thomas, recently diagnosed as suffering from mental health problems, was placed on section 3 of the Mental Health Act 1983. He approached the advocacy project for advice regarding both diagnosis and medication. He had recently been admitted and was very confused as to what a diagnosis of schizophrenia entailed and the purpose and side effects to continuing medication. He was also unsure as to what section 3 meant. The advocate explained his rights under the Mental Health Act 1983 and its purpose, i.e. duration, appeal. In addition, information literature was provided regarding the diagnosis and possible medications, including potential side effects. Thomas disagreed with the diagnosis and after discussion with the consultant in the ward round, the advocacy project assisted him in an application to a tribunal and subsequent choice of solicitor who would represent him.

USER INVOLVEMENT

It has been suggested that the two most stressful events in life are getting married and moving house (Ryan 1999). Many of us experience this in our lives and can recall the stress that such occasions bring. Many of us will be able to recall major life events, clearly and graphically, that demonstrate the experience of some form of posttraumatic stress. For some of us, this will have been extended into posttraumatic stress disorder (PTSD).

Imagine having to go into hospital because of the stress caused by this major life event, which manifests itself as a psychotic episode or depression. What if during your stay in hospital you found that the admitting nurse did not have time to listen to your attempts to explain why you had come into hospital and that you didn't think you should really be there. The nurse was under a lot of pressure. There were numerous interruptions and they did not seem very sympathetic. The doctors did not explain the treatment clearly. No one could tell you when you were going to go home. Your children were distressed at leaving you in this strange environment; all they want is for you to go home with them. They scream and cry for you as your partner drags them off to the car at the end of visiting. The medication makes you feel drowsy and you can't think straight. You begin to put on weight due to the medication, which no one told you might happen. You feel uncomfortable, have no energy, can't sleep at night because of the noise in the corridors and doors banging. Someone is bothering you constantly for cigarettes every day, even though you don't smoke. There was a fight in the day room which frightened you and you are now scared to come out of your room in case that odd-looking chap, who keeps swearing and shouting, attacks you.

When you get a chance to speak to the doctor you go into the room and there are 15 people in there. You know only the ward nurse and the doctor who saw you on admission. The man you believe to be the consultant asks you a range of questions, which means you have to make personal disclosures about yourself in front of a room full of strangers. You feel obliged to talk because you feel you might get home quicker. What you really want to do is to run out and hide but you know this will not help. The doctor ends by telling you something about your treatment, to which you nod and say 'thank you' and leave the room trying not to break into a run. You have not understood a word he said.

Does any of this sound familiar? Is it possible that if you did not have PTSD before you went into hospital, you certainly might have now? A recent study by Morrison et al (1999) found that 44% of the patient sample developed PTSD symptoms as a result of a psychiatric admission. One of the contributory factors in the report is that hospitalization and treatment involve a global loss of control for the individual. Is it any wonder that the user movement has grown over the years and that so many user groups are active throughout the country, attempting to improve the experience of treatments, based upon their experience of the past?

There are four main levels at which service users function well and have developed expertise.

1. Strategic involvement: the decision-making processes that change and develop services now and for the future.
2. Individual care planning involvement: when a patient should have all the relevant information about treatment and outcomes.
3. Training: service users need to get involved in moulding the staff of the future, to ensure that attitudes change and this unwitting thoughtlessness disappears.
4. Representation, canvassing of opinion and feedback of information.

There is a phrase often used by mental health workers that can be viewed as a way of trying to diminish the opinion or dissatisfaction expressed by a service user representative. It is a statement used to maintain the status quo in keeping the mental health service user in their place, as a patient. 'I don't think that they (the service user) are truly representative of the patient group.'

What does this mean? Does it mean they are not ill enough? Or that they have not been in hospital for long enough? Or does it mean that now they are recovered, they do not qualify? Or they have the wrong illness? Surely if someone has had experience of mainstream services, i.e. being in hospital, they are qualified to comment and represent others? Although it could be asked what this representation actually means. The user groups that we have worked with collect information on issues from service users that health professionals would never obtain. They distribute information and hold conferences and workshops to gain opinions on new approaches and then take that information back to the mental health forums. Surely, this is as representative as you can get!

What of the representatives? Patients often get involved in user representation because they have a cause of their own to pursue and when this is seen through, the interest goes away. However, there are those special few who believe in the cause and, despite mental ill health, are prepared to try to compete with the well-versed professionals, challenge views and opinions and relate unique experiences. Our experiences of joint presentations with service users at major national conferences and local mental health forums, on issues such as disability allowance, medication information for patients, the care programme approach and staff induction programmes, have never ceased to amaze us. These special people will stand up in front of a crowd of professionals, which can range from anything from a dozen to 100 or 200 strong. Yet they bare their soul, revealing the most intimate details which on occasions reduces them to tears, to try to get people to listen and act to make things better for others in the name of user involvement. It takes a special person to do that.

Sir William Macpherson proposed that attitudes can lead to behaviour which brings about discrimination (DoH 1999a). Attitude is always going to be one of the hardest dispositions to overcome, especially in an environment that has been set up to contain people who may have committed hideous crimes, as a result of disorder of personality or severity of mental illness.

The involvement of service users in the interview process, mainly of nursing staff at present, is an issue that is producing heated debate and bringing attitudes to the forefront which contradict moral values. This form of debate should continue, for without the debate we cannot go forward. However, the debate must be tackled from a considered position and not from one of prejudice, unwitting or otherwise. For example, the suggestion that service users should interview prospective nursing staff in a forensic environment was put forward for debate at the Royal College of Nursing forensic community psychiatric nurses forum in 1998. The debate unfortunately produced a motion that contained prejudice, naiveté and accusations of populist politically correct thinking and, therefore, supported a misguided attack on user empowerment.

Thus, it appears that the rules of service user engagement which Perkins (1996) suggests are clear.

◆ User involvement must not mean fitting users into existing staff agendas and structures, but the development of user-generated agendas and structures.
◆ Involving service users is a process, not a one-off exercise. Building up trust involves a long-term commitment and is a development in its own right, requiring dedicated worker time and funds.
◆ Users are not a uniform group: the diversity of opinions, experience, backgrounds and interests present amongst users can be enormously valuable.
◆ If user involvement is to be effective there must be constituencies of users who can be consulted – patient councils, users, forums – rather than a token user on existing committees.
◆ Users' forums should be properly funded. We cannot expect users to help develop mental health services without paying for it.
◆ Users' forums should be independent of mental health service staff control, but at the same time properly supported and resourced.
◆ Mechanisms for involving service users must recognize and accommodate the specific problems and disabilities that users may have.
◆ Service users must not be excluded because they cannot meet the demands of the situation

themselves. If nothing ever happens when you express your opinions, you will quickly give up doing so.

◆ Users' forums must have access to high-level support within the organization. Mental health service users are a devalued group and are unlikely to be taken seriously without the backing of the upper echelons.

◆ There already exist independent user organizations and user trainers with a wealth of experience that can be tapped.

◆ All service users should have easy access to independent support, advice and, where necessary, advocacy from someone who understands their situation. This should be a properly funded service.

User groups and individuals nationally have developed many initiatives which are extremely successful, such as crisis cards, direct power, Avon self-assessment, telephone helplines and advocacy. The range of initiatives can be adapted for use in all mental health services, from community to secure environments.

For example, the Avon self-assessment (Avon mental health measure) has been developed by MIND for people using services in the community or in the wider adult acute mental health services. It allows them to collect information about themselves and build a profile of their needs and ability to cope at different times, in response to different events of everyday living. The user is able to express their unusual thoughts and experiences, their mood swings or obsessive thoughts and show how these affect their abilities to cope with life. It allows them to explain their tolerance to treatments and to state which treatments they consider to be the most effective. This form of self-assessment could benefit people not only in the community but in forensic settings and would help to nurture an involvement in the care process.

To a lesser extent direct power would assist users to develop their own care plans and support networks but this would require more adaptation than the Avon for forensic patients.

As can be seen, the resource to help patients achieve self-determination in the care process does exist. Moreover, it is impossible for the user movement to work in isolation. Indeed, many of the major mental health-related organizations have recognized the need to develop partnerships and philosophies of working with users. These include the production of documents that encourage the move towards user involvement. Examples include:

◆ *Patient partnerships: building a collaborative strategy* (NHSE 1996)
◆ *Pulling together* (Sainsbury Centre for Mental Health 1997).

Each of the above documents recommends good practice for user involvement and they are excellent. Further, there are examples throughout the UK of involvement at all levels in mental health.

However, is there a need to take the good practice still further, by establishing legislation to make discrimination against people with mental illness an offence? The legislative models for this already exist in equal opportunities law. Should individuals who are discriminated against because of mental health problems be protected by the Disability Discrimination Act 1995? Sulek (1999) has already written about a case that was tested under this and although the employment appeal tribunal found in favour of the individual, the tribunal declared that the individual's mental health problem did not constitute a disability. His illness, although having a clinical diagnosis, had not been a long-term one. It is therefore possible that some people may be able to take recourse through the Disability Discrimination Act 1995.

Is there a need for an equal rights commission to uphold the rights of people with mental health problems, to improve the situation for those who are trapped by poverty, unemployment, poor housing and discrimination by local communities? Aside from legislation, which is unlikely, partnership and the user movement are very necessary.

ADVOCACY

The concept of advocacy has been well recorded and the literature available is vast and varied. The United Kingdom Advocacy Network (1994) has produced a code of practice for advocacy, the basic premise being that mental health workers must listen to, and work with, mental health service users. Further, they must acknowledge the user's understanding of what works well for them and what does not and allow them to make informed choices as a result of having an independent source of information, ensuring rights and dignity are protected at all times.

Based on this widely accepted and now well-established postulation, it is still surprising that advocacy has not yet become an intrinsic part of the mental health system. Mental health advocacy services have come a long way in the past few years, working as intermediaries and enabling communication and effective dialogue between service users, professionals and others. It is well developed in pockets of excellence, not least in the high security services. However, despite its recognition it is not as powerful as could be expected.

Advocacy is still fraught with many problems, especially in relation to adequate funding being made available. Projects usually have single paid workers and some volunteers, making isolation a major issue. Stress and solitary working practices create dilemmas, affecting the ability to empower patients.

Very little has been done to explore the effectiveness of advocacy. There are a few examples of evaluation by notable people or organizations but it is questionable whether expertise has been developed. Therefore, advocacy itself and academia need to work in partnership to evaluate developments and effectiveness. The expectation is that by now a national advocacy organization should have been formed to draw together natural allies; providing advocacy and establishing the organization; gaining credibility through consistency of working; campaigning for local and governmental recognition – something UKAN, CAB and MIND have not yet achieved.

One of the main influences in the success or failure of advocacy is the attitude that mental health workers show towards it. It is suggested that the opportunity to explore the ethical and moral issues which surround advocacy should be taken. Moreover, this should examine the issues which mental health workers find difficult. For instance, just when the mental health worker thinks they are doing everything they can for a patient, which they believe is in the patient's best interests and which is based on an acceptable body of knowledge and good practice, someone comes along and says 'Hey, that is not really what the patient wants'! Mental health workers then have to reexamine their stance. Are they going to listen to the advocate when affronted by this approach? Is it seen as confrontational? Is it constructive?

A criticism which is consistently found in many reports produced by advocacy workers and services is the lack of referrals to advocacy by professionals. It could be expected that nurses, in particular, would be able to grasp and engage with the concept of advocacy quite easily, recognizing the similarities of the patients' struggle for autonomy and their (the nurses) continual fight for their own autonomy, accountability and independence from the medical model and to be recognized as professionals in their own right. However, this is not always the case.

Trandel-Korenchuk & Trandel-Korenchuk (1983) provide examples of the inequalities in the nurse–physician relationship, of the social, economic and educational differences and the class bias that has created the need for nurses to become independent and autonomous, and suggest the relationship between power and authority should be explored.

Trandel-Korenchuk & Trandel-Korenchuk (1983) intimate that if the authority a doctor holds exceeds its limits, the nurse must question whether to obey. It is also suggested that, whilst it seems obvious that the word of an expert in a position of authority should be taken for granted, should that person in authority be able to make decisions for other people?

A parallel can be drawn between the nurse–patient relationship and the doctor–patient relationship. Is a doctor or a nurse more virtuous or knowledgeable about ethics than the patient? Should the nurse or doctor make decisions independently of the patient? Or is it that when goals are shared by the person in authority with the people they command, the authority is validated by the shared goals (Trandel-Korenchuk & Trandel-Korenchuk 1983).

Good practice might involve the mental health worker, when considering patient care, saying to themselves, 'I may have the knowledge and the ability, but just to ensure that I have not forgotten or overlooked anything, I will involve the advocate and we can all sit down and discuss the treatment together to arrive at a solution'. The referral to advocacy does not mean that the mental health worker is wrong; on the contrary, the involvement of advocacy lends more power to the therapeutic approach. It shows that the mental health worker is able to establish a credible plan of care, through confidence in their ability to deliver effective treatment that can be supported by current knowledge and relevant practice. Contact with advocacy should be actively encouraged to ensure that the user's needs and interests are known; that service provision is directed to meet the expressed need; that communication improves; and that mental health workers and users work together gradually to increase the effectiveness of services (Trivedi 1996).

Advocacy is often seen as a threat by mental health workers, as well as a source of stress and pressure for those workers in more intense settings, such as acute inpatient, medium secure and high security hospitals. In many cases mental health workers are under threat of criticism and, as we find from the Department of Health (1999b), let down by the system, unsupported, working within unclear boundaries and blurred parameters. The question still remains: how do you maintain therapeutic optimism and keep staff interested when you are working with people who will never go anywhere, because of the political imperatives or the dangerousness (Jackson 1999)?

The answer to Jackson's question is even more difficult to formulate but an important element of that answer, which will always feature in a huge range of approaches, must be user involvement and advocacy. Indeed, it would appear that the need for advocacy is greater in secure environments, not just from a political point of view but also because of patients' needs to make a meaningful contribution. Ashworth Hospital Authority Citizens' Advice Bureau (1996) stated this quite clearly: that it should be each patient's basic right to understand the reasons for a particular

course of action, and in some way feel confident that their views have been heard through participation in a two-way process of communication, whatever the final outcome.

The establishment of good practice through the use of advocacy is important in all areas of mental health and is comparable with the principles of user involvement. Rae (1993) recommended that advocacy, in all its forms, should be established in Ashworth Hospital, with each approach being just as important as the next.

The inherent danger in mental health is to regard people as being incapable due to their illness. This view is traditionally held by the general public and has been difficult to eradicate from some mental health workers. It seems that workers regard suggestions from patients about their own care as insulting to them or undermining their professionalism. The assumption that advocacy is required in health care implies that the process of becoming a patient results in a reduction of autonomy and that the patient's rights or interests may not be respected. Therefore, the assumption must be that the system or delivery of health care is wrong (Willard 1996).

If this is accepted as fact, then there are only two ways forward: one is time and the other is legislation to help make up the time and establish the practice of advocacy, leading to autonomy as an individual's legal right. The Mental Health Act 1983 went some way towards this by ensuring that people's civil rights are upheld. Many consider that the Mental Health Act 1983 did not go far enough and that a new Act should concentrate more on such issues, by embracing the concept of people's rights and advocacy with confidence and incorporating referral to advocacy for all patients who are sectioned, prescribed ECT or placed on supervised discharge. The issue of consent to treatment is a prime example. If a judgement is made by a medical doctor that a person is incapable of understanding the treatment proposed, a second opinion is sought from another medical doctor. This second doctor has the same training, same knowledge base and ultimately draws the same conclusion. Based on the practice of psychiatry that exists now this may be correct, but where does the patient come into this?

What independent view or support does the patient receive at this time? Is enough time spent with the patient to allow them to understand or make a decision?

The Mental Health Act 1983 is implemented for the few rather than the many, although the principles within the Act need to be maintained for all mental health patients. Civil rights issues clearly exist for service users, as they are at risk of having their viewpoint discounted on the grounds that their illness automatically means that they 'lack insight'. This issue is not new; having the capacity to make decisions is an ongoing debate within mental health care. The Code of Practice (DoH & Welsh Office 1999: para 15.10) defines clearly the basic principles of capacity to make treatment decisions. The Law Commission (1991) outlines that the presumption should always be that 'a person is capable until proved otherwise, and capacity is judged in relation to the particular decision, transaction or activity involved'. The need is for the person to understand rather than have wisdom. The test of competence, therefore, depends on a three-stage criterion.

◆ Understanding and remembering essential information about treatment.
◆ Believing essential information about treatment.
◆ Weighing it in the balance of alternatives to arrive at a choice.

Some of the advocacy and patient empowerment publications question the whole concept of empowerment, believing that unless mental health workers are empowered, patients will never be empowered. This may be so but a contrary argument may be that mental health workers already have the power and need to share it to form partnerships. However, 'power suggests corruption, power is vulgar, and without power there is no need for empowerment' (Jenkins 1997). Gibson (1991) maintained that this position can be reversed by a social process of recognizing, promoting and developing people's abilities, so that they can be helped to meet their own needs, solve their problems and mobilize the necessary resources to control their own lives.

If mental health workers are to contribute to this process, a clear understanding of the concept of power is necessary. Gibson (1991) argued that without this, mental health workers will merely perpetuate the professional dominance of their predecessors. Trivedi (1996) suggested that the word 'empowerment' may be replaced by the less confusing and more practical concept of enablement. Moreover, people may be enabled, rather than empowered, to take control of their own lives. Traditionally, professionals have enjoyed a dominance over their patients, yet their task is to empower people who have been dependent for most of their lives. Tyne (1994) believed that professionals such as mental health workers, who have traditionally enjoyed exercising power, will not readily curtail this activity. It is something of an illusion to believe that disabled people can become consumers and able to make rational choices and important decisions about their lives.

A particular problem with advocacy is that it developed from the early movements of anti-psychiatry groups. Advocacy therefore still has a long way to go to become an integral part of the mental health scene. Advocacy is well established in its methods and styles of working, through independent professional, peer, citizen and self-advocacy. Unless legislation arrives, linked with a common body of knowledge for advocacy services, based on governmental recognition, it will take longer for integration to develop. In an ideal world there should be no need for advocacy but let us not be fooled; advocacy will need to be around for as long as mental illness and mental health services exist.

In the 21st century, advocacy needs to be incorporated into mental health legislation. There needs to be commitment from government to fund a national advocacy body and time, training and cultural changes within mental health services that must embrace and engage user involvement at all levels and in all types of service, from primary to forensic care. Until there is a commitment to total user involvement and advocacy service, users will continue to suffer through lack of knowledge of their rights and responsibilities and the inability to effectively express their needs.

Box 11.4 raises a number of important questions about acting on someone's behalf. For instance, what if the man had not accepted the advocate's assistance in applying for a tribunal? Should the advocate have applied on his behalf, given that he clearly wanted to leave the hospital? What if he had not been willing to sign the letter written on his behalf? He may not have been willing to sign for any number of reasons unconnected with his need for a tribunal. In this case, could the advocate have applied on his behalf?

These particular questions are to do with issues of detention of the confused and need to be addressed by the Mental Health Act Commission and the Tribunals Office.

When this man became an informal patient and was no longer communicating his views or wishes, the advocate was left with the dilemma of whether to continue to act for him, according to the model of advocacy then in use. However, the absence of instruction left the advocate with no basis for action. With the proposed model outlined, the

---

Box 11.4 Case study – a confused man

A confused man had been admitted to hospital under section 2 of the Mental Health Act 1983. Since admission, he had persistently asked to go home and did not seem able to retain information about how and why he had been detained. He was referred to the advocacy project by ward staff who were concerned about the reasons for detaining this man.

The worker's initial task was to convey something to this man about the function and status of an advocate, i.e. that the worker was not a nurse/doctor/social worker. For people who are finding it difficult to retain information or who have overriding and urgent concerns that make them very anxious, explanations of the concept of advocacy may be more or less incomprehensible or irrelevant and this may of course impede an individual's use of an advocate. With this man, this was indeed the case and it was up to the worker to demonstrate her role in her approach (one of respect and non-judgement, not diagnosing, not having control of resources or treatment options; by the kind of questions asked and general demeanour). Happily this man did appear to grasp some key points about the advocacy service: that the worker could help him do something about leaving the hospital and was taking this desire seriously, that she was 'on his side' and not part of the institution that was detaining him. The advocate explained about the man's right to a tribunal and whilst he was not in a position to grasp precisely the notion of 'tribunal', he could

appreciate in general terms what a tribunal meant: that it could, but by no means would, discharge him; that it was an opportunity to obtain a review of his care and treatment and future options by a group of independent people; and that he could have independent representation to put his case forward. However, to obtain a tribunal, the patient concerned must write a request and send it to the tribunal office, something that this confused man was not able to do.

The advocate then asked the advice of the tribunal office, who stated that asking to go home is tantamount to requesting a tribunal (or that they would take it as a request, as this is not common knowledge or common practice amongst others who can assist someone in asking for a tribunal, such as ward staff). Their advice to the advocate was to write a letter to them and to get the patient to sign it. This was duly done and the man concerned did sign the request. When a tribunal date was set the consultant psychiatrist cancelled the section. As the man was too confused to be allowed to leave the unit unattended (indeed, it would have been a failure of the duty of care on the part of the care team to allow him to leave), his rights as an informal patient were academic and he remained effectively detained. He had now been in hospital for a number of weeks and had withdrawn considerably. He was no longer asking to go home and was not willing to communicate with the advocate.

advocate could then consider representing the wish to go home that the man had articulated earlier and which presumably had not changed. The advocacy worker could also have remained involved with future decision making on his behalf, as the situation meant that the rights of this man, as an informal patient, were subsumed under the unwillingness or inability of services to give him the kind of support he needed to take the risk of leaving. Just because he was no longer saying so, this does not mean that he no longer wanted to go home (Jones 1995). Who else but an independent advocate could work with the patient, on his behalf, to expound his wish to go home?

PATIENT COUNCILS

Patient councils, or clients'/users' councils, are terms used to describe a group of people who either volunteer or are selected by other users within an inpatient or residential service to represent a collection of views. The first patient council to be nationally recognized is believed to have started at Mapperly Hospital in Nottingham in the mid 1980s. By the early 1990s forensic mental health services also began to facilitate their development, with examples being found in high security and medium secure services. Experiences from these schemes, however, found that the more articulate client group, in particular those with personality disorders, tended to be the more prominent and dominant members, whilst those with mental illness and the more vulnerable diagnoses tended to be underrepresented. Nonetheless, patient councils have been successful in achieving alterations in numerous areas of care, from environmental change to policy amendment.

To enable patient councils to function in an effective and meaningful way, managers and clinicians need to consider a number of issues.

◆ A set of mutually agreed guidelines should be developed by managers and the council which clearly identify the communication channels, boundaries and responsibilities of each group.

◆ The ground rules for the functioning of the council should be developed solely by council members.

◆ As a guide, it is suggested that these meetings should occur not less than monthly to ensure continuity and participation in ongoing service issues.

◆ All patients within the service should be made aware of the council and given the opportunity to participate. Representation from all wards and clinical areas should be encouraged.

◆ An adequate room such as a board room or committee room with access to refreshments should be made available. This can be difficult for a number of patients requiring staff escorts for legal and/or issues of risk and special arrangements may need to be made.

◆ Administrative facilities to enable effective functioning and organization of the council need to be considered. These may include access to word-processing facilities, photocopier, telephone and filing cabinet.

◆ A chairperson for the council needs to be identified. He or she can be drawn from group membership or be an independent advocate or support worker. Most councils would liaise with a nominated person from the clinical services who holds a position of influence. This enables views and suggestions of the council to be considered and actioned where appropriate, through local management or clinical groups. In some instances the chairperson of the patient council may hold membership on a management forum.

◆ Notice boards specifically designated for use by the patient council should be available in all clinical areas to enable them to display posters, minutes, information and agendas relevant to the council. The maintenance of these boards is usually the council's responsibility.

◆ Staff should not attend council meetings unless they are invited to talk about specific issues or answer council's questions and queries. Good practice suggests that attendance at these meetings by managers (where invited) can enable quick responses and changes to occur, where appropriate.

◆ Managers and clinicians may request specific items to be placed on agendas, although the agenda should always be set by the council itself.

◆ It may be necessary to provide training to some members of the council, usually by an independent advocate, and this should be facilitated where possible.

◆ Patients may wish to continue their involvement in the patient council after discharge and this should be encouraged and facilitated. The views of this group can often provide additional insight for council members and bring a fresh perspective to relevant issues.

◆ If the clinical service is unable to respond to issues raised by the council, a sound rationale should be provided by those making decisions. It should be remembered that the purpose of the patient council is not to rubber stamp or agree to service suggestions but to influence and shape change in running and planning services.

TRAINING ISSUES FOR SERVICE PROVIDERS AND USERS

To enable the effective and efficient introduction of any user scheme, whether it be a self-help group, an independent advocacy scheme, peer advocacy or a patient council, the preparation of both staff and users is essential. Without this, it is likely that the introduction of the user concept will meet fierce resistance, particularly from those whom the schemes are likely to challenge and criticize. A practicable and pragmatic approach should acknowledge the perceived misconceptions and potential negative attitudes and beliefs that staff may hold when developing the training programme.

Empowering users, either through individual or group advocacy and user schemes, means encouraging and facilitating them to make decisions, a contrast to the traditional expectations placed upon them. Training and development opportunities need to reflect this to enable development of appropriate skills such as: non-verbal and verbal communication; problem-solving techniques; idea generation; and negotiation. Training options for both staff and users need to be carefully thought through.

During the past few years, many people who use or have used services have been successfully involved in training managers, clinicians and other users. A variety of training models exist and have been utilized effectively. Training programmes may include contributions from recognized voluntary and advice groups such as citizens' advice bureaux. Other models may include joint training between professionals, managers and trained advocates. This model often includes looking at source materials, such as mental health law, from diverse perspectives (Royal College of Psychiatrists 1999). Experiential groups facilitated by trained advocates have also proved successful. A number of users also provide training from their own perspectives and experience.

There is no right or wrong training model. The training package must be developed for those it is intended to serve. It must take account of local cultures, policies and guidelines and the philosophy of the organization. Most importantly, any training programme or event must clearly explore and reflect on the beliefs held by those participating. It must challenge attitudes but adopt a sensitive approach to enable the concept of empowerment to be clearly understood.

The Mental Health Task Force (1994) has developed a training pack called *Building on experience*. This is aimed at mental health service users working as trainers, speakers and workshop facilitators. The pack is intended to develop skills to enable more users to build on personal experiences that can be used to enable them to train others.

AVOIDING THE PITFALLS

Anecdotal evidence suggests that there are many pitfalls to be avoided if user involvement is to be developed in a meaningful and effective way.

◆ The development of advocacy schemes and user groups that are not sufficiently financially independent of trust or health organizations. It is essential that funding mechanisms are not dependent upon trusts or individuals within such organizations, whom schemes may wish to challenge or criticize. Where trusts have directly financed schemes, it is appropriate for these funds to be managed by an independent organization, such as CAB or MIND.

◆ The recruitment of any individuals, for example advocates, should not be the responsibility of someone who is employed by the trust, which may compromise the contractual obligations of that individual. There are a number of particular clinical spheres, for example forensic mental health, where input into the recruitment process by skilled and knowledgeable professionals is believed to be essential due to the complex nature of some of the individuals using those services.

◆ The appointment or involvement of those who are not necessarily concerned with the issues but who have personal grievances.

◆ The implementation of user involvement schemes or advocacy services without undertaking training and awareness programmes with staff.

◆ A clear recognition of the level at which the organization is prepared to accept involvement. Is it concerned with specific individual patients' issues or is it concerned with influence at all levels of decision making?

◆ Appropriate support and supervision of those involved to prevent the development of inappropriate intimate relationships with patients.

◆ The recognition of unhelpful organizations which may conflict with appropriate clinical management of individuals.

◆ The appointment of untrained or inexperienced advocates, particularly in difficult areas of mental health such as forensic services.

That was the intention and we hope we succeeded. It is the continuing debate that will move the proposition along.

In order to achieve the formulation of opinion, this chapter has been a little short on definition but lengthy on example and experience. However, it would be useful to end by trying to create not a definition but the meaning of involvement and its related topics covered here, to help continue the debate.

We need to be clear what 'involvement' means. For example, you might find yourself involved in a road accident when you are hit by a number 42 bus. Of course, you did not have any control over this accident or the injuries you sustained, but it happened to you.

Ask yourself what might have been different if:

◆ you had been told that the bus was heading towards you (information supplied)

or

◆ you were asked what you thought of the accident about to happen (consultation took place)

but you were still not able to do anything about it and you were hit by the bus.

This is where empowerment steps into the picture. Involvement means not only having the information along with the opportunity but, most essentially, being able to do something about it. Health and social care provision is one awfully big bus.

CONCLUSION

The mind reflexively interprets other people's words and gestures by doing whatever it takes to make them sensible and true. If the words are sketchy or incongruous, the mind charitably fills in missing premises or shifts to a new frame of reference in which they make sense. (Pinker 1997)

This is the psychological process outlined by Pinker which he names the 'principle of relevance'. In other words, did this chapter make you think? Have you formulated opinions? Did it raise the issues of debate as you read each portion?

REFERENCES

Ashworth Hospital Authority Citizens Advice Bureau 1996 Patients advocacy service report 95/96. Ashworth Hospital Authority, Maghull

Beauchamp TL, Childress JF 1994 Principles of biomedical ethics, 4th edn. Oxford University Press, Oxford

Byrne P 1997 Psychiatric stigma: past, passing and to come. Journal of the Royal Society of Medicine 90(11): 618–621

Davis A 1988 Radical perspectives on the empowerment of Afro-American women: lessons for the 1980's. Harvard Educational Review 58(3): 348–353

Department of Health 1991 The patient's charter. HMSO, London

Department of Health 1994 The health of the nation: key area handbook, mental illness, 2nd edn. HMSO, London

Department of Health 1999a The Stephen Lawrence inquiry: report of an inquiry by Sir William Macpherson of Cluny. Stationery Office, London

Department of Health 1999b The Report of the Committee of Inquiry into the Personality Disorder Unit, Ashworth Special Hospital. Stationery Office, London

Department of Health & Welsh Office 1999 Mental Health Act 1983: code of practice. Stationery Office, London

Drinkwater J 1982 Violence in psychiatric hospitals: developments in the study of criminal behaviour. Wiley, New York

Edwards M 1997 Powerlessness, oppression and women. Mental Health Nursing 17(3): 10–12

Gallo KM 1994 First person account: self stigmatization. Schizophrenia Bulletin 20(2): 407–410

Gibson CH 1991 A concept analysis of empowerment. Journal of Advanced Nursing 16: 354–361

Gilbert H 1995 Choosing treatments: patient empowerment. King's Fund, London

Goldman CR, Quinn FL 1988 Effects of patient education program in the treatment of schizophrenia. Hospital and Community Psychiatry 39(3): 282–286

Haney P 1988 Providing empowerment to the person with AIDS. Social Work 33(3): 251–256

Hegar R, Manzeker IJ 1988 Moving towards empowerment: practice based in public child welfare. Social Work 33(6): 499–502

Jackson C 1999 Sinned against not sinners. Mental Health Care 2(6): 189

Jenkins R 1997 Issues of empowerment for nurses and clients. Nursing Standard 11(46): 44–46

Jones H 1995 MIND in Brighton and Hove: research report. MIND, London

Kirp D, Epstein S 1989 AIDS in America's school houses: learning the hard lessons. Phi Delta Kappan 70(8): 585–593

Law Commission 1991 Mentally incapacitated adults and decision making: an overview. Consultation paper no 119. HMSO, London

Mental Health Task Force 1994 Building on experience. NHS Executive, London

Minkler M, Cox K 1980 Creating critical consciousness in health: applications of Freire's philosophy and methods to the health care setting. International Journal of Health Sciences 10(2): 311–322

Morrison AP, Bowe S, Larkin W, Nothard S 1999 The psychological impact of psychiatric admission: some preliminary findings. Journal of Nervous and Mental Disease 187(4): 250–253

Murphy E 1991 After the asylums: community care for people with mental illness. Faber and Faber, London

NHS Executive 1996 Patient partnerships: building a collaborative strategy. Department of Health, London

Perkins R 1996 Working with mental health service users: effectively managing mental health. Sainsbury Centre for Mental Health, London

Pinker S 1997 How the mind works. Allen Lane, London

Prior L 1988 The architecture of the hospital: a study of spatial organisation and medical knowledge. British Journal of Sociology 39(1): 87–113

Pugh R, Eastwood N 1997 Long term medication in depot clinics and patients' rights: an issue for assertive outreach. Psychiatric Bulletin 21: 273–275

Rae M 1993 Freedom to care. Ashworth Hospital Authority, Maghull

Read J, Baker S 1996 Not just sticks and stones: a survey of stigma, taboos, and discrimination experienced by people with mental health problems. MIND, London

Read J, Wallcraft J 1992 Guidelines for empowering users of mental health services. MIND, London

Richards K 1982 A mind disordered: the public view … lay attitudes towards mental illness. Nursing Mirror 55(15): 55–56

Royal College of Psychiatrists 1999 Patient advocacy. Council report CR7. Royal College of Psychiatrists, London

Ryan A 1999 Managing crisis and risk in mental health nursing. Stanley Thornes, Cheltenham

Sainsbury Centre for Mental Health 1997 Pulling together: the future roles and training of mental health staff. Sainsbury Centre for Mental Health, London

Sayce L 1998 Stigma, discrimination and social exclusion: what's in a word. Journal of Mental Health 7: 331–343

Sulek J 1999 The Disability Discrimination Act 1995: the case of Goodwin v the Patent Office. Open Mind Jan/Feb: 25

Taylor MS, Dear MJ 1981 Scaling community attitudes toward the mentally ill. Schizophrenia Bulletin 7: 225–240

Tempier R 1996 Long term psychiatric patients' knowledge about their medication. Psychiatric Services 47(12): 1385–1387

Trandel-Korenchuk D, Trandel-Korenchuk K 1983 Nursing advocacy of patients' rights: myth or reality? … part 2. American Journal of Primary Health Care 8(4): 37, 40–42

Trivedi P 1996 Partners, not adversaries: planning resources and care in cooperation with users of mental health services. Nursing Times 92(21): 59–60

Tyne A 1994 Taking responsibility and giving power: disability and society practice. NHS Executive, London

United Kingdom Advocacy Network 1994 Advocacy: a code of practice. NHS Executive, London

Webb R, Tossell D 1991 Social issues for carers: a community care perspective. Edward Arnold, London

Wilcocks A 1968 Public attitudes to mental health education (editorial). British Medical Journal 1(5584): 69–70

Willard C 1996 The nurse's role as patient advocate: obligation or imposition? Journal of Advanced Nursing 24: 60–66

Williams B, Wilkinson G 1995 Patient satisfaction in mental health care. British Medical Journal 166: 559–562

Withington J, Renoden M 1997 Sharing medication information with patients. Mental Health Care 1(1): 22–24

Wolff G, Pathare S, Craig T, Leff J 1996 Community knowledge of mental illness and reaction to mentally ill people. British Journal of Psychiatry 168(2): 191–198

FURTHER READING

Edwards M 1997 Powerlessness, oppression and women. Mental Health Nursing 17(3): 10–12

Hatfield B, Huxley P, Hadi M 1992 Accommodation and employment: a survey into the circumstances and expressed needs of users of mental health services in a northern town. British Journal of Social Work 22: 61–73

Kerr G, Gilbert D, Mawhinney S 1997 Advocating advocacy. Open Mind 84: 12–13

Sheldon K 1996 Positive voice for change. Nursing Times 92(20): 63

Thompson P 1999 Meadowbrook advocacy project. Salford Citizens Advice Bureau, Salford

Whitehill I 1996 General reflections. Nursing Times 92(21): 61

Chapter Twelve

Interpersonal relationships: staff development, awareness and monitoring issues

Colin Dale

INTRODUCTION

The concept that mental health practitioners behave in particular ways as a consequence of feelings and attitudes towards individuals and specific groups of patients is nothing new. In her seminal work on interpersonal relationships, Stockwell (1972) introduced the first empirical study into 'the unpopular patient'. Forensic mental health services by their very nature care for these 'unpopular patients', many of whom are vulnerable people who may be emotionally fragile, thought disordered or have relationship difficulties. Furthermore, studies have repeatedly shown that high percentages of forensic populations can be expected to fulfil formal diagnostic criteria for one or more personality disorders (Gunn et al 1991, Maden et al 1995); the very patients who are most difficult to care for and treat. Regardless of patients' formal psychiatric diagnoses, shared psychopathological characteristics exist amongst the population detained in forensic mental health services, which require a consistent response from the health-care professionals managing this group. Milieu therapy has been highlighted as a potential approach which has shown some success in personality-disordered populations (Dolan & Coid 1993) but has been criticized in its application in secure environments (DoH 1999). The feelings, attitudes and behaviour of clinicians risk being compromised by the very nature of interpersonal transactions which are part of their role; therefore safeguards are necessary to protect individual clients, members of staff and the integrity of the organization.

One of the core functions of care and treatment in forensic mental health services is to enable patients to form, maintain and end satisfying personal relationships, in a manner which is meaningful to the individuals concerned and which ensures the safety and security of both parties. Complications which arise when the organization

127

as a whole fails to accommodate the patients' psychopathologies are clear (DoH 1999). Unremitting examples of harrowing, disabling incidents and untoward traumatic events have characterized the care for this group in recent years, as evidenced by a plethora of public enquiries (DoH 1992, 1999).

Nurses' awareness of their own personal needs, reactions to the patient and the effects of this relationship are all necessary in achieving therapeutic relationships with forensic patients (Schafer 1999). The greatest therapeutic impact can be made by nurses, who have more extensive contact with the forensic patients than other health-care professionals. Conversely, they may engage in patterns that replicate pathology-producing situations (Peplau 1989). The goal is not that nurses be perfect but that they be aware of imperfections and capable of exploring them (Schafer 1999).

INTERPERSONAL
RELATIONSHIPS AND
BOUNDARIES

The theory of interpersonal relationships

In her seminal work on psychiatric nursing, Peplau (1952: 16) defined nursing as:

> ... a significant, therapeutic, interpersonal process. It functions cooperatively with other human processes that make health possible for individuals in communities ... Nursing is an educative instrument, a maturing force, that aims to promote forward movement of personality in the direction of creative, constructive, productive, personal and community living.

The interaction between the thoughts, feelings and activities of the patient and those of the nurse lies at the very centre of the nursing process (Peplau 1952, 1989).

Killian & Clark (1996: 102) begin to explore some of the more complex interpersonal issues associated with nursing in forensic services. These authors describe the challenges associated with applying humanistic interventions instead of more mechanistic ones in forensic nursing:

> The exchange of physical boundaries for the security provided by relationships that patients develop with nurses, places a large demand upon nursing staff. They have to provide emotional and practical (physical) containment whilst allowing at the same time, for optimum conditions of therapeutic interaction.

Levinger (1980) describes five stages that relationships pass through.

1. Acquaintance or initial attraction
2. Building up the relationship
3. Consolidation or continuation
4. Deterioration or decline
5. Ending

Levinger suggests that at each of the stages, there may be positive factors which promote the development of the relationship or negative factors that inhibit its development or cause it to fail. Brehm (1992) points out that there is little empirical evidence to support the view of fixed stages in the development of interpersonal relationships. However, there is little dispute that relationships do change and develop and Gross (1996: 384) suggests that, 'It is useful to think of this as involving a beginning, a middle and an end'.

Social exchange theory (Berscheid & Walster 1978, Blau 1964, Homans 1974, Thibaut & Kelley 1959) suggests that people are fundamentally selfish and concerned only with getting as much out of a relationship as possible. However, critics of the theory (e.g. Rubin 1973) argue that humans are capable of altruism as well as selfishness. Certainly, within a forensic environment, care staff are consistently exposed to patients with a psychological presentation, involving a high percentage with personality disorder, either as a primary or secondary diagnosis, where some of the key characteristics involve disrupted and pathological abuse of relationships.

Relationships can be compared by the types of rules that apply generally to them and Argyle & Henderson (1985) describe how the rules of each relationship reflect the nature and type of relationship. Argyle (1994) describes the main types of relationship as:

◆ friends (where satisfaction is derived from common interests and social and emotional support)
◆ love
◆ kinship
◆ workmates.

Of these relationships, the care staff/patient relationship in forensic settings with the long-term nature of contact (an average of eight years in high security services) most closely approximates to that of a work relationship with in some cases an element of friendship. Argyle & Henderson (1985) described rules for co-working which included:

◆ cooperate with physical conditions
◆ help when asked
◆ cooperate despite dislike
◆ don't denigrate to supervisor
◆ ask for help and advice
◆ don't be overinquisitive about private life.

In modern forensic services some staff have struggled to come to terms with this new form of relationship with people who have been kept at a remote distance and dealt with as subhuman, from the descriptions of some services in public inquiries (DoH 1992, Special Hospitals Service Authority 1993). The removal of traditional barriers, such as uniforms, and the insistence on the introduction of modern therapeutic techniques have left some care staff ill equipped to deal with situations where they are forced to interact with articulate and at times disruptive individuals, who will often use systems, such as complaints procedures, in a manipulative way (DoH 1999).

The nature of nursing within forensic services is predominantly concerned with interpersonal relationships with patients and has its primary base in their social environment. It is for these reasons that the patients' developmental experiences are of such immediate concern to nursing (Aiyegbusi 1997). Nurses are the most likely targets of interpersonal violence by patients, followed by fellow patients, and this is consistently reported in

research studies about risk, violence and assaultiveness (Dale et al 1999a).

Duck (1988) suggests that conflict is inevitable in all relationships but it is how these conflicts are handled that determines whether this leads to a growth or a breakdown in the relationship. Conflict most often arises when relationship 'rules' are broken (Argyle et al 1985), with deception probably being the most important of these (Gross 1996).

The therapeutic relationship is the primary intervention within forensic mental health services and is founded upon a basis of trust, respect and the appropriate use of power. Boundaries within the treatment setting must be clear and not transgressed, otherwise an ambiguous, confusing and possibly frightening environment is created for patients and staff. On these issues, texts are clear: don't get overinvolved; don't have secrets from the team; seek out consultation or supervision (Dale et al 1999b).

Personal relationships

Reports and inquiries into forensic mental health services have highlighted a core attitudinal problem which has a direct bearing on an organization's ability to respond sensitively to the issue of personal relationships (DoH 1999, Special Hospitals Service Authority 1993). In forming and maintaining a personal relationship, a patient is often expressing their own sexuality. Sexuality is a term which encompasses the individual's self-concept, their unique characteristics and sexual identity and is not merely concerned with sexual behaviours.

The plight of women patients in forensic mental health services was a feature of the 1992 Ashworth Inquiry (DoH 1992: 230), where in evidence, one of the senior consultants from the hospital stated:

The hospital is male dominated, and with that goes the attitude of the whole of society in the way that males tend to perceive women conventionally, that women are objects, sexual objects particularly that can be used, that have definite roles within society and if they transgress those roles, they are, in fact, more villified than if a man did a similar thing.

It is suggested in the report that language is an important indicator of attitude and an example given is that women in Ashworth were commonly referred to as 'girls'. The inquiry report stated that:

> We believe that it is perfectly possible to establish mutually warm and trusting therapeutic relationships, with the informality appropriate to the situation, without resorting to banter which can be easily misinterpreted and may carry connotations of teasing and disrespect to patients in a dependent social position. We are not proposing that relations between patients and nurses should be governed by a rigid formal code of social behaviour, but that language should reflect a courteous valuation of patients as adult people deserving respect. (DoH 1992: 230)

During the inquiry period difficulties were discovered in opposite-sex staff working on wards and the report went on to suggest: 'It is clear that many staff could not handle appropriately the emotional tensions, particularly sexual attractions and fears, which arise both between patients and between patients and staff' (DoH 1992: 230).

The plight of women patients in forensic mental health services is given further credence by the report into the deaths of three black men at Broadmoor Hospital which stated that:

> Infantalisation seems to be part of the Broadmoor culture and again little seems to have changed since the Watts inquiry team. It is the same culture that refers to female patients as girls and produces glossy brochures for staff featuring cartoon characters that perpetuate and indeed make acceptable the whole process of infantilisation through patronizing attitudes. Such attitudes inevitably result in a failure to recognize the needs of individual patients and consider the various possibilities associated with cultural and ethnicity related issues. (Special Hospitals Service Authority 1993: 61)

The report went on to suggest that 'Staff seemed to take the moral high ground looking on patients as a lower class. They do not see them as equals and this is a clear obstacle to developing meaningful staff/patient relationships' (Special Hospitals Service Authority 1993: 61).

Boundaries

In the forensic mental health environment the issue of boundaries in interpersonal relationships is fundamental to the therapeutic process, both for the protection of the staff member and to aid the progress of the patient. Melia (1997) describes two main themes that need to be managed, particularly when dealing with the personality disordered: relationships and splitting, and secrets. At the outset, the relationship between the patient and clinical team members is relatively neutral with clear boundaries dictated by professional standards and cultural expectation. The process of assessment and treatment, however, can challenge the social construct of a neutral relationship, as the discussion will often relate to the most intimate and intrusive components of the patient's life, experience and feelings. This can be particularly difficult for the nurse who will spend long periods of time with the patients.

Gutheil & Gabbard (1993) note three degrees or levels of challenge to relationship boundaries: boundary crossing, boundary violation and sexual misconduct. They further note that the care environment can predict the violation of boundaries and this is particularly so in forensic mental health services, given the complex nature of offending behaviours that has led individuals to be admitted.

Splitting is a process which makes an individual or group feel different (normally better or worse) than their peers or those around them. In practice, the negative splitting behaviours are often quickly picked up; for example, a patient may claim a specific staff member (or staff group) is victimizing him by not facilitating a request that he claims others do (even if this is contrary to the ward/hospital policies). In this, the patient is both exerting a pressure on the staff member who is attempting to maintain consistent practice to alter or 'bend' the rules and also creating conflict between staff members.

More destructive than this, however, are the seductive components to splitting, which are more easily missed and can have a greater effect; for example, when the patient invests an apparent trust and confidence in a particular member of the care team. This is further complicated and distorted when the patient invites the team member to maintain 'secrets', often in the name of confidentiality. This can be particularly divisive when more than one discipline is involved and can lead to major conflicts amongst the clinical care team (Melia 1997).

Forensic patients often bring to their relationships high levels of emotional need and vulnerability and the experience of abuse and manipulation. Previous dysfunctional relationships add to the proclivity to distort and misinterpret the behaviour and signals given out by others. Most offenders are prepared to trust and reveal personal feelings and experiences in this context but may expect an equal investment on the part of the worker (Dale et al 1999b). It is easy to see the potential for role boundaries to slide should the worker lose focus and concentration, when daily walking the tightrope of care and control. Staff need to have clearly defined professional boundaries between themselves and their patients. Development and maintenance of these boundaries is the ongoing responsibility of the individual staff member, their line manager and their colleagues within the multidisciplinary team.

Boundaries within professional practice are used to define acceptable conduct and limits of practice. Most of the literature, particularly within psychotherapy, has focused upon the area of sexual misconduct, this being an extreme example that identifies the relationship complexities in mental health care. Epstein & Simon (1990) describe other areas where boundary violation and exploitation can occur which include: excessive familiarity; dependency; non-clinical business dealings; and breaches of confidentiality. In a recent Canadian study of nurses' views on professional boundaries, the nurse participants were in agreement about a taboo on sexual contact but less clear on other boundaries (Gallop et al 1998). Pilette et al (1995) assert that role definitions assign to the nurse the responsibility of 'separating

and containing his/her needs separately from the patient's needs'.

Gallop et al (1998) further suggest that professionals contemplating the appropriateness of various activities should ask themselves: 'Would I do/say this in front of my supervisor? Would I tell my supervisor/colleague what I have done/said and if not, why not?' Secrecy is usually a central tenet of boundary violation and often starts with a small slip, such as excessive self-disclosure, and proceeds on to a special relationship that may include secrecy.

Gutheil & Gabbard (1993) outline a number of areas where boundary violations can occur:

◆ Role
◆ Time
◆ Place and space
◆ Money
◆ Gifts, services and related matters
◆ Clothing (excessively revealing or frankly seductive clothing worn by the staff may represent a boundary violation with potential harmful effects on patients)
◆ Language
◆ Self-disclosure. Self-disclosure represents a complex issue. Clearly, the staff may occasionally use a neutral example from their own lives to illustrate a point. Sharing the impact of a borderline patient's behaviour on the staff may also be useful. However, the staff's self-revelation of personal fantasies or dreams, social, sexual and financial details, special holiday plans or expected births or deaths in the family is usually burdening the patient with information and opening the therapist up to potential future difficulties
◆ Physical contact. Some staff can argue that some benign physical contact can be positive, particularly when working through a difficult patch with a patient, but in today's rarefied atmosphere, it must be clear and open and preferably documented to prevent any misconstruing of this.

Boundary crossing may be benign or harmful; it may take many forms and may pose problems related to both treatment and potential liability. The differences in impact may depend on whether clinical judgement has been used to make the decision, whether an adequate discussion and exploration has taken place and whether documentation adequately records the details. Heightened awareness of the concept of boundaries, boundary crossings and boundary violations will both improve patient care and contribute to effective risk management.

EMOTIONAL OR SEXUAL RELATIONSHIPS BETWEEN STAFF AND PATIENTS

It is now becoming increasingly acknowledged, particularly in psychotherapeutic work, that there is a real danger of emotional and sexual involvement for the two parties involved in a caring situation. Gottlieb (1990) reports a 275% increase in complaints by clients of such abuse in 4 years of study. Furthermore, Holroyd & Bradsky (1977) indicate that there is a general consensus that such relationships are harmful.

Staff too are not immune from the potentially damaging effects of the therapeutic encounter. The case study in Box 12.1 raises a number of issues with regard to providing care in forensic services.

The tragic case in Box 12.1 highlights a number of issues for supporting and supervising staff in forensic mental health-care settings and the difficulties and intensities of interpersonal relationships. It is interesting to consider this case in relation to dangerousness. Indeed, a number of factors could be considered under a heading of professional dangerousness. Dangerousness is not confined to individuals and families. It can equally be applied to professionals and agencies. The Department of Health (1988: 12) indicated that professional dangerousness may be illustrated by a member of staff being allowed to:

◆ operate alone and unsupported
◆ collude with an individual in order to avoid the real issues (e.g. 'it would damage my

---

Box 12.1   Anonymized case study

A patient discharged from a forensic psychiatric hospital because he was no longer considered dangerous was convicted of subsequent murder.

The former patient smashed a bottle over a young girl's head and strangled her. The court heard that the former patient led a double life. He lived during the week with a nurse whom he had met whilst a patient in a forensic psychiatric hospital and at weekends he stayed with another woman.

The former patient had previous convictions for indecent assault and had spent 6 years in a forensic psychiatric unit following a conviction for rape and was ordered to the hospital without limit of time. Six years later he was transferred to a mental hospital and then discharged by a review tribunal. 'It was felt he was no longer a threat to women.' Two years after he was released, the ex-patient met a trainee health worker through the former nurse he now lived with.

The ex-patient was seen flirting with the trainee at a social event at her place of work. As

she left he jumped into her taxi and went with her to another party. She was dead by morning.

The nurse he lived with, who resigned from her job at the forensic unit to be with the ex-patient, told police that she was aware of his background. 'But I have never seen him to be violent towards anyone, or me' she said. 'I would describe him as passive, in fact he told me the forensic unit was the best place for him. It had given him space to work things out in his own mind and made him feel safe.' She had not delved into the reasons why he committed crime. He said it was the way he was treated as a child – his mother had remarried when he was 12.

The victim had not known of the ex-patient's background. Doctors said the ex-patient was 'charming, seductive and personable' towards women, 'But when a woman rejected or disbelieved him he became aggressive.'

The ex-patient pleaded guilty to the murder.

relationship' is a phrase commonly used by a dangerous professional)

◆ act without a theoretical base or a systematic, structured approach to intervention
◆ maintain unrealistic optimism about an individual against all the evidence
◆ become overinvolved and overidentified with an individual so that he or she cannot see the wood for the trees and misses the significance of patterns of behaviour by focusing only on the contents of events in crisis
◆ avoid recognizing and dealing with his or her own personal feelings and values, including cultural or religious values
◆ avoid contact with the individual due to unacknowledged fears for personal safety.

Relationships between agencies can also reflect dangerous patterns. The Department of Health (1988: 13) provides examples of interagency dangerousness.

1. Undefined boundaries of roles and responsibilities.
2. The absence of clear written procedures to guide intervention.
3. The existence of hidden agendas that affect formal activity.
4. The presence of competition and hostility between professionals.
5. The avoidance of a disagreement about the management of cases.

Such patterns of behaviour can often be observed within a case conference; therefore, the significance of this needs to be understood and carefully handled by the person chairing the conference.

RECRUITMENT AND SELECTION

A major problem within forensic mental health services is the supervision, support and training of staff to work in such environments. Indeed, in the report of the inquiry into the death of Joseph Watts, Mr Watts' stepmother stated that 'I know it is nice to have a new hospital and all the rest, but if you have the same staff it is no different'

(Special Hospitals Service Authority 1993: 57). The issue of staff training and development commences at the very start of employment, including the recruitment and selection of staff in the first place. The Special Hospitals Service Authority (1993: 53) reported that:

Nursing staff are usually recruited from the local community, and this results in a workforce to whom inner city life may be alien. The majority of members of staff are white. Many have a working class rural background. A significant number have a history of military service. All these factors play a part in determining the value judgements of the nursing community at the hospital and how nursing staff perceive patients who have a background of unemployment and crime.

Critically important, therefore, in forensic mental health services is good staff selection, which considers not only the skill mix and criteria of skills needed but also the qualities expected from members of staff, thus enabling them to effectively deal with the extreme pressures and demands of forensic mental health environments. In order to achieve the best results in matching individual aptitudes and characteristics to the demands of caring for clients who present with extensive problems, detailed specifications should be formulated highlighting the precise requirements expected from an employee. Moreover, sophisticated ways of filtering out unsuitable individuals should be explored and developed, with rigorous probing at interview, covering issues that may reveal instability, aptitude and personality traits. Observing how applicants relate to clients and members of staff, together with knowledge about previous employment, should be considered. The rigid application of equal opportunity policies must be sensibly balanced to safeguard the welfare of clients. Furthermore, competencies need to be considered during individual staff review. Evidence for good practice and/or underperformance should be cited on the staff review document, indicating also the action to be taken to rectify the deficit, with a review date.

Below are the competencies which have been identified as providing a potential framework for staff working in forensic environments (Dale et al 1999b).

◆ *Self-awareness*. Showing evidence of reflective statements/practice; identification of own interactive strengths/weaknesses; strengths/weaknesses in professional knowledge base; triggers to defensive responses; ability to challenge the practice of others; demonstrate professional approach to patients; and awareness of own attitude to offence behaviours.

◆ *Perception of role*. Showing evidence of clarity about primary purpose of relationship.

◆ *Ability to communicate*. Showing evidence of: the ability to listen/synthesize information; unambiguous verbal communication with patients; unambiguous verbal communication with colleagues; awareness of own non-verbal forms of communication; accurate and concise written communications; and the ability to work as part of a team.

◆ *Empathic approach to patients*. Showing evidence of insight into the patient's perceptions of being in secure care; his/her maladaptive behaviour(s); the need for treatment; and the risks to the patient of asking for help/treatment.

◆ *Negotiation of relationship boundaries*. Showing evidence of a patient-centred opinion on therapy/security issues; the ability to create and maintain trust; genuineness, warmth and trust; ability to evaluate practice in the here and now; understanding of dynamics in relationships; willingness/ability to challenge others; and evidence of appropriate limit setting.

◆ *Reality-based risk taking*. Showing evidence of shared decision making with patients; allowing the patient to experiment; constructive use of influence/role modelling.

◆ *Achievement/motivation*. Showing evidence of setting the environment for the patient to achieve.

◆ *Sense of humour*. Showing evidence of appropriate use of humour to create rapport and lower tension.

◆ *Ability to seek support*. Showing evidence of recognition of anxiety in self and other members of staff; ability to seek support for self and others.

INDUCTION ISSUES

This rigorous selection process leads to the importance of new staff understanding what is expected of them and being prepared to meet with the clinical and professional expectations. Therefore, it should be the responsibility of the manager of each discipline to ensure that all aspects of patient/staff relationships are discussed and fully understood by the new employee, taking into account their respective codes of conduct. In relation to personal and sexual relationships, the role of the health-care worker should be to encourage patients to form and maintain meaningful relationships. Ashworth Hospital (1994) indicates six areas that could be included.

1. Identifying with patients the aspects of their personal relationships which can promote growth and a sense of well-being.
2. Protecting patients from unrealistic relationship expectations and unwanted intimacy.
3. Enabling patients to develop, maintain and end friendships and other relationships.
4. Exploring assumptions, beliefs and attitudes regarding gender, personal power in relationships, sexuality, sexual lifestyles, intimate relationships, both personal and sexual in nature.
5. Recognizing that patients can benefit from personal relationships in a variety of ways, including: increased awareness of self and others; giving and receiving affection and support; sharing ideas and feelings in confidence; increasing self-esteem by being needed.
6. Acknowledging both the dignity and dangers of risk taking inherent in clients developing personal and sexual relationships.

Forensic mental health professionals, whilst pursuing their role, need to be aware of how to provide an appropriate environment of care, whilst giving patients opportunities to associate with others, for the purposes of forming and maintaining appropriate personal relationships. The ambience created by staff members needs to be positive and supportive and one which maximizes the individual's dignity and opportunities for meeting with others and also exercising personal privacy. The clinical environment needs to be arranged so as to afford patients the facility to associate with each other and to find solitude as required (Ashworth Hospital 1994).

EDUCATION AND TRAINING

Almost all reports, both internal and external, into forensic mental health services call for some form of additional education and training as part of the solution to the problem (Blom Cooper et al 1995, DoH 1992, Special Hospitals Authority Service 1993). Knowledge, skills and attitudes in relation to interpersonal relationships have been sadly lacking in many of these recommendations, yet should form a key focus for training and development. There is clearly a heightened need for all clinical staff to gain a better understanding of sexuality issues and greater awareness in skills development in handling relationships with clients, especially when some client groups are likely to have been abused in the past and the psychodynamics associated with this could be demanding for inexperienced staff.

Professional preparation will facilitate a better understanding in coping with transference and the personal exploration of feelings, beliefs and attitudes to human relationships and sexuality. This preparation will enable the professional carer to explore the relationship between personal experiences, beliefs and professional persona and behaviour. Moreover, professional, legal and ethical considerations need to be explored, with heightened awareness leading to improved patient care and contributing to effective risk management. As was noted within the Ashworth Inquiry (DoH 1992: 231):

A good deal more though needs to be given by management to the education needs of staff working on opposite sex wards. Where staff are placed on opposite sex wards, a properly prepared programme of education and training should be given in advance of placement.

Education and training should be provided for all staff on the type and nature of the client group they will be working with. Particular reference should be given to the intense nature of the therapeutic relationships and professional boundaries that must be maintained.

In the 1980s the Family Planning Association developed practically based training materials designed for group activity to facilitate the exploration of key problems in institutional care (particularly with people with a learning disability), which allowed staff to debate perceived problems in a safe environment (Heather 1987). These materials helped staff to get in touch with their own attitudes and prejudice in relation to sexuality, particularly in relation to disability, illness and setting. Any staff groups utilizing such material need some expert facilitation and opportunities should be provided for all staff who work in a unit, irrespective of their position within the hierarchy, to share their views and perceptions. Such facilitated sessions could be a precursor for policy formation for a unit, based on a shared understanding of the issues and a discussion of the implications which lie behind them. These issues need to be debated within the context of a philosophical value base for the unit, which could utilize the work of Wolfensberger and others into normalization, more recently referred to as social role valorization (Wolfensberger 1972).

An understanding of human relationship difficulties and stages of development of human bonding will undoubtedly be valuable. Staff will need to be able to understand the motivation of patients to establish a relationship in an impoverished environment.

The prerequisites for working in this area are: being non-judgemental; being able to demonstrate genuineness, warmth and empathy, thus leading to the formation of trust between the carer and the patient. These skills are what Egan (1986) would describe as prehelping skills in relation to his three-stage model of counselling, which has become the accepted model in most counselling training within the UK. Notably, this is the framework that Relate uses within its counselling training programme. Whilst it would undoubtedly be valuable for staff to have the full array of skills as outlined in the Egan (1986) model, the standard should be set to develop the skills at the prehelping and stage one level of the model to be able to work successfully with forensic patients.

STAFF SUPERVISION

Working with forensic patients can be anxiety provoking and depressing and an essential part of professional training involves learning how to deal with the emotional byproducts of treating patients. Cognitive understanding is not enough to deal adequately with these problems; support and introspection are also necessary. Therefore, it is vitally important that staff working in forensic services are adequately supervised through a formal contract between supervisee and supervisor. Moreover, supervision should address any difficulties which they may have in their interpersonal relationships, not only with patients but also with their colleagues. Chapter 19 deals with the process of supervision in some detail.

CONCLUSION

This chapter has attempted to outline some of the fundamental problems currently facing forensic mental health-care services. Drawing on the criticism of various inquiry reports and focusing on the complex attitudinal baseline that currently exists in many services, emphasis has been placed on the key difficulties which have been highlighted.

The complexities of the psychopathologies of the patient population, and their commonly disturbed development and upbringing, present a significant challenge for all staff required to form and maintain relationships with them. It also places some staff, particularly care staff who have more prolonged contacts with this group, at particular risk of being drawn into inappropriate, damaging or abusive relationships.

Untrained and unsupervised staff who work in forensic mental health services are especially vulnerable to difficulties and this can manifest itself in a number of ways. This clearly has ramifications for a service regarding the monitoring of

professional boundaries as well as the protection of the individuals and, in fact, the safety of the entire environment where these problems are developing.

A key solution lies with the training and education of staff and meeting head on many of the negative attitudinal and belief systems held by current employees, as well as thinking how new employees may be selected and prepared for their role. Part of this training strategy is the development of appropriate supervision and support systems to ensure that staff are helped, as far as possible, to be able to offer appropriate guidance to patients in this complex area, as well as ensuring that their own safety and security are not compromised in the process.

REFERENCES

Aiyegbusi A 1997 Personality disorder and nursing at Ashworth Hospital: a position paper. Evidence to the Inquiry into the Personality Disorder Unit at Ashworth Hospital Authority. Unpublished

Argyle M 1994 The psychology of interpersonal behaviour, 5th edn. Penguin, London

Argyle M, Henderson M 1985 The anatomy of relationships. Penguin, London

Argyle M, Henderson M, Furnham A 1985 The rules of social relationships. British Journal of Social Psychology 24: 125–139

Ashworth Hospital 1994 Personal and sexual relationships. Guidelines for clinical practice. Ashworth Hospital, Liverpool

Berscheid E, Walster E 1978 Interpersonal attraction, 2nd edn. Addison-Wesley, Reading, MA

Blau PM 1964 Exchange and power in social life. Wiley, New York

Blom Cooper L, Hally H, Murphy E 1995 The falling shadow (one patient's mental health care 1978–1993). Duckworth, London

Brehm SS 1992 Intimate relationships, 2nd edn. McGraw-Hill, New York

Dale C, Woods P, Allen G, Brennan W 1999a Violence in high secure hospital settings: measuring, assessing and responding. In: Kemshall H, Pritchard J (eds) Good practice in working with violence. Jessica Kingsley, London

Dale C, Wallis EV, Taylor P 1999b Professional, contractual and volunteer relationships: maintenance of strengths, and prevention and management of breach. In: Taylor P, Swan T (eds) Couples in care and custody. Butterworth Heinemann, Oxford, ch 13, pp 159–187

Department of Health 1988 Protecting children – a guide for social workers undertaking a comprehensive assessment. HMSO, London

Department of Health 1992 Report of the Committee of Inquiry into Complaints about Ashworth Hospital. HMSO, London

Department of Health 1999 The Report of the Committee of Inquiry into the Personality Disorder Unit, Ashworth Special Hospital. Stationery Office, London

Dolan B, Coid J 1993 Psychopathic and antisocial personality disorders: treatment and research issues. Gaskell, London

Duck S 1988 Relating to others. Open University Press, Milton Keynes

Egan G 1986 The skilled helper, 3rd edn. Brooks/Cole, Monterey, CA

Epstein RS, Simon RI 1990 An early warning indicator of boundary violations in psychotherapy. Bulletin of the Meriger Clinic 54: 450–465

Gallop R, McCay E, Austin W, Bayer M, Peternelj-Taylor C 1998 A survey of psychiatric nurses regarding working with clients who have a history of sexual abuse. Journal of the American Psychiatric Nurses Association 4(1): 9–17

Gottlieb MC 1990 Accusation of sexual misconduct: assisting in the complaint process. Professional Psychology: Research and Practice 21(6): 451–461

Gross R 1996 Psychology: the science of mind and behaviour, 3rd edn. Hodder and Stoughton, London

Gunn J, Maden A, Swinton M 1991 Treatment needs of prisoners with psychiatric disorders. British Medical Journal 303: 338–341

Gutheil TG, Gabbard GO 1993 The concept of boundaries in clinical practice: theoretical and risk-management dimensions. American Journal of Psychiatry 150(2): 180–196

Heather B 1987 Sharing: a handbook for those involved in training in personal relationships and sexuality, 2nd edn. Family Planning Association, London

Holroyd JC, Bradsky A 1977 Psychologists' attitudes and practices regarding erotic and non-erotic physical contact with patients. American Psychologist 32: 843–849

Homans GC 1974 Social behaviour: its elementary forms, 2nd edn. Harcourt Brace Jovanovich, New York

Killian M, Clark N 1996 The multidisciplinary team – the nurse. In: Cordess C, Cox M (eds) Forensic

psychotherapy: crime, psychodynamics and the offender patient: part II mainly practice. Jessica Kingsley, London, ch II-8-ii, pp 101–106

Levinger G 1980 Towards the analysis of close relationships. Journal of Experimental Social Psychology 16: 510–544

Maden T, Curle C, Meux C, Burrow S, Gunn J 1995 Treatment and security needs of special hospital patients. Whurr, London

Melia P 1997 Boundaries and inter-relatedness: practice issues within the personality disorder service. Ashworth Hospital Authority response to the Fallon Inquiry. Ashworth Hospital, Liverpool

Peplau HE 1952 Interpersonal relations in nursing. Putnam, New York

Peplau HE 1989 Interpersonal relationships in psychiatric nursing. In: O'Toole AW, Welt SR (eds) Interpersonal theory in nursing practice: selected works of Hildegard E. Peplau. Springer, New York, pp 5–20

Pilette PC, Berck CB, Achber LC 1995 Therapeutic management of helping boundaries. Journal of Psychosocial Nursing 33(1): 40–47

Rubin Z 1973 Liking and loving. Holt, Rinehart and Winston, New York

Schafer P 1999 Working with Dave: application of Peplau's interpersonal nursing theory in the correctional environment. Journal of Psychosocial Nursing and Mental Health Services 37(9): 18–24, 58–59

Special Hospitals Service Authority 1993 Report of the Committee of Inquiry into the Death in Broadmoor Hospital of Orville Blackwood and a Review of the Deaths of Two Other Afro-Caribbean Patients: 'Big, Black and Dangerous'. Special Hospitals Service Authority, London

Stockwell F 1972 The unpopular patient, vol. 2. Royal College of Nursing, London

Thibaut JW, Kelley HH 1959 The social psychology of groups. Wiley, New York

Wolfensberger W 1972 The principle of normalisation in human services. National Institute in Retardation, York University, Ontario

FURTHER READING

Argyle M 1994 The psychology of interpersonal behaviour, 5th edn. Penguin, London

Taylor P, Swan T (eds) Couples in care and custody. Butterworth Heinemann, Oxford

The application of values in working with patients in forensic mental health settings

Paul Williams   Colin Dale

INTRODUCTION

This chapter brings together work on the application of values, considerations of clinical need and requirements for secure provision in the care of patients in forensic mental health settings. The extremely difficult path trodden by professionals in such settings is identified and acknowledged. Guidelines are suggested that may help such professionals in their individual and collective decision taking and in such contexts as professional supervision, maintenance of professional standards and quality monitoring. The issues and suggestions are discussed under three main headings: professional values; cultural values; and patients' values. The contexts provided by clinical needs and needs for secure provision are discussed and a model is presented which links these considerations together to provide a holistic approach to the application of values in this field.

It is assumed throughout that the context of forensic mental health work is an interdisciplinary one, in which nurses play a prominent role since they have the most direct contact with the patient. It is also assumed that everyone involved is able and willing to share and evaluate their experiences in a completely non-defensive way, to offer the best professional service to the patient and to society. Throughout the chapter, suggestions are made for questions that forensic mental health professionals can ask to review and improve their practice.

PROFESSIONAL VALUES

Six specific professional values are identified for discussion here. These values are inherent in all mental health work but they have been chosen as having particular relevance to and presenting particular challenges in work with mentally disordered offenders.

1. Respect for the patient as a human being, regardless of behaviour, offending history or diagnosis.
2. Acceptance and application of current concepts of ill health and needs for care and treatment operated by the medical and psychiatric professions.
3. Not judging patients.
4. Applying an equally high quality of care to every patient.
5. Treating all patients with equality and fairness.
6. Maintaining confidentiality.

Value 1 Respect for the patient

This is an overarching stance that depends on the other values for its adoption. It will be returned to after consideration of these more specific values.

Value 2 Acceptance of current concepts of ill health

This involves accepting that the task of the forensic mental health professional is to deliver their skills and resources to whoever is deemed to require them. It is of course good practice, indeed essential practice, for reservations about treatment needs or the effectiveness of treatment to be communicated to senior colleagues and fellow members of the multidisciplinary team. However,

---

Box 13.1

◆ Is there any patient whose diagnosis of illness or disorder I question?

◆ Has this affected in any way my provision to that person of professional skills or resources?

---

the professional should resist the temptation to judge the worthiness of an individual to receive treatment for illness or mental disorder, where this has been determined by competent and authorized others.

In forensic mental health work, the issue can arise particularly in two circumstances: first, where the professional may feel that the patient is pretending to be ill to avoid punishment; and second, where the professional may question whether personality disorder is a true mental disorder. Box 13.1 provides some questions the professional needs to ask.

Value 3 Not judging patients

This value can particularly be called into question when the behaviour of the patient is manipulative or violent or when the offences the patient has committed are of a singularly vicious or unpleasant nature. The terms used here do have judgemental undertones but the judgement is of the behaviour or the offence, not the person.

This value is one of the most difficult for some professionals to adopt. Those with young children of their own, for example, may find it almost impossible to adopt this value in relation to patients who have committed gross sexual acts with children or have tortured or murdered children.

The labelling of patients by their offence is likely to reinforce negative judgements of them as people: a paedophile, a murderer, a rapist, an arsonist. Even some terms of medical or psychiatric origin may have acquired negative judgemental connotations about the person; a psychopath, for example.

Equally, one of the challenges of work in some forensic mental health settings is that there is likely to be a level of day-to-day violence, often directed at staff (Williams 1999a). The skills of professional work in such environments include the deescalation of potential violent events, the safe management of violence when it occurs and effective debriefing of staff, patient(s) and others affected after the violence has occurred (Turnbull & Paterson 1999). The professional must resist the temptation to judge that the patient is deliberately vindictive towards them personally.

Even more difficult may be the tendency of some patients to exploit and manipulate any perceived weakness or relaxation of vigilance on the part of staff or fellow patients (DoH 1999). A professional may feel that a good therapeutic relationship of trust has been built up with a patient, only to have that trust seriously violated by abuses, excesses or offences, often carried out with secrecy and pretence. The professional must again resist the sense of being let down, allowing them to feel that the patient is deliberately acting against them personally.

In all these circumstances, however heinous the offence or however difficult and distressing the patient's current behaviour, the professional's perception of them must be solely as a patient with care and treatment needs. However, this is a counsel of perfection and it is sensible practice to allow professionals with personal difficulties in relating to certain patients to request not to work with them. There are always staff who have a vocation for working with very difficult patients and it is best that these people should actually care for them. Box 13.2 provides some questions the forensic mental health professional needs to ask.

Value 4 Applying equal quality of care

This value requires that the professional eschews any temptation to punish or neglect or otherwise deny the highest standards of care and treatment to any patient. This is again particularly difficult in the case of patients who have committed horrific offences or show current violent, manipulative or exploitative behaviour to self, colleagues or other patients. Attribution of blame to the patient may result in a belief that the patient 'deserves' harsh treatment or 'does not deserve' favourable treatment. The professional must resist such feelings. Box 13.3 provides some questions the forensic mental health professional needs to ask.

Value 5 Fairness to all patients

This introduces the additional element that the professional should not show unfair favouritism towards any patient for reasons of personal feelings rather than professional need. Favouritism is not the same as individualization and the needs of patients for the professional's time and skills, for resources or for encouragement, for conversation and for positive regard will vary depending on their individual background and condition. Professionalism does not merely mean making these things available equally to all; however, they should be made available on the basis of professional assessment rather than personal feelings.

Where relationships are based on personal feelings rather than professional assessment, the risk of feelings of let-down discussed under Value 3 are greatly increased. The scenario is the opposite of that described under Value 4. As well as creating inherently unfair situations, unfair behaviour

---

Box 13.2

◆ Is there any patient to whom I feel such antipathy that I cannot regard them solely as a patient?

◆ If so, should I request not to work with that patient or patients with similar behaviour or history?

Box 13.3

◆ Are there any occasions on which I behave towards a patient in a punitive or neglectful way as a response to their offence history or current behaviour?

◆ How can I improve my skills of avoiding this?

Box 13.4

◆ Is there any patient with whom I feel so closely involved that it may affect my professional assessments of their needs or my reactions to their behaviour?

◆ If so, can I adopt a more professional relationship or should I cease contact with that patient?

Box 13.5

◆ Have I been asked, inside or outside work, to divulge confidential information about any patient or have I ever been tempted to reveal such information?

◆ Have there been circumstances and/or situations when I have discussed confidential patient information in a public setting where it is possible to be overheard?

◆ If so, do I need any advice or training in the handling or resisting of such situations?

Box 13.6

◆ Do I respect all patients in my care as human beings or are there any areas of belief or feelings that detract from this, for which support, advice, training or other action may be required?

---

can cause tensions with other patients and damage group processes.

A professional relationship with a patient is one that has therapeutic potential but is not so close as to affect the correct actions of the professional nor their reactions to setbacks. Too close a relationship with a patient may be a legitimate reason for moving a professional from work and even contact with that patient. Box 13.4 provides some questions the forensic mental health professional needs to ask.

Value 6 Confidentiality

This value means that the professional will not disclose information about any patient to unauthorized persons. This can be difficult when treating patients who are well known for their offences. High-profile offenders may attract persistent long-term media attention and professionals may be approached inside or outside the work setting to disclose information about such patients. In addition, information may be sought by victims and their associates, by people local to where the offence took place or other people affected by the offence. Motives for seeking the information, either by the media or others, and subsequent use of the information were it to be given, are highly unlikely to benefit the patient or be in his or her interests. Over and above that, information held on patients by professionals should be inherently confidential under the terms of any medical assessment or treatment. However difficult, professionals in forensic mental health settings must adhere strictly to this rule of confidentiality. Box 13.5 provides some questions

the forensic mental health professional needs to ask.

The overarching review

Returning to Value 1, the general question can now be asked, as shown in Box 13.6.

CULTURAL VALUES

Consideration of the relevance of general cultural values to the care and treatment of patients in forensic mental health settings rests on the premises that offenders who are sentenced or committed to detention in hospital are there for treatment and care, not punishment, and for those who are detained in prison as punishment, it is their removal from society that constitutes the punishment, not the conditions in which they live.

Given this, the well-being of offenders, their self-esteem, their comfort, their reputation, the quality of their relationships and the potential for their successful rehabilitation into society can all be enhanced by applying the criteria of positive cultural values to them (Wolfensberger 1998).

The application of general positive cultural values to enhance the life experiences of people at risk of poor or negative experiences has been explored in human services through the concepts of 'normalization' and 'social role valorization' (Race 1999). These ideas have been extremely influential in services for people with learning disabilities and, to a lesser extent, in services for older people, people with mental health problems and other groups, underpinning the major moves in recent decades from institutional to community-based provision. The ideas have been little thought through and applied in situations of detention or in forensic mental health services (Riding 1997, Williams 1999b).

Some experiences are almost universally valued in our culture; they are positively regarded and sought after by most people for themselves. Osburn (1998) lists some which will form the basis of discussion here.

◆ Having a home and family
◆ Having friends
◆ Being accorded dignity and respect
◆ Being accepted, having a sense of belonging, participating in and having a say in the affairs of one's community
◆ Living in a place that accords with certain standards
◆ Having education and having one's abilities developed
◆ Having opportunities for work and self-support

These can be taken as major aspirations of the principle of 'normalization' for people who have lost, are at risk of losing or have never had these things.

The theory of social role valorization takes these ideas further by postulating that positive experiences like those listed flow from having a role in society which is valued (Wolfensberger 1998). If people can be helped to have, and be seen to have, valued social roles, many of the positive experiences will become available to them. Indeed, defined roles that are socially valued go along with each of the experiences listed.

◆ Parent, son or daughter, uncle or aunt, grandparent
◆ Neighbour, friend, companion
◆ Citizen, person
◆ Community member, contributor
◆ Resident, home owner, tenant
◆ Student, learner, developing person
◆ Worker, taxpayer, self-supporter

Some of these roles are likely to be impossible for some people to achieve. To the extent that this is true, social role valorization would suggest that it is all the more important to develop those positive roles that are possible. Pursuit of positive roles is made difficult, but all the more necessary, by the fact that forensic mental health patients are already in the highly negative roles of offender, detainee, prisoner, mentally disordered person or sick person.

The theory of social role valorization suggests that the acquisition and maintenance of social roles depend on two things: positive perceptions by others (image); and possession of the necessary skills, resources and supports (competence). In relation to each role considered, therefore, it needs to be asked how others' perception of the person in that role and their competence in carrying out the functions of the role can be enhanced. Both image and competence are likely to be influenced by the environment, the contacts and relationships people have, the activities they engage in and such things as personal appearance, possessions and the language people use about the person (Wolfensberger & Thomas 1983).

Roles involve relationships and it is the aim of social role valorization in relation to patients in forensic services to achieve good relationships between them and other people in society, thus opening up opportunities for good experiences and successful rehabilitation. There are, however, four important contexts for this work in forensic mental health settings. First, the establishment and maintenance of relationships may be an area of particular lack of skill for many patients; for example, it is known that a high proportion of psychiatric patients in forensic services are not in a stable relationship with a spouse or partner (Williams 1999a). Second, relationships with certain people in the patient's life may be very poor (Heads et al 1997). Third, there may be clinical considerations in the fostering of relationships; for example, if some relationships have been abusive in the past, if certain relationships are likely to be therapeutically unhelpful to the patient or if there are elements of delusion in the patient's perception of the relationship. And fourth, there may be security considerations in that certain relationships may be likely to involve behaviour by the patient or another party that is abusive, exploitative, violent, dangerous, criminal or unacceptable (DoH 1999). These considerations should always be taken into account in working towards the creation and/or maintenance of potential roles that may be relevant.

Space precludes discussion here of the complete range of possibilities for pursuit of social role valorization that may exist in forensic mental health settings. As examples, just three roles will be considered: those of family member, citizen/community member and resident.

Family member

The patient can be helped by supporting them in family roles. They can be encouraged and helped with actions that are supportive to family relationships, such as:

◆ sending cards and presents on birthdays and anniversaries
◆ keeping in frequent touch by letter or telephone
◆ providing hospitality to family members when they visit
◆ keeping mementos of family, such as photographs
◆ having a record of extended family members, regularly updated
◆ being supported to attend family occasions such as weddings and funerals
◆ talking about family relationships
◆ having references made to positive family roles in accounts of the patient.

Box 13.7 provides some questions the forensic mental health professional needs to ask.

Box 13.7

◆ Can I strengthen the family role of any patients I work with?
◆ Do I need any additional advice, information, skills, resources to do this?

Citizen/community member

Functions that reinforce a patient's role as citizen and member of ordinary society might include:

◆ membership of societies, clubs or community organizations
◆ voting
◆ voluntary contribution to community agencies through work or gifts
◆ maintaining contact with friends
◆ using community facilities for leisure or shopping
◆ retaining membership of and attendance at church, synagogue or mosque.

Possibilities for some of these may be severely restricted by other factors, especially the need for security, and some may be prevented by the legal status of the patient. A general principle, however, is that the more restricted the opportunities, the more important it is that the professional encourages and supports those functions that are appropriate and possible. There may often be possibilities for staying in touch with community agencies and networks, even when physical presence is impossible.

Patients will also be members of the community within the forensic mental health setting and positive roles can be encouraged in relation to that community. This may help the quality of the patient's relationships and their self-esteem and confidence and may constitute helpful preparation for similar roles outside. Examples of functions supporting such roles might be:

◆ participation in patient councils and other self-advocacy structures

Box 13.8

◆ Can I strengthen the positive role of any patients I work with in relation to the outside community?

◆ Can I strengthen the positive role of any patients I work with in relation to the internal community?

◆ Do I need any additional advice, information, skills, resources to do either of these?

Box 13.9

◆ Can I encourage and support a more homelike environment for any patients that I work with?

◆ In what ways can I further encourage and support behaviours and skills associated with home-keeping?

◆ Do I need any additional advice, information, skills, resources to do either of these?

◆ assistance in the care of fellow patients
◆ befriending fellow patients
◆ participation in internal social, leisure or cultural events, especially as performer or organizer
◆ contribution to upkeep of the communal environment
◆ helping to operate internal resources such as shops
◆ participating in internal religious events.

Box 13.10

◆ Which valued social roles are appropriate and relevant to pursue for each of the patients in whose care I am involved?

Box 13.8 provides some questions the forensic mental health professional needs to ask.

Resident

Perception of the patient as resident (that is, someone whose home is, at least temporarily, in the forensic mental health setting), rather than as prisoner or as (merely) a patient, can be helped by encouraging behaviours and conditions that go with that role. Relationships can be improved through such perceptions, and competencies useful for rehabilitation can be practised. To the extent that other considerations, for example security, allow, there can be encouragement of such things as:

◆ comfort in furnishings, lighting, temperature, noise level, quality of food
◆ homelike decor in living rooms and bedrooms
◆ possessions appropriate to one's home, with adequate storage and security
◆ keys to one's personal spaces
◆ minimization of sharing of toilet and washing facilities

◆ avoidance of unnecessary disturbances, especially at night
◆ participation in cooking, cleaning and maintenance of the environment
◆ choice of who one lives with.

If the patient still has a home in the outside community, it may also be helpful to consider ways of encouraging and supporting functions of the resident or home-owner role in relation to that outside home, such as contributions to maintenance or making or purchasing items for the home prior to discharge.

Box 13.9 provides some questions the forensic mental health professional needs to ask.

Overall review of the application of cultural values

To identify patient needs in relation to support of valued social roles that may be relevant to them, there needs to be an individualized assessment of such needs. A life-history approach may help in this (Gillman et al 1997, Williams 1999b). Here, an overarching question for the professional is suggested in Box 13.10.

PATIENTS' VALUES

Patients' own values can be divided into those that are positive and should be respected and those that are unacceptable and should not be colluded with.

Diversity and positive values

Patients come from all backgrounds of class, gender, age, sexual orientation, lifestyle, language, religion, culture, place of origin or residence and physical characteristics. Antidiscriminatory practice involves not showing favouritism and not denying care, treatment or attention to anyone on the basis of such differences (Thompson 1998). Respect for patients' own positive values, however, takes us further than this minimal requirement. Oppression is often experienced by members of minority or 'different' groups not only as a constant risk of negative discrimination against them but as a lack of welcome in the social situations they encounter. A professional response that counters oppression therefore needs to involve an active welcoming of diversity (Thomas & Woodruff 1999).

Differences are likely to be reflected in specific positive values that are important to the individual. Part of welcoming the diversity that people bring to social situations is being knowledgeable about and sensitive to the positive values associated with their identity. Such values may concern dress, cleanliness, religious practices, strongly held beliefs, privacy, appropriate language, preferences for music, images in the environment, forms of greeting, sexual practices, display of symbols of identity and so on. Box 13.11 provides some questions the forensic mental health professional needs to ask.

Unacceptable values and beliefs

On the other hand, it is in the nature of forensic mental health work that patients may present with value systems or strongly held beliefs that are socially unacceptable. The application of those values may have been behind the offences the patient committed, which may include instances of extreme harm to other people. Indeed, the task of forensic mental health work, particularly with

---

Box 13.11

◆ What is the diversity of characteristics and identities amongst the patients I care for?

◆ Do I know the positive values that are associated with these identities?

◆ Are there additional ways in which I can help people to feel welcome by respecting these values?

◆ Do I need advice, information, support or resources in doing this?

---

those with a diagnosis of personality disorder, is often to challenge the value beliefs of patients and to seek their replacement with more socially acceptable frameworks for action.

The professional needs, therefore, to have a clear perception of the values and beliefs held by the patient that are unacceptable and therefore must not be colluded with (Vaughan & Badger 1995). Such values may centre around violence, paedophilia, hatred of specific individuals or of minority groups, obsessions with harming or harassing others, dangerous or exploitative sexual practices and so on. They may be expressed in conversation, possessions or imagery collected by the patient or in actual behaviour. They may be pursued with ingenuity and secrecy and through the willing or unwilling enlistment of others.

Non-collusion with patients in any expression of such values and beliefs requires careful attention to boundaries and the nature of relationships with patients. It is beyond the scope of this chapter to cover these in more detail but it is suggested that active ongoing review of these aspects is necessary for all forensic mental health professionals. Box 13.12 provides some questions the forensic mental health professional needs to ask.

THE CONTEXT OF CLINICAL AND SECURITY NEEDS

There are two important contexts for work with patients that is based on consideration of values:

Box 13.12

◆ Am I fully aware of any unacceptable values or beliefs held by the patients in my care?

◆ Am I confident of my ability not to collude in any expression of these values?

◆ Am I confident of my ability to work with patients to replace such value systems with more acceptable ones?

◆ Am I able to set appropriate boundaries in my work with patients?

◆ Do I have a relationship with any patient that runs a risk of collusion in the expression of unacceptable values?

◆ Do I need any help and support in these areas?

their clinical condition and consequent clinical needs, and the need for secure provision for the protection of the patient or others.

Clinical needs are likely to provide a context particularly for work based on cultural values (pursuing valued roles). A patient may be so overwhelmed by distress, depression, hallucinations, delusions or other manifestations of mental disorder that such work may have to wait until these have been ameliorated.

Security measures, particularly for the protection of other people, are likely to be the primary consideration for patients who have committed offences of extreme harm to others or are considered dangerous. For some patients, it is only in an environment where the risk of dangerous, violent, abusive and exploitative behaviour is minimized that therapeutic work can take place. Where there is such a need, it is to be expected that maintenance of this security will be a priority for professionals, as essential underpinning for their care and treatment of patients. The difficulties of forming and sustaining relationships that involve stringent security measures, whilst at the same time facilitating therapeutic work with the patient, have been fully outlined by the UKCC & University of Central Lancashire (1999) (and covered in some detail in Chapter 23). The need

for such relationships to be guaranteed to be in place is emphasized by the Department of Health (1999).

A MODEL FOR VALUES-LED WORK WITH PATIENTS IN FORENSIC MENTAL HEALTH SETTINGS

Based on these considerations, a model can be suggested for planning and sustaining professional work in forensic mental health settings that applies a range of values-led approaches. A pyramid is presented which places values-led applications and considerations of clinical and security needs in relation to each other (Fig. 13.1). Each level of activity requires that those below are firmly in place. The higher the level of activity that is possible, the greater the benefit to the patient and the greater the chances of successful rehabilitation.

CONCLUSION

Historically, forensic mental health services have suffered from an absence of clear direction in what the services were seeking to achieve. All too often, the services have been reactive to pressures from the media, politicians and the general public and have consequently become riddled with contradictory customs and practices, some from a treatment basis, others with a security or custodial foundation. It is the contention of the authors that this is a consequence of the absence of a clearly articulated philosophy of practice and values.

Values, as outlined in this chapter, should not be regarded as peripheral or academic considerations for the musing of academics or to beautify business plans with mission statements or fine words. Rather, they are the centrality of practice which should shape and direct it so that when challenges and criticisms are voiced, they can be

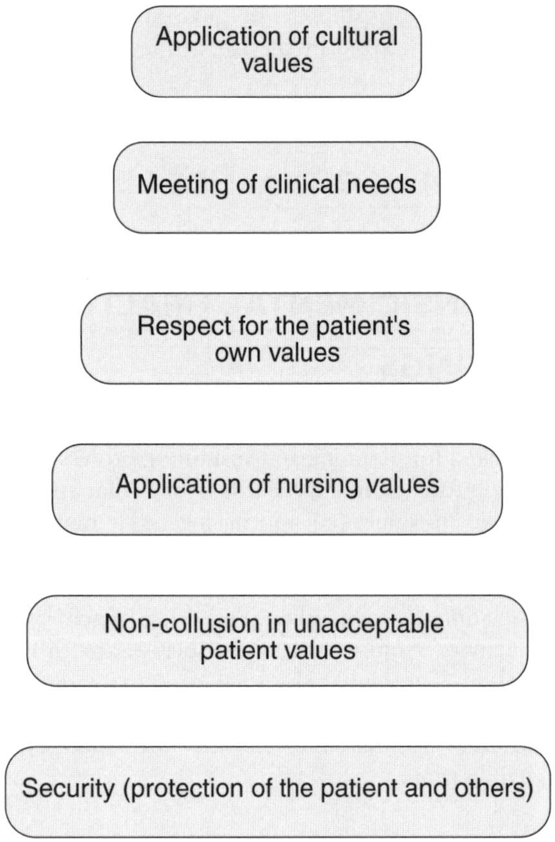

Figure 13.1 A values-led model for planning and sustaining professional work in forensic mental health settings.

squarely faced and defended. This should avoid the perpetual 'blowing in the wind' of services being modified to accommodate competing forces and demands.

The values and philosophical basis for the forensic mental health service should be widely shared and agreed with all stakeholders (users, staff, relatives, friends, purchasers, politicians and media) at the earliest opportunity and exemplars reinforced consistently. No one should be left in any doubt about the working practice of the service and its core beliefs and once articulated, they should inform all policies, procedures and publications which emanate from the service.

REFERENCES

Department of Health 1999 The Report of the Committee of Inquiry into the Personality Disorder Unit, Ashworth Special Hospital. Stationery Office, London

Gillman M, Swain J, Heyman B 1997 Life history or 'case' history: the objectification of people with learning difficulties through the tyranny of professional discourses. Disability and Society 12: 675–693

Heads T, Taylor P, Leese M 1997 Childhood experiences of patients with schizophrenia and a history of violence: a special hospital sample. Criminal Behaviour and Mental Health 7: 117–130

Osburn J 1998 An overview of social role valorisation theory. International Social Role Valorisation Journal 3: 7–12

Race D 1999 Social role valorisation and the English experience. Whiting and Birch, London

Riding T 1997 Normalisation: analysis and application within a special hospital. Journal of Psychiatric and Mental Health Nursing 4: 23–28

Thomas R, Woodruff M 1999 Building a house for diversity: new strategies for today's workforce. American Management Association, New York

Thompson N 1998 Promoting equality: challenging discrimination and oppression in the human services. Macmillan, Basingstoke

Turnbull J, Paterson B 1999 Aggression and violence: approaches to effective management. Macmillan, Basingstoke

United Kingdom Central Council for Nursing, Midwifery and Health Visiting, University of Central Lancashire 1999 Nursing in secure environments. UKCC, London

Vaughan P, Badger D 1995 Working with the mentally disordered offender in the community. Chapman and Hall, London

Williams P 1999a A review of recent academic literature on the characteristics of patients in British special hospitals. Criminal Behaviour and Mental Health 9: 296–314

Williams P 1999b An exploration of the application of social role valorisation in special hospitals. Journal of Psychiatric and Mental Health Nursing 6: 225–232

Wolfensberger W 1998 A brief introduction to social role valorisation, 3rd edn. Syracuse University Training Institute, New York

Wolfensberger W, Thomas S 1983 PASSING: programme analysis of service systems' implementation of normalisation goals. National Institute on Mental Retardation, Toronto

FURTHER READING

Bynoe I (ed) 1994 Values for change: mental health services in a secure environment. Institute for the Study and Treatment of Delinquency, London

Clarke L 1999 Challenging practice in mental health nursing: a critical approach. Routledge, London

Flynn R, Lemay R (eds) 1999 A quarter-century of normalisation and social role valorisation: evolution and impact. University of Ottawa Press, Ottawa

Hollin C 1995 Working with offenders: psychological practice in offender rehabilitation. Wiley, Chichester

Horne M 1999 Values in social work. Ashgate, Aldershot

Kaye C, Franey A (eds) 1998 Managing high security psychiatric care. Jessica Kingsley, London

Chapter Fourteen

Mental illness

Mike Musker   Phil Woods   Colin Dale

INTRODUCTION

Patients with a mental illness make up the majority of those detained within forensic mental health services. Mental illness is one of the subcategories of mental disorder under the Mental Health Act 1983; however, it is the only specific disorder which is not defined.

Schizophrenia is the most common form of mental illness found in forensic mental health services (Maden et al 1995). Symptoms vary considerably in nature and severity but generally perception is distorted and thinking, interpretation, behaviour and feelings are modified.

Patients with a mental illness in forensic mental health services, especially within high security, present particular challenges to health professionals as many are treatment resistive, highly institutionalized and a drain on resources with their associated long-term rehabilitation and lengthy, or even continual, follow-up needs

when discharged back into the community. This chapter will explore briefly the demographics of this group within forensic mental health care, before moving on to diagnostic and assessment issues. However, the primary focus is on treatment and care as these are the primary issues for practice.

DEMOGRAPHICS

The Department of Health (1999a) reports that, from court and prison disposals admitted under part 2 of the Mental Health Act 1983 during the period 1998–99, there were 1860 formal admissions to NHS facilities (including high security hospitals) and mental health nursing homes. On 31 March 1999, 80% of the formally detained patients had a legal category of mental illness. Conflating this data, 65% of patients in high security hospitals had a legal category of

151

mental illness (men 67%, women 55%). Further, from the 121 admissions to high security hospitals during the 1998–99 period, 78% had a category of mental illness. Eighty-eight percent of all court and prison disposals under the Mental Health Act 1983 had a legal category of mental illness.

The Department of Health (1999b: 134), in a more comprehensive publication from the same data set, reports that from the 846 (65%) patients with a classification of mental illness detained on 31 March 1999, there is some variation in the numbers in each individual high security hospital, relative to each hospital's total patient population: 289 (69%) are in Ashworth Hospital; 314 (74%) in Broadmoor Hospital; and 243 (53%) in Rampton Hospital.

Previously, Taylor (1997) reported that in the three English special hospitals, 59% had a legal classification of mental illness in 1986 and 66% in 1994. Furthermore, the average length of stay in 1994 was 8 years for men with mental illness and 9 for women. Thomson et al (1997) reported that at Carstairs 74% had a diagnosis of psychosis whilst Taylor (1997) found that a diagnosis of psychosis accounted for 56% of the special hospital population of England and Wales. For the total English special hospital population, Taylor et al (1998) found that of those with psychosis, 34% had an index offence of homicide, other violence 52%, sexual offence 7% and arson or property offence 7%.

In relation to ethnicity, Shubsachs et al (1995) found that in a special hospital Afro-Caribbean men were more likely to have a legal classification of mental illness (87% compared with 52%). Amongst the mentally ill, the Afro-Caribbean group was more likely to be diagnosed as schizophrenic (61% compared with 34%).

Singleton et al (1998) reported on psychiatric morbidity amongst prisoners. Assessing the prevalence of functional psychosis in the past year (i.e. schizophrenia, manic depression), they found rates of 7% for the male sentenced, 10% for the male remand and 14% for female prisoners. Further, they report that schizophrenic or delusional disorders were more common than affective disorders.

DIAGNOSTIC AND ASSESSMENT ISSUES

As with any of the other mental disorders defined under the Mental Health Act 1983, there are two main diagnostic approaches used. First, there is the ICD-10 (World Health Organization 1992) in which mental illness is categorized as follows.

◆ Schizophrenia, schizotypal and delusional disorders (F20 schizophrenia, F21–29 other non-organic functional psychoses)
◆ Mood (affective) disorders (F30 manic episode, F31 bipolar affective disorder, F32–33 depressive episodes and disorders [mild, moderate and severe])
◆ Neurotic, stress-related and somatoform disorders (F40 phobias [agoraphobia, social phobia and specific isolated phobia], F41.0 panic disorder, F41.1 generalized anxiety disorder, F41.2 mixed anxiety and depressive disorder, F42 obsessive-compulsive disorder, F43.1 posttraumatic stress disorder)

Second, there is the DSM-IV (American Psychiatric Association 1994), a multiaxial system which assists clinicians to plan treatment and predict outcome. This includes five axes.

◆ Axis I. Clinical disorders and other conditions that may be a focus of clinical attention
◆ Axis II. Personality disorders and mental retardation
◆ Axis III. General medical conditions
◆ Axis IV. Psychosocial and environmental problems
◆ Axis V. Global assessment of functioning

Both these systems are highly criticized for usage in clinical practice and at times are said only to be useful for research purposes. Therefore, the assessment processes are crucial if care and treatment are to be effective.

There are many assessment tools available to assist in the treatment and care planning and subsequent rehabilitation of those with severe and enduring mental illness. One such instrument, the Behavioural Status Index (Woods et al 1999), is described in Chapter 9. Woods (2000) and Woods

& Reed (2000) also provide case studies on its application within forensic mental health care. Another useful resource is Barnes & Nelson (1994) which brings together many useful assessment instruments and related information on their usage and application in the assessment of psychoses.

CARE AND TREATMENT ISSUES

Those classified with a mental illness under the Mental Health Act 1983 have profound, severe and enduring mental illness. Many have chronic symptoms, yet are in acute phases of illness; many have complex interpersonal difficulties, social functioning problems or complex offending behaviour patterns. Many have had extensive previous contacts with differing levels of mental health services prior to contact with the forensic mental health services. Associated care and treatment can therefore be complex and difficult.

The co-occurrence of mental illness with other disorders, most notably personality disorder (see Chapter 16) and substance misuse (see Chapter 18), within this population increases the complexity of treatment and management. There is also evidence to suggest that for at least some of this population, previous attempts at treatment have been unsuccessful in ameliorating symptoms, and therefore it is quite common to see people on large amounts of antipsychotic medication (often above BNF limits) and atypical neuroleptics (e.g. clozaril and risperidone).

The care and treatment of offenders with a mental illness needs to focus on both the illness symptoms and offending behaviour. Offending behaviour programmes are complex and will be explored in Chapter 20. It is vital that any treatment is part of a comprehensive programme of care, tailored to meet the needs of the individual concerned. Treatment needs to consider the disorder itself as well as the main focus of treatment in a forensic mental health setting – the reduction of risk or dangerousness – and must aim at reducing this and/or offending behaviour.

Many patients still have positive symptoms despite long-term treatment for these. These include hallucinations, delusions, disturbance of thought processes as shown by incoherent speech, being illogical, etc. and bizarre patterns of behaviour. Hallucinations may be visual but most are auditory. They may give orders such as self-injury or injury to others. Delusions are genuinely held irrational beliefs which are unresponsive to logical argument. For example, people may believe that they possess special information, have been wicked or evil, are being victimized or that someone is determined to hurt them. Evidence now suggests that patients with delusions, particularly of a paranoid nature, are more likely to act on these delusions and be violent (Taylor et al 1998).

Many also have profound negative symptoms. These include blunted emotions, profound lack of interest or energy and apathy; marked social withdrawal; reduction in spoken communication; lack of drive and interest in work, friends, family or career; low self-esteem; self-neglect; and loss of activities which were previously a source of pleasure. Sometimes these symptoms are misunderstood and related to 'difficult behaviour'. Sometimes they only appear as a result of medication.

Pharmacotherapy

Medication management is still a key area in the promotion of mental health (Gournay & Gray 1998). Pharmacotherapy falls into two main groups: the neuroleptics (including chlorpromazine and depot injections) and the new atypical neuroleptics (including amisulpiride, clozapine, zotepine, olanzapine, risperidone, quetiapine, sertindole).

These new atypical neuroleptics are demonstrating marked positive effects on some patients who are considered to have an intractable or difficult-to-treat form of psychosis, including aggression (Glazer & Dickson 1998, Spivak et al 1997). Following clozapine treatment, some patients have described waking from a 100-year dream (Burnett 1994). Forensic consultants have reported that clozapine has enabled them to move many 'difficult-to-treat' individuals back into the community (Ward 1996). Although clozapine is an expensive drug the overall cost of care can be dramatically reduced owing to a reduction in hospitalization (Meltzer 1997). Problems with this drug, however, are the risk of agranulocytosis and therefore the need for regular blood screening. Furthermore, it cannot be given in a depot form and therefore requires considerable supervision in non-inpatient settings.

Psychosocial interventions

McKeown & McCann (2000) report that there is considerable evidence to support the efficacy of psychosocial interventions with schizophrenia. They go on to report the specific application of these to mentally disordered offenders.

The Thorn initiative (named after Sir Jules Thorn) has led to an increase in the practice of psychosocial interventions and cognitive-behavioural therapy, to support or even provide an alternative to the biological approach of medication for patients with enduring mental health problems. Psychosocial intervention focuses on a detailed assessment of the client and their carers; education about schizophrenia; utilization of communication and problem-solving strategies; and specific cognitive-behavioural treatments.

The model assumes that psychotic symptoms are related to stress vulnerability and that psychotic episodes arise when stressors breach the patient's tolerance threshold. Patients are encouraged to develop psychological and environmental interventions to provide inoculation against the stress that contributes to their psychotic symptoms. Additionally, the role of the family is seen as a major dynamic in the patient's health.

In forensic environments a patient has to live with other dangerous individuals who may be violent, manipulative bullies or just generally stressful to live with. For carers, managing such an environment can be as important as the interpersonal relationship with the patient. High expressed emotion (being hostile, hypercritical or overprotective) has been described as the charged emotional environment within the patient's home. It could be suggested that the ward environment could be equally charged with expressed emotion, the nurses

and fellow patients being the protagonists. It is the carer's task to provide feedback in an empathic, non-demanding way that will defuse tense situations, reduce personal conflicts and create a relaxed atmosphere within ward environments (Davison & Neale 1998).

A key part of this treatment is psychoeducation, which involves teaching the patient and their family about the illness, treatment and their legal status. Cognitive-behavioural therapy is utilized in helping an individual cope with specific problems, getting them to refocus and analyse problems in new ways. For example, patients suffering from hallucinations are encouraged to deal with their voices using alternative methods such as thought stopping, belief modification, a personal stereo or even an ear plug in the dominant ear (Dawber 1997). Delusions are also open to belief modification.

It is beyond the scope of this chapter to provide an in-depth example of psychosocial intervention in practice and the reader is directed to McKeown & McCann (2000) and McCann & McKeown (2000) as excellent examples of this.

Cognitive-behavioural therapy

In Great Britain over the past few years researchers have begun to develop cognitive-behavioural interventions for patients with psychosis. These have been considered to be part of a broader normalizing strategy for patients to accept their disturbing experiences (Kingdon & Turkington 1994); to enhance their coping skills (Tarrier et al 1993); or as treatment for delusions or hallucinations (Bentall et al 1994, Chadwick & Birchwood 1994, Chadwick & Lowe 1990, Garety et al 1994), although Bentall suggests more success in relation to work with delusions as opposed to hallucinations.

Cognitive and behavioural approaches are perhaps the most widely used at present in forensic services. These programmes usually offer a skills- or social skills-based approach to therapy. Behavioural therapy has been shown to be more successful, although this only addresses current environmental antecedents and consequences of behaviour. Cognitive-behavioural approaches question an individual's maladaptive irrational thoughts, thus providing new cognitions to replace these. Cognitive therapy works at a dual level of manifested behavioural problems and inferred schema.

It is beyond the scope of this chapter to provide comprehensive accounts of the treatment methods currently being tried with severe and enduring mental illness. Bentall & Haddock (2000) provide insight into cognitive-behavioural therapy for auditory hallucinations and Ewers et al (2000) cover cognitive-behavioural therapy for delusions in a forensic setting.

Behaviour therapy

At the extreme end of care, there are individuals who are frequently violent or malevolent in their approaches to others. The majority of patients admitted to forensic care have a history of violence and not all of this violence can be attributed to ill health, examples being bullying or intimidation. Even when someone is psychotic, they still have some level of accountability for their actions.

When examining why assaults occur, it is often found that the patient is reacting to some form of aversive stimulus, such as being asked to take medication or to complete a task, rather than responding to psychotic phenomena. Behavioural approaches attempt to identify the specific function of a target behaviour. This is done by completing a functional analysis, examining antecedents, the target behaviour in detail and the consequences of such behaviour. There are two key methods of behaviour modification: a reinforcement model of applying positive and negative consequences in order to increase the frequency of appropriate behaviour, and a token economy system. These are particularly useful with patients who demonstrate severe challenging behaviour. An assessment of the patient's likes and dislikes is made and used to provide reinforcers. Each target behaviour is identified and strategies are developed as part of a personal behaviour schedule. The care team discusses and ratifies the plan, in particular identifying the consequences for each behaviour in order to support the nurses who have to implement it. The most important aspect of implementing behavioural approaches is the consistency of the nursing teams, particularly across shifts. The frequency, intensity and duration of each target behaviour must be measured at regular intervals in order to assess the effectiveness of the programme.

Group therapy

Anger management, mental health education, sex offender work, substance abuse education, social skills training, counselling, arson groups and predischarge preparation are all key areas that can be built into most patients' care pathways. Individuals may need to attend more than one group during their stay in hospital for reinforcement of that particular aspect of care. For example, a patient with problems of sex offending or arson may have to attend group therapy on an annual basis, as they are likely to experience a long stay. It is preferable that groups are closed, limiting disclosure of traumatic experiences to only a few fellow patients and carers. Most groups should be gender specific, avoiding problems such as a rape victim involved in group work with someone who has carried out sexual offences but who may share an index offence of arson. The Mental Health Act Commission, in its Eighth Biennial Report, has expressed its concern for women patients, stating there should be separate facilities for women patients, and the Commission offers a variety of recommendations and safeguards to provide for their dignity and safety (Mental Health Act Commission 1999). The Department of Health (1999c) has further indicated that patients with mental illness should be treated separately from those with personality disorder.

In many areas of secure care, it is not feasible to physically separate the personality disordered from the mentally ill, or even to separate by gender, owing to the small numbers of patients in some units. The list below provides more specialized areas that could be considered when developing a rehabilitation programme:

◆ Individual psychotherapy/counselling
◆ Psychotherapy groups
◆ Attention process training

◆ Relationships group
◆ Reason and rehabilitation group
◆ Muslim group/Asian group
◆ Daily living skills
◆ Relaxation and anxiety management
◆ Empathy training skills group
◆ Assertion group.

Insight

The assessment of insight is high on the treatment agenda in forensic mental health services. Insight is a protean concept which has exercised the academic imagination for many years now. This is mainly owing to the problematic issues surrounding its measurement. It is still not entirely clear what constitutes 'good' or 'bad' insight in relation to clinical values or outcomes (Markova & Berrios 1992).

There are notorious difficulties attendant on theorizing about insight and its relationship to patients (Jaspers 1959) and in defining and classifying the concept (Richfield 1954). Amador et al (1993) indicate the research difficulties attendant on such conceptual ambiguities, arising mainly when assessment methods fail to consider its complexity by treating insight as a unitary concept.

David (1990) suggests that insight involves three significant notions:

1. the patient's capacity to recognize that he or she is, or has been, mentally ill
2. his/her ability to relabel unusual mental events as pathological
3. his/her degree of self-awareness.

Consequently, within the academic arena, insight has been examined from various perspectives, asking key questions such as: What is insight? How do we help patients gain insight? With what activities or attributes does it correlate?

By contrast, in the clinical arena insight has tended to be an extremely narrow concept and viewed rather unidimensionally in mainstream psychiatric practice (Perkins & Moodley 1993). The exception is in the field of psychotherapy, where it is not viewed as a unitary, clearly delineated attribute which is either present or absent but rather as a *continuum* of thinking and feeling which is affected by numerous variables.

The assessment of insight and its consequential treatment in forensic mental health care needs to consider one or all of the following areas (Woods et al 1999): tension, anger, strategies for reducing tension, features of personal and shared antecedent events leading to treatment, ascription of respons   ibility and treatment and problem solving. The importance of insight is that those patients who achieve it can seek help once known early symptomatology begins to manifest itself. Also, the individual is likely to be more compliant in relation to self-medicating when they accept that they are unwell and therefore require ongoing treatment.

Communication and social skills

Another key area for assessment and treatment within forensic mental health services is communication and social skills. Considerable advances in clinical knowledge regarding assessment and treatment of interpersonal difficulties have been made over the years. Perhaps of special significance in this context are certain behavioural guidelines proposed some years ago which suggest that consideration should initially be given to the measurement of the *content* of interpersonal behaviours, as opposed to the *consequences* of such behaviours. A second principle asserts that social skills are situation specific. Third, it is important that the assessor possesses the ability accurately to read social situations and response patterns for dealing with these. Fourth, it is essential to understand the relationship between single responses and behavioural sequences. Fifth, the assessor must be able to differentiate social skill deficits from performance inhibition. Finally, the assessor should understand the social 'pay-offs' created by physical appearance (Arkowitz 1981).

Mental disorder has long been associated with poor communication and social skills functioning. Specific deficits are those cited by Bellack et al (1990), who found marked social isolation and life role functioning deficits and prominent prodromal symptoms. Argyle (1988) reported specific social skill deficits such as inappropriate facial expression, gestures, posture and poor social meshing.

The social behaviours of people with mental disorders are neither simple nor uniform and may manifest as either excessively frequent or reduced patterns of 'acceptable' behaviours (Pantelis & Curson 1994). Both Robertson (1988) and Taylor (1985) point out that, at the time of offending, many psychotic offenders are disorganized, socially isolated and homeless. Robertson further suggests that 'social incompetence' is a central related factor in offending behaviour. For example, a high proportion of sexual offenders have deficits in their levels of social functioning, leading to the well-recognized precipitating factor of social inadequacy (Abel & Osborne 1992). It is highly unlikely that this social incompetence will suddenly diminish when such patients are admitted to hospital.

The assessment of communication and social skills and consequential treatment in forensic mental health care needs to consider one or all of the following areas (Woods et al 1999): habitual facial expression; various aspects of proxemics; paralinguistic features; aspects of conversational interaction; potential conflict; self-presentation and interpersonal skills.

CONSENT TO TREATMENT

Issues of consent to treatment are a critical consideration within forensic mental health services, given the vulnerability of the patients in relation to their compulsory detention under the Mental Health Act 1983 and more limited access to communications and advocacy systems.

The requirements governing consent to treatment are outlined in part 4 of the Mental Health Act 1983. Treatment must be for mental disorder, under the direction of the Responsible Medical Officer (RMO), and for medical treatment and not restraint.

Consent is defined in the Mental Health Act 1983 Code of Practice (DoH & Welsh Office 1999: 15.13) as 'the voluntary and continuing permission' of a patient based on an 'adequate knowledge' of the proposed treatment and an understanding of its nature, purpose and likely effects as well as the likely consequences of it not being given, the likelihood of its success and whether there are alternatives to it. Under the Mental Health Act 1983 the RMO should only deem a patient to be consenting to a proposed treatment if all these conditions are satisfied, as one of the main issues pertaining to consent to treatment is the authenticity of consent.

For those with severe and enduring mental illness, treatment refusal can be part of the disorder itself. However, at all costs patients should be given the opportunity to consent to treatment. It should not be automatically assumed that a second opinion is required.

A number of voluntary organizations, as well as the Mental Health Act Commission, have called for written information on psychiatric treatments to complement that which should be provided orally by RMOs when they discuss proposed treatments with patients and seek their consent to such proposals. The current availability of this is minimal (Mental Health Act Commission 1999: 167). The revised Code of Practice (DoH & Welsh Office 1999: 16.10) now requires that patients who are treated with ECT should receive a leaflet which helps them understand and remember advice about 'its nature, purpose and likely effects' as a matter of good practice.

Section 58(3) of the Mental Health Act 1983 requires that for certain treatments (the administration of medicine for mental disorder beyond 3 months in any continuous period of detention and ECT at any time), the RMO must certify on a Form 38 that the patient has the capacity to consent and does so or a Second Opinion Appointed Doctor must authorize the treatment on a Form 39 (curiously, the patients do not themselves sign Form 38s indicating their consent to treatment). In addition to this, the Mental Health Act Commission (1999) reports that it is not uncommon for patients, particularly those who have consented to ECT undergoing an anaesthetic, to be asked by hospitals to sign hospital consent forms.

Consent may be withdrawn by the patient at any time and it is not uncommon for patients' opinions on consent to fluctuate (real consent is the continuing permission of a patient rather than a one-off agreement). This is a particular issue for nursing staff administering medication where consideration of the patient's expressed wish needs to be given each time treatment is administered authorised under Form 38. Form 38s should be regularly reviewed by the RMO and regarded as effective for a maximum of 1 year.

The Code of Practice now specifically requires that a record of discussions between a patient and the RMO should be placed in the patient's medical notes (DoH & Welsh Office 1999: 16.9a, 16.13). The Mental Health Act Commission monitored such recordings during 1998 and found that nearly half showed no corroborative record of a discussion between the patient and the RMO in the 7 days before the doctor's signing of the Form (Mental Health Act Commission 1999: 169). It also found that patients were being authorized for treatment under the Act when held under sections not covered for consent for treatment regulations (e.g. sections 5.2 and 5.4).

Common law allows that treatment to save life or prevent a deterioration in the patient's physical or mental condition may be given without the patient's consent but where doubt may exist then it is recommended that practitioners seek legal advice without delay.

The Mental Health Act Commission has a statutory responsibility for appointing registered medical practitioners (referred to as Second Opinion Appointed Doctors or SOADs), to consider authorizing non-consenting detained patients' treatment with medication for mental disorder after an initial 3 months of treatment or with ECT at any time. The SOAD has a statutory duty to consult a qualified nurse who has been professionally concerned with the patient's care and a person similarly qualified who is neither a nurse nor a doctor.

Between March 1997 and March 1999 there were 15 470 requests for a second opinion. Slightly over half of the second opinions were required because the patient was judged to be incapable of informed consent and the remainder were refusing treatment; 89.5% of the completed

second opinions were for the category of mental illness and 5.2% dual diagnosis (Mental Health Act Commission 1999: 176).

Treatments normally requiring either a patient's consent or a second opinion can be given in an emergency without either safeguard provided that certain criteria listed in the Mental Health Act 1983 are met. The least stringent criterion allows for treatments to be continued pending the visit of a SOAD if discontinuation of treatment would cause serious suffering to the patient. The initiation of any treatment under section 62 must meet the criterion of being immediately necessary, either to save the patient's life or to prevent a serious deterioration of the patient's condition or to either alleviate serious suffering by the patient or to prevent the patient behaving dangerously (there is a requirement for hospitals to both record and monitor this). Treatments giving rise to special concern (such as psychosurgery) require consent and a second opinion.

CONCLUSION

It is evident from this chapter that the care and treatment of those with a mental illness within forensic mental health care is neither easy nor uniform. They make up the largest group of patients and many have lifelong severe and enduring mental illness. Many are treatment resistant and hard to rehabilitate owing to profound institutionalization.

There is evidence to suggest that many patients with mental illness in high security hospitals do not need that level of security but despite many years of hospitalization and pharmacotherapy, still have positive symptoms of their illness (Maden et al 1995).

The core issue for the care and treatment of this group is risk and the association this has with their offending behaviour and illness symptoms. Many will need ongoing follow-up when discharged to the community. Thus they are a frequent drain on resources and often areas of lesser security are reluctant to take on their care and treatment.

REFERENCES

Abel GG, Osborne C 1992 The paraphilias: the nature and extent of sexually deviant criminal behaviour. Clinical Psychiatry 15(3): 675–687

Amador XF, Strauss DH, Yale SA, Flaum MM, Endicott J, Gorman JM 1993 Assessment of insight in psychosis. American Journal of Psychiatry 150(6): 873–879

American Psychiatric Association 1994 Diagnostic and statistical manual of mental disorders, 4th edn. (DSM-IV) APA, Washington

Argyle M 1988 Bodily communication, 2nd edn. Routledge, London

Arkowitz H 1981 Assessment of social skills. In: Hersen M, Bellack AS (eds) Behavioural assessment: a practical handbook, 2nd edn. Pergamon, Oxford

Barnes TRE, Nelson HE (eds) 1994 The assessment of psychoses: a practical handbook. Chapman and Hall, London

Bellack AS, Morrison RL, Wixted JT, Mueser KT 1990 An analysis of social competence in schizophrenia. British Journal of Psychiatry 156: 809–818

Bentall R, Haddock G 2000 Cognitive-behaviour therapy for auditory hallucinations. In: Mercer D, Mason T, McKeown M, McCann G (eds) Forensic mental health care: a case study approach. Churchill Livingstone, Edinburgh, ch 4 pp 67–75

Bentall RP, Haddock G, Slade PD 1994 Cognitive behaviour therapy for persistent auditory hallucinations: from theory to therapy. Behaviour Therapy 25: 190–201

Burnett S 1994 A new lease of life. Nursing Times 90(31): 57–59

Chadwick P, Birchwood M 1994 The omnipotence of voices: a cognitive approach to auditory hallucinations. British Journal of Psychiatry 164: 190–201

Chadwick P, Lowe CF 1990 The measurement and modification of delusional beliefs. Journal of Consulting and Clinical Psychology 58: 225–232

David AS 1990 Insight and psychosis. British Journal of Psychiatry 156: 798–808

Davison GC, Neale JM 1998 Abnormal psychology, 7th edn. Wiley, New York

Dawber N 1997 Current approaches and interventions for schizophrenia. Nursing Standard 11(49): 49–56

Department of Health 1999a Statistical bulletin, 1999/25. Department of Health, London

Department of Health 1999b Inpatients formally detained in hospitals under the Mental Health Act 1983 and other legislation. Department of Health, Statistics Division, London

Department of Health 1999c Report of the Committee of Inquiry into the Personality Disorder Unit, Ashworth Special Hospital, vol 1. Stationery Office, London

Department of Health, Welsh Office 1999 Mental Health Act 1983: code of practice. Stationery Office, London

Ewers P, Leadley K, Kinderman P 2000 Cognitive-behaviour therapy for delusions. In: Mercer D, Mason T, McKeown M, McCann G (eds) Forensic mental health care: a case study approach. Churchill Livingstone, Edinburgh, ch 4, pp 77–89

Garety PA, Kuipers L, Fowler D et al 1994 Cognitive behavioural therapy for drug-resistant psychosis. British Journal of Medical Psychology 67(3): 259–271

Glazer WM, Dickson RA 1998 Clozapine reduces violence and persistent aggression in schizophrenia. Journal of Clinical Psychiatry 59 (suppl 3): 8–14

Gournay K, Gray R 1998 The role of new drugs in the treatment of schizophrenia. Mental Health Nursing 18(2): 21–24

Jaspers K 1959 General psychopathology (trans. Hoenig J, Hamilton M 1963). Manchester University Press, Manchester

Kingdon DG, Turkington D 1994 Cognitive-behavioural therapy of schizophrenia. Lawrence Erlbaum, Hove

Maden T, Curle C, Meux C, Burrow S, Gunn J 1995 Treatment and security needs of special hospital patients. Whurr Publishers, London

Markova IS, Berrios GE 1992 The meaning of insight in clinical psychiatry. British Journal of Psychiatry 160: 850–860

McCann G, McKeown M 2000 Family work. In: Mercer D, Mason T, McKeown M, McCann G (eds) Forensic mental health care: a case study approach. Churchill Livingstone, Edinburgh, ch 4, pp 91–98

McKeown M, McCann G 2000 Psychosocial interventions. In: Chaloner C, Coffey M (eds) Forensic mental health nursing: current approaches. Blackwell Science, Oxford, ch 12, pp 232–251

Meltzer HY 1997 The clozapine story. In: Hertzman M, Feltner DE (eds) The handbook of psychopharmacology trials: an overview of scientific, political, and ethical concerns. New York University Press, New York

Mental Health Act Commission 1999 8th biennial report. HMSO, London

Pantelis C, Curson DA 1994 The assessment of social behaviour. In: Barnes TRE, Nelson HE (eds) The assessment of psychoses. Chapman and Hall, London, pp 135–155

Perkins R, Moodley P 1993 The arrogance of insight. Psychiatric Bulletin 17: 233–234

Richfield J 1954 An analysis of the concept of insight. Psychoanalytical Quarterly 23: 390–408

Robertson G 1988 Arrest patterns among mentally disordered offenders. British Journal of Psychiatry 153: 313–316

Shubsachs A, Huws R, Close A, Larkin E, Falvey J 1995 Male Afro-Caribbean patients admitted to Rampton Hospital between 1977 and 1986 – a control study. Medicine, Science and the Law 35: 336–346

Singleton N, Meltzer H, Gatward R, Coid J, Deasy D 1998 Psychiatric morbidity among prisoners in England and Wales. Stationery Office, London

Spivak B, Mester R, Wittenberg N, Maman Z, Weizman A 1997 Reduction of aggressiveness and impulsiveness during clozapine treatment in chronic neuroleptic-resistant schizophrenic patients. Clinical Neuropharmacology 20(5): 442–446

Tarrier N, Beckett R, Harwood S 1993 A trial of two cognitive-behavioural methods of treating drug-resistant residual psychotic symptoms in schizophrenic patients I: outcome. British Journal of Psychiatry 162: 524–532

Taylor P 1985 Motives of offending among violent and psychotic men. British Journal of Psychiatry 147: 491–498

Taylor P 1997 Damage, disease and danger. Criminal Behaviour and Mental Health 7: 19–48

Taylor P, Leese M, Williams D, Butwell M, Daly R, Larkin E 1998 Mental disorder and violence: a special hospital study. British Journal of Psychiatry 172: 218–226

Thomson L, Bogue J, Humphreys M, Owens D, Johnstone E 1997 The State Hospital survey: a description of psychiatric patients in conditions of special security in Scotland. Journal of Forensic Psychiatry 8: 263–284

Ward M 1996 Forensic use of clozaril: personal experience. Clozaril Newsletter 14: 3

Woods P 2000 Social assessment of risk: the Behavioural Status Index. In: Mercer D, Mason T, McKeown M, McCann G (eds) Forensic mental health care: a case study approach. Churchill Livingstone, Edinburgh, ch 12, pp 333–339

Woods P, Reed V 2000 Use of the Behavioural Status Index in therapeutic programmes with high-risk clients. Mental Health Care 3(6): 194–196

Woods P, Reed V, Robinson D 1999 The Behavioural Status Index: therapeutic assessment of risk, insight, communication and social skills. Journal of Psychiatric and Mental Health Nursing 6(2): 79–90

World Health Organization 1992 The ICD-10 classification of mental and behavioural disorders: clinical descriptions and diagnostic guidelines. WHO, Geneva

FURTHER READING

Bellack AS, Mueser KT, Gingerich S, Agresta J 1997 Social skills training for schizophrenia: a step-by-step guide. Guilford Press, London

Faulk M 1994 Basic forensic psychiatry, 2nd edn. Blackwell Science, London

Gunn J, Taylor PJ 1993 Forensic psychiatry: clinical, legal and ethical issues. Butterworth Heinemann, London

Chapter Fifteen

Learning disability

Mike Musker

INTRODUCTION

This chapter will examine the secure care provision for those diagnosed with learning disability and how this has developed over recent years. It considers the current population of the high security hospitals and the dramatic changes within this arena. The diagnostic, care and treatment issues for this population will also be presented.

The inadequate provision of secure services has been highlighted since the Butler Report (Home Office & DHSS 1975) when it was suggested that there is a need for up to 2000 medium secure beds. Other reports have since reflected on the failure to appropriately place those with learning disability who have secure needs into an appropriate setting (DHSS 1974, DoH & Home Office 1992, Halstead & Cassidy 1994, Maden et al 1995). Over the past 5 years there has been a drive to move patients diagnosed with learning disability in high security hospitals back into medium secure settings or to long-term care services in the community (Dickens 1998). There is a new air of optimism with the development of the National Service Frameworks and the way local authorities are planning to increase medium secure services that are needs led. There has been an increase in new medium secure services, both in the private and public sector, that will cater for learning disability patients in the long term, rather than the former arbitrary 2-year limit. This supports the five recommendations made by the Reed Committee (DoH & Home Office 1992) of: care based on individual need; where possible in the community; near the patient's home; the level of security matching the patient's dangerousness; and care aimed at rehabilitation and independent living.

DEMOGRAPHY OF CLIENT GROUP

One of the most comprehensive studies on needs-led secure care provision was completed by Maden et al (1995). The section on learning disability concluded that the chronicity of some service users' level of dangerousness meant that it would be difficult to transfer them from a maximum security to a medium security setting for some time. It was noted that it would be difficult to provide the standard of care and quality of life programmes as received in the high security hospitals for this group, in a smaller setting. One of the main reasons for this is

161

that the size, variety of occupational therapy/ clinical therapy and high staffing ratios provided at maximum security level would be difficult to duplicate in some smaller units.

Of the learning disability sample studied by Maden et al (1995) (n=72), 15% had previously been admitted to a high security hospital and many others had lived in an institutional setting for most of their lives. The study reported that up to 40% of service users with a mental impairment diagnosis in high security settings could be placed in less secure environments by the year 2000. Additional calculations resulted in the approximation that only 25% of the mentally impaired high security hospital population required maximum security (Dickens 1998).

This advice matched the strategic thinking of the Special Hospitals Service Authority (1995: 5), who recognized that the numbers of this population had been reducing significantly since 1986 (in 1986 the figures were 141 mentally impaired men and 38 mentally impaired women, 44 severely mentally impaired men and 45 severely mentally impaired women. By 1994 these figures had reduced to 67 mentally impaired and 22 severely mentally impaired men and 22 mentally impaired and 10 severely mentally impaired women). At the same time, referrals for admissions for this group had also dwindled (in 1986 there were 36 referrals for patients with a mental impairment diagnosis and four referrals for severe mental impairment; by 1994 these figures had reduced to six and nil respectively; Special Hospitals Service Authority 1995: 7).

As a consequence of this the Special Hospital Service Authority determined that maximum security learning disability services were to be provided by unifying this service at one location in Rampton Hospital. The reorganization and relocation project was finalized in 1999 with the result that almost all learning disability patients are now based at Rampton. This approach of utilizing out-of-area treatment causes major problems for family members who live in other parts of the country and may result in difficulties with implementing the service users' rehabilitation back into their own community. This initiative curiously contradicted one of the main Reed recommendations (DoH & Home Office 1992) of being 'near the patient's home'.

The Special Hospitals Service Authority had already declared in 1990 that they would not admit any more service users with a diagnosis of 'severe learning disability' to high security hospitals. This statement only confirmed what had become accepted clinical practice in the 1980s, which is reflected in the referrals and rejection statistics over a 4-year period between 1984 and 1988 when 22 out of 23 referrals for people with mental impairment to high security hospitals were rejected (cited in Gunn & Taylor 1993).

The case register is a research tool which attempts to track service users as they move through the high security hospital system and involves interviewing (or gaining information concerning) all service users when they are admitted. According to the case register, in 1999 there were 123 learning disabled patients in high security hospitals, the majority being based at Rampton Hospital. It is apparent from Table 15.1 that most of this group are male (105 service users) and the largest group has a single diagnosis of mental impairment (68 service users).

The way service users receive a classification of mental impairment is based on the Mental Health Act 1983 and although the term is defined in the Act, it remains ambiguous.

Table 15.1 Learning disabled within high security care in 1999

Type of illness	Males	Females	Total
Mental impairment	59	9	68
Personality disorder and mental impairment	20	6	26
Severe mental impairment	11	1	12
Mental illness and mental impairment	8	0	8
Not known	3	2	5
Mental illness and severe mental impairment	4	0	4
Totals	105	18	123

(Source: Special Hospitals Case Register 1999; statistics provided by case register worker Julie Mason, Ashworth Hospital)

◆ *Mental impairment* is defined as a state of arrested or incomplete development of mind (not amounting to severe mental impairment) which includes a significant impairment of intelligence and social functioning and is associated with abnormally aggressive or seriously irresponsible conduct.

◆ *Severe mental impairment* is defined as a state of arrested or incomplete development of mind which includes severe impairment of intelligence and social functioning and is associated with abnormally aggressive and seriously irresponsible conduct.

The only change between the two definitions is from 'significant' to 'severe'. The actual difference between significant and severe is not stated but in practice these are accepted as significant impairment being IQ 60–70 and severe impairment as IQ below 60 (Stone et al 2000). As is reflected in practice, the use of intelligence quotients to determine a person's diagnosis, care and treatment can be a haphazard affair. The picture is further confused by the complexities of dual diagnosis, usually in the form of additional mental health problems or a personality disorder. Maden et al (1995) found that amongst the learning disability population about a third of those patients surveyed had positive signs of psychosis. It is often the case that the individual's personality disorder or mental health problems are far greater than those caused by the learning disability. In these cases the person may be better placed within the mental health services or more specialized personality disorder services.

Those diagnosed with mental impairment in the criminal justice system have been commonly associated with the crimes of arson or sexual offences (Turk 1989). This can involve children and may often arise out of a naïve childlike interest, which in the worst-case scenarios can lead to fatal encounters (Gunn & Taylor 1993).

One of the problems with sexual offences and learning disability is that it is difficult to assess the level of risk without an actual trial in the community. The notion of mental impairment indicates a reduced ability to learn or mature in this area; consequently professionals are understandably wary concerning discharge and rehabilitation programmes. People with a mental impairment may display problematic behaviours such as openly masturbating or by performing inappropriate homosexual and heterosexual behaviours. Many are used to this leading to punishment, resulting in the development of further maladaptive problems in the dimension of their sexual needs (Craft 1987). Once a person has entered the institutional system their sexual needs are unlikely to be addressed, other than by sex education and counselling.

This group of people is easily managed in the forensic care system and does not require high staffing ratios, but they are likely to require care in terms of decades rather than years. It is the longitudinal aspects of such care programmes that require consideration during new policy development and service planning. It is thought that levels of learning disability in prisons are between 2% and 10%. Around 10% of clients in the Probation Service have an IQ of less than 75 and it is approximated that 8% of people entering police stations have confirmed learning disabilities (Mason 1999).

Woods & Mason (1998) studied 20 years of admissions to Ashworth high security hospital (n=1464), finding that the mean age on admission was 26 years for those with a mental impairment, compared with those without mental impairment who had a mean age of 30 years. Many patients with mental impairment were admitted in their teenage years (26%), whilst a few patients had been admitted as young as 13 years old. The ratio of male to female admissions for those diagnosed with mental impairment was 4:1.

The two main reasons for admission for people with mental impairment were physical attacks on others (44.9%) and property damage (17.8%), demonstrating that the key risk area from this group is physical assault. In the study by Maden et al (1995), the largest victim groups leading to admission were recognized as fellow patients (49%), nurses or doctors (43%), and official visitors (12%), some individuals having attacked a combination of victim groups. The commonest reason for admission was repeated assaults.

DIAGNOSTIC ISSUES

Learning disability is usually described as a significant impairment of intelligence and social functioning acquired before adulthood (it is also known as mental handicap and mental retardation). The people to whom it applies prefer the term learning difficulty. (NHSE 1998)

The Mental Health Act 1983 classifications of mental impairment and severe mental impairment reflect past methods of assessing learning disabilities based solely on performance in intelligence tests, which resulted in categorization of disability as profound, severe, moderate or mild. It is now recognized, however, that people with learning disabilities form a diverse group and the extent of their disability depends on the interaction between intellectual abilities, social functioning and personal development.

The Special Hospitals Service Authority (1995: 7) set out its criteria for people with a learning disability who might need high security. In relation to the definition of learning disability, it listed the criteria as low IQ, communication disorder, impaired social functioning and documented delay in intellectual development. In relation to need for high security, it listed the criteria as diagnosable personality/mental disorder; assessment of dangerousness and could not be cared for in other circumstances.

When transferring service users between services, however, the term 'challenging behaviour' is often used to imply level of need. This term is a descriptive and graphically evocative phrase, although it does not convey anything of clinical value about the individual. It evokes images of the problems that may be encountered rather than identifying the potential that may be discovered and utilized within the person involved. However, many local authorities are recognizing the need to develop expertise in the area of behavioural approaches for people with learning disabilities and training is being focused toward this developing field. A common definition for challenging behaviour is as follows.

Challenging behaviour refers to behaviour of such an intensity, frequency or duration that the physical safety of the person or others is placed in serious jeopardy, or behaviour is likely seriously to limit or deny access to and use of ordinary community facilities. (Emerson et al 1987)

There seem to be four systems of labelling people with learning disabilities: legislative, taxonomic (ICD-10 and DSM-IV; both use mental retardation), needs based and politically acceptable terminology (Gates 1997). The drive for political correctness creates confusion when trying to develop service provision both locally and at a national strategic level (Emerson et al 1994).

Aetiological factors for learning disability are genetic disorders, congenital disorders, epilepsy, brain damage and social factors. The causative factors of conditions such as autism are less well known. The criminogenic relationships between specific disorders remain unclear, although low intelligence is likely to be a factor in many crimes (Gunn & Taylor 1993). Various studies have attempted to demonstrate a causal relationship between crime and epilepsy or chromosomal links, such as XYY. Other factors include poor literacy, communication, memory and general interpersonal skills (Murphy & Clare 1995). There is a small minority of patients with sensory deficits in secure care, including auditory and visual impairment (Dickens 1998). Special provision needs to be made for this group, the most cost-effective way being to commission outside specialist services when required, ensuring individuals receive support regardless of their location.

Many patients with mental impairment are at increased risk of mental health problems due to varying skill deficits, particularly in the areas of communication and relating to others, and this has a concomitant effect on the person's repertoire of problem solving skills (Murphy & Clare 1995). When working with this client group in a secure environment, it becomes apparent how professionals are expected to be multiskilled in managing learning disability, mental health and personality disorder, usually within one ward. The closure of many mental handicap institutions and the diminishing population of service users within secure care is gradually deskilling experienced RMNH nurses, as service users with challenging behaviours are being transferred to more diverse settings (Dickens 1998).

CARE AND TREATMENT ISSUES

Maden et al (1995) found that patients with learning disabilities in high security hospitals had a range of other psychiatric problems and their perceived therapeutic needs were thus not dissimilar to the needs of other patient groups, namely:

◆ nursing care
◆ medication
◆ occupational therapy
◆ escorted leave
◆ individual psychotherapy
◆ group psychotherapy
◆ behavioural treatments
◆ interaction with opposite sex
◆ sexual assessment.

The need for psychotherapy for this patient group was highlighted in particular.

Caring for people with learning disabilities in forensic mental health environments usually involves managing some form of challenging behaviour. This is a generic term that covers a multitude of behavioural deficits or ways in which the individual challenges the service. The service user group is often of mixed abilities with a varying range in cognitive abilities and understanding. The legal classification is made using the person's intelligence quotient but this may not reflect the person's social functioning. Some service users who have not had a functional education are often 'streetwise' and there can be a marked gap between their abilities and those of their fellow service users within an inpatient setting. A common problem is bullying, or stealing property and power struggles between patients for the status of 'top dog'.

The management of the mentally impaired in prisons is open to the same practical problems, in that they mix with more able individuals who may

prey upon them (Gunn & Taylor 1993). People with moderate learning disabilities can irritate others, exposing them to assault, and much of their management is in providing protection whilst trying to extinguish their 'nuisance' behaviours. There is a range of challenging behaviours, from severely challenging to moderately challenging, and these may fall into the following categories (Emerson et al 1994).

1. Severely challenging
   ◆ Physical aggression
   ◆ Self-harm
   ◆ Destroying property (own and others)
   ◆ Temper tantrums
   ◆ Wandering
   ◆ Antisocial behaviour
   ◆ Inappropriate sexual behaviour.

2. Moderately challenging
   ◆ Objectionable personal habits (e.g. regurgitating, eating or throwing faeces)
   ◆ Overactivity/hyperactivity
   ◆ Disturbing noises/speech
   ◆ Stereotypical behaviour.

There are two definitive areas where the learning disabled patient may not have challenging behaviours but the service user poses a serious and long-term danger to the public and these are arson and sexual offences. This category could be cared for in long-stay medium secure facilities, dependent on the level of risk they pose to the public, as they require only a limited number of staff but undoubtedly require constant supervision.

Offending in the learning disabled is usually the consequence of undersocialization, poor internal controls and faulty social learning; educational underachievement, lack of social and occupational skills and poor self-image are frequently additional factors (Day 1993). Cullen (1993: 146) suggests that:

It seems that poor self-control and an absence of more appropriate repertoires, together with behaviour which is under the control of immediate rather than longer term contingencies, are all at the core of the problem for many offenders with learning disabilities.

Other learning disabled patients within the forensic care system have not committed an offence but their level of violence and potential for property damage is so great that they require high staffing levels in order to manage them safely. Problems include stabbing carers, biting or just extreme violence, for which they have not been formally charged with a criminal offence. Managing these severe challenging behaviours is an area of expertise that requires not only high staffing numbers but highly skilled residential staff, who are supported by regular training in control and restraint and a well-structured controlled environment. A necessary adjunct to this type of service requires supportive mechanisms such as team building, debriefing sessions and 'me' time for all involved (Mason & Chandley 1999).

The aims of treatment are to assist maturation, facilitate adequate levels of self-control, instil a sense of personal worth and personal responsibility, establish acceptable social behaviour and improve social, occupational and educational skills (Day 1993).

Most learning disability units and medium secure facilities are not geared up to cope with severe challenging behaviour and the level of injuries caused by the service users results in some individuals filtering up to the high security hospital system. The current proposals to devolve responsibility for commissioning services for individuals who require forensic mental health services to regional levels will hopefully lead to more specialized community services, maintaining patients who pose challenging behaviours in less secure environments nearer their homes (Emerson & Hatton 1994, Felce et al 1998). Numerous research projects are emerging in the field of risk assessment in order to support such strategies, questioning the nature of accountability and levels of responsibility (Morgan 1998).

Mansell (1993) mapped out the future of learning disability care for those with challenging behaviour. He identified how mental health services tended to offer a generic institutional-type care, being almost a jack of all trades and a master of none. He suggested five key areas for developing good practice in the future development of specialized services for people with learning disabilities and challenging behaviour, which should essentially be centrally promoted by managers and needs led.

1. *Commitment.* Where senior managers need to be seen as 'developers' who promote long-term planning of specialized services rather than 'removers' who diminish such local services.

2. *Individualization.* Shaping services to meet the needs of service users, which will be identified through complex assessment profiling of the individual, such as functional analysis, research and evidence-based assessments and physiological investigations.

3. *Specialized services.* These should be shaped around the knowledge of the specific challenging behaviours presented by the individual and managed as a multidisciplinary team using the individualized research above.

4. *Good management.* First-line managers need to be effective in shaping the interventions put forward by the team, ensuring good team-working, clear communication between staff and a balance in the implementation of models of care between rigid structure and promoting autonomy. As the report says, the lives of the individual will often look 'quite ordinary'.

5. *Relationships and networking.* Working with challenging behaviour often means high stress levels for carers. Utilizing family members and care teams in the decision-making process is essential and can both ease pressure and provide support in the care process.

CONCLUSION

The future for secure provision for those with learning disability will be determined by a committee at local authority level, who will develop relationships with local trusts, medium secure units and high security hospitals to describe the developments of future services. The national learning disability strategy is being developed with input from 24 local authorities and their respective health authorities, where possible utilizing advisory and user groups. All finances will be channelled via these new fundholders and they will have the power to ensure a needs-led service and value for money for their client group. It is hoped that these approaches will break down the historical interorganizational barriers of moving patients from large institutions and into community-based services toward independent living (DoH 1999).

Networking across professional boundaries is also beginning to develop with interdisciplinary training and reinforcement of the care programme approach. One effective strategy has been the use of 'resettlement nurses', who specialize in networking between institutions across the secure care spectrum, smoothing the way for service user transfers and relocation. They are able to provide effective communication between care teams, arrange for caseworkers to meet up with clients and facilitate linkages for effective transfer of care programmes (Musker 1998).

There has been a slight backlash toward community care in that it is expensive and lacks resources and many have declared that it has failed (DoH 1998). This could result in policy makers moving toward the middle ground of developing small to large group homes for people with challenging behaviour. The lessons of other national projects, such as the All-Wales Strategy, NIMROD (New Ideas for the Care of Mentally Retarded in Ordinary Dwellings) and the AOL (An Ordinary Life) initiative, which explore planning and funding of services on a local level, are being learned.

Felce et al (1998) suggest that alternatives are feasible in well-organized and supported community services. It is important that there are enough places for those who come into contact with the criminal justice system, so that problems may be addressed at the court diversion stage or even before, rather than being warehoused in the criminal justice system. According to the Minister for Health John Hutton, such aspirations are apparent as he assures us that agencies are working together to ensure the principles of 'social inclusion, citizenship and ordinary community living' for service users with a learning disability.

The challenges for the future suggest that the numbers of people with learning disabilities requiring high security services are minimal yet the national focus of Rampton Hospital for this group remains. Could these services be relocated without losing the developed expertise in the management of this group?

The use of different labelling systems may affect the way that services are planned and care is delivered. The management of this group of people at a more local level will challenge the ingenuity and skills of the professions involved.

REFERENCES

Craft A 1987 Mental handicap and sexuality: issues and perspectives. Costello, Kent

Cullen C 1993 The treatment of people with learning disabilities who offend. In: Howells K, Hollin CR (eds) Clinical approaches to the mentally disordered offender. Wiley, London

Day K 1993 Crime and mental retardation: a review. In: Howells K, Hollin CR (eds) Clinical approaches to the mentally disordered offender. Wiley, London

Department of Health 1998 Modernising mental health services: safe, sound and supportive. Department of Health, London

Department of Health 1999 Learning disability strategy: letter from John Hutton. MISC (99)(56). Department of Health, London

Department of Health, Home Office 1992 Review of health and social services for mentally disordered offenders and others requiring similar services (Reed Committee). Cm 2088. HMSO, London

Department of Health and Social Security 1974 Revised report of the working party on security in NHS psychiatric hospitals (Glancy Report). DHSS, London

Dickens D 1998 Learning disability in the special hospitals. In: Kaye C, Franey A (eds) Managing high security psychiatric care. Jessica Kingsley, London, pp 123–135

Emerson E, Hatton C 1994 Moving out: relocation from hospital to community. HMSO, London

Emerson E, Barrett S, Bell C et al 1987 Developing services for people with severe learning difficulties and challenging behaviours. Institute of Social and Applied Psychology, University of Kent, Canterbury

Emerson E, McGill P, Mansell J 1994 Severe learning disabilities and challenging behaviours. Chapman and Hall, London

Felce D, Grant G, Todd S et al 1998 Towards a full life: researching policy innovation for people with learning disabilities. Butterworth Heinemann, Oxford

Gates B 1997 What is learning disability: a question of semantics or political correctness. Journal of Learning Disability 1(2): 51–52

Gunn J, Taylor PJ 1993 Forensic psychiatry: clinical, legal and ethical issues. Butterworth Heinemann, London

Halstead SM, Cassidy L 1994 Assessment of need for services for mentally disordered offenders and others with similar needs in South West Thames Regional Health Authority: learning disability (mental handicap). Survey of detained patients by county and by District Health Authority. St George's Hospital Medical School, London

Home Office, Department of Health and Social Security 1975 Report of the Committee on Mentally Abnormal Offenders. Cm 6244. HMSO, London

Maden A, Curle C, Meux CJ, Burrow S, Gunn J 1995 The treatment and security needs of special hospital patients. Whurr, London

Mansell JL 1993 Services for people with learning disabilities and challenging behaviour or mental health needs. HMSO, London

Mason J 1999 Responding to people with learning disabilities in the probation service. British Journal of Forensic Practice 1(2): 16–21

Mason T, Chandley M 1999 Management of violence and aggression for nurses and healthcare workers. Churchill Livingstone, Edinburgh

Morgan S 1998 Assessing and managing risk. Pavillion Publishing, Brighton

Murphy GH, Clare ICH 1995 Capacity to make decisions affecting the person. In: Bull R, Carson D (eds) Psychology in legal contexts. Wiley, Chichester, pp 97–128

Musker M 1998 Implementing the care programme approach. In: Thompson T, Mathias P (eds) Standards and learning disability. Baillière Tindall, London

National Health Service Executive 1998 Health services for people with learning disabilities. HSC EL(98)3. NHS Executive, London

Special Hospitals Service Authority 1995 Service strategies for secure care. SHSA, London

Stone JH, Roberts M, O'Grady J, Taylor AV, O'Shea K 2000 Faulk's basic forensic psychiatry, 3rd edn. Blackwell Science, Oxford

Turk J 1989 Forensic aspects of mental handicap. British Journal of Psychiatry 155: 591–594

Woods P, Mason T 1998 Mental impairment and admission to a Special Hospital. British Journal of Developmental Disabilities 44(87): 119–131

FURTHER READING

Emerson E, McGill P, Mansell J 1994 Severe learning disabilities and challenging behaviours. Chapman and Hall, London

Gunn J, Taylor PJ 1993 Forensic psychiatry: clinical, legal and ethical issues. Butterworth Heinemann, London

Maden A, Curle C, Meux CJ, Burrow S, Gunn J 1995 The treatment and security needs of special hospital patients. Whurr, London

Stone JH, Roberts M, O'Grady J, Taylor AV, O'Shea K 2000 Faulk's basic forensic psychiatry, 3rd edn. Blackwell Science, Oxford

Chapter Sixteen

Personality disorders

Phil Woods

INTRODUCTION

There is little doubt that of all the diagnoses, personality disorder raises more emotions within forensic mental health professionals than most others. Some professionals are convinced the disorder is untreatable, whilst others believe that it is; others even believe that its association should be removed from mental disorder. This chapter will explore the epidemiology of personality disorder within forensic services, both prisons and secure mental health units; diagnostic issues, encompassing assessment and measurement; care and treatment issues within the interpersonal context. Underpinning the chapter will be current research and development, in which the author is an active participant through the national forensic mental health research and development programme.

Within the UK personality disorder diagnosis is clouded by the legal category of psychopathic disorder. The Mental Health Act 1983 defines psychopathic disorder as: 'a persistent disorder or disability of mind (whether or not including significant impairment of intelligence) which results in abnormally aggressive or severely irresponsible conduct'.

Psychopathic disorder has three meanings: first, it is a legal classification, as noted above; second, it is a clinical diagnostic construct or category in some classifications; and third, in the vernacular it is a term of derogation (Moran 1999: xi) and has become associated with fear and trepidation in the eyes of the lay person. It has also acquired a disparaging overtone in clinical work, particularly when a patient is identified as 'a psychopath' or as 'psychopathic', with the implication that the patient is untreatable. The term has survived increasingly widespread criticism as recorded in many official reports and professional publications and has attracted cogent arguments for its replacement. More recently, the review of the Mental Health Act 1983 calls for its replacement by the term 'personality disorder' (DoH 1999: 3). Notwithstanding this debate, however, the term 'psychopathy' remains and is closely associated with the diagnostic classifications of antisocial personality disorder and dissocial personality disorder.

DEMOGRAPHICS

Any forensic mental health service, whether in the health or social care sectors or criminal justice system, will find a high proportion of its population has one or more personality disorder. Moreover, many patients diagnosed with a mental illness have co-morbid personality disorder. As personality disorder within the UK is clouded by the legal classification of psychopathic disorder this makes it difficult to be clear about the extent of the problem, with many researchers referring to legal classification, others personality disorder and yet others to both.

The most recently published review of the prevalence rate of personality disorders within forensic services is that by Moran (1999). However, this review was specifically commissioned to report on the prevalence of antisocial personality disorder and its diagnostic equivalents of psychopathy, sociopathy and dissocial personality disorder, the most frequently occurring and studied of all the personality disorders in forensic services.

Studies have repeatedly shown that a high percentage of any forensic population can be expected to fulfil formal diagnostic criteria for one or more personality disorders. Within a representative 5% sample of the sentenced male prison population, Gunn et al (1991) found the prevalence rate of personality disorder to be 10%. Singleton et al (1998), in the most recent survey of psychiatric morbidity amongst prisoners, report a high prevalence of personality disorder: for the male remand 78%, for the male sentenced 64% and for female prisoners (both remand and sentenced collectively) 50%. Further, they report antisocial personality disorder as having the highest prevalence rate: 63%, 49% and 31% respectively.

In relation to the remand population in the UK, Bowden (1978) found a prevalence rate of 12% for psychopathic disorder and 24% for personality disorder; Taylor & Gunn (1984) found a 13.8% prevalence rate for personality disorder; Dell et al (1991) found a 17% prevalence rate for psychopathic disorder; Watt et al (1993) found a 13% prevalence of personality disorder; and Birmingham et al (1996) a 7% personality disorder prevalence rate.

Within high security hospitals, Mbatia & Tyrer (1988), in a sample of 103 consecutive admissions, judged 77% to have a personality disorder. Maden et al (1995) found 24% with a primary diagnosis of personality disorder. Based on 1990 figures of all four high security hospitals, Hamilton (1990) reported an overall rate for psychopathic disorder of 24%. Blackburn et al (1990) reported that 68% of their sample met the criteria for at least one personality disorder and only 12% displayed an absence of deviant personality traits. Thompson et al (1997), in a study at the State Hospital Carstairs, found that 5.4% had a primary diagnosis of antisocial personality disorder. Smith et al (1991) examining female admissions to a regional secure unit found that 33% were said to be personality disordered.

DIAGNOSTIC ISSUES

An effective diagnosis has to be based on systematic assessment. Personality disorder research has predominantly focused on assessment, examining the numerous self-report and interview schedules which assist in the classification of personality disorders (e.g. Clark et al 1997, Maffei et al 1997, Perry 1992, Zimmerman 1994). Comparisons are frequently made with the current diagnostic categories or the factor structures of abnormal and normal personality (e.g. Blais & Norman 1997, Livesley et al 1994, Parker 1998, Strack & Lorr 1997).

Moran (1999: 2) comments on how, by their very nature, the personality disorders present a multitude of measurement problems, as they are diagnosed in an interpersonal context and are almost totally dependent on the characteristic patterns of social interaction. Grubin & Duggan (1998) indicate that a core assessment battery of instruments should relate to specific treatment targets (pre- and posttest), e.g. diagnosis, impulsivity, hostility, empathy, defence style and additional, more specific instruments are available to address arson, sex offending and self-harm. Meux & McDonald (1998) suggest that assessment is the gatekeeper to treatment (and often the progress through it) and it should assist in determining treatability. There is general agreement that current assessment methods are probably inadequate and that assessment cannot be separated from treatment issues. Meux & McDonald (1998) make some key points:

> It is important to use both dimensional and categorical approaches; it should involve multidisciplinary collaboration; assessment methods should provide vertical descriptions of disorder within the individual (biological; cognitive; behavioural; and social issues) as well as protective factors (intrapersonal and environmental factors) and Axis I co-morbidity; as interview, observation and history are the most reliable forms of assessment these should form the bulk of the process.

It is important that hypothesis generation through assessment should include aetiology (predisposing factors) – any variable that may have made the individual vulnerable to develop the problem; precipitating events – any specific trigger event which appears to generate the problem; and maintaining factors. Turkat & Maisto (1985) indicate that the modification of social behaviour involves four key areas which are specific to assessment: social attention, information processing, response emission and feedback.

Dolan & Coid (1993: 278) suggest a standard assessment of psychopathic disorder, recommending a two-dimensional conceptualization of psychopathic disorder consisting of personality disorder, clinical syndromes and behavioural disorder. First, for the assessment of personality disorder, they recommend use of one or both of the following: standardized diagnostic approaches or structured clinical interview. Second, for the assessment of clinical syndromes (axis I) they recommend: a detailed psychiatric history of all major mental disorder, paraphilias and substance abuse; and inclusion of a lifetime perspective, age of onset and any time of resolution for any of the symptoms. Third, for behavioural disorder, they recommend a detailed assessment in relation to culturally determined norms of: criminal history; non-criminalized antisocial/aggressive behaviours; the ability to form and maintain relationships; and occupational functioning. They suggest a longitudinal approach to record the time of appearance and

resolution of different forms of behaviour disorder. Nurses can contribute significantly to the latter.

Widiger & Frances (1994: 34) indicate that clinicians who use the five factor model (FFM) will be able to provide a reasonably comprehensive description of adaptive as well as maladaptive traits. The FFM includes: neuroticism; extraversion; openness to experience; agreeableness; and conscientiousness (Digman 1990).

One of the main problems inherent in the diagnosis of personality disorder is whether or not a dimensional or a categorical approach should be used. However, in the absence of any answer to this vigorous academic theoretical debate, personality disorders are diagnosed either through the Diagnostic and Statistical Manual of Mental Disorders (DSM-IV) (American Psychiatric Association 1994) or the International Classification of Disease 10 (ICD-10) (World Health Organization 1992).

DSM-IV

The American Psychiatric Association (1994) developed a multiaxial system to assist clinicians to plan treatment and predict outcome. There are five axes included in the DSM-IV.

- ◆ Axis I. Clinical disorders and other conditions that may be a focus of clinical attention
- ◆ Axis II. Personality disorders and mental retardation
- ◆ Axis III. General medical conditions
- ◆ Axis IV. Psychosocial and environmental problems
- ◆ Axis V. Global assessment of functioning

The diagnosis of personality disorders according to DSM-IV (p 630) requires an evaluation of the individual's long-term patterns of functioning and the particular personality features must be evident by early adulthood. The personality traits that define these disorders must also be distinguished from characteristics that emerge in response to specific situational stressors or more transient mental states.

The clinician should assess the stability of the personality traits over time and across different situations. Although a single interview with the person is sometimes sufficient for making the diagnosis, it is often necessary to conduct more than one interview and to space these over time. Assessment may also be complicated by the fact that the individual may not consider the characteristics that define a personality disorder to be problematic. To help overcome this difficulty, supplementary information from other informants may be helpful.

The DSM-IV manual lists general diagnostic criteria for a personality disorder as follows.

◆ An enduring pattern of inner experience and behaviour that deviates markedly from the expectations of the individual's culture. This pattern is manifested in two (or more) of the following areas: cognition (i.e. ways of perceiving and interpreting self, other people and events); affectivity (i.e. the range, intensity, lability and appropriateness of emotional response); interpersonal functioning; impulse control.

◆ The enduring pattern is inflexible and pervasive across a broad range of personal and social situations.

◆ The enduring pattern leads to clinically significant distress or impairment in social, occupational or other important areas of functioning.

◆ The pattern is stable and of long duration and its onset can be traced back at least to adolescence or early adulthood.

◆ The enduring pattern is not better accounted for as a manifestation or consequence of another mental disorder.

◆ The enduring pattern is not due to the direct physiological effects of a substance (e.g. a drug of abuse, a medication) or a general medical condition (e.g. head trauma).

DSM-IV describes 10 specific personality disorders grouped into three clusters based on descriptive similarities.

◆ Cluster A – includes paranoid, schizoid and schizotypal personality disorders.
◆ Cluster B – includes antisocial, borderline, histrionic and narcissistic personality disorders.
◆ Cluster C – includes avoidant, dependent and obsessive-compulsive personality disorder.
◆ There is also personality disorder not otherwise specified.

ICD-10

ICD-10 classifies personality disorders to include a variety of clinically significant conditions and behaviours, each of which is classified according to clusters of traits which correspond to the most frequent or conspicuous behaviour manifestations. General diagnostic guidelines are given as:

Conditions not directly attributable to gross brain damage or disease or to another psychiatric disorder, meeting the following criteria: markedly disharmonious attitudes and behaviour, involving usually several areas of functioning, e.g. affectivity, arousal, impulse control, ways of perceiving and thinking, and style of relating to others; the abnormal behaviour pattern is enduring, of long standing, and not limited to episodes of mental illness; the abnormal behaviour pattern is pervasive and clearly maladaptive to a broad range of personal and social situations; the above manifestations always appear during childhood or adolescence and continue into adulthood; the disorder leads to considerable personal distress but this may only become apparent late in its course; the disorder is usually, but not invariably, associated with significant problems in occupational and social performance.

ICD-10 classifies personality disorders into 10 specific categories.

◆ Paranoid personality disorder
◆ Schizoid personality disorder
◆ Dissocial personality disorder
◆ Emotionally unstable personality disorder (either impulsive or borderline type)
◆ Histrionic personality disorder
◆ Anankastic personality disorder
◆ Anxious (avoidant) personality disorder
◆ Dependent personality disorder
◆ Other specific personality disorders
◆ Personality disorder, unspecified

Hare's Psychopathy Checklist (PCL – Revised)

The most widely used measure of psychopathy is the Hare Psychopathy Checklist (Hare 1991). Hare took 16 criteria, first delineated by Cleckley

(1941), as characteristic in the diagnosis of psychopathy and, with further refinement, developed a 20-item checklist consisting of characteristic traits found typically in psychopathy and which can be used in making a diagnosis according to Hare's scheme.

1. Glibness/superficial charm
2. Grandiose sense of self-worth
3. Need for stimulation/proneness to boredom
4. Pathological lying
5. Conning/manipulative
6. Lack of remorse or guilt
7. Shallow affect
8. Callous/lack of empathy
9. Parasitic lifestyle
10. Poor behavioural controls
11. Promiscuous sexual behaviour
12. Early behaviour problems
13. Lack of realistic long-term goals
14. Impulsivity
15. Irresponsibility
16. Failure to accept responsibility for actions
17. Many short-term marital relationships
18. Juvenile delinquency
19. Revocation of conditional release
20. Criminal versatility

The checklist is scored on a simple 0, 1, 2 rating depending on whether the characteristic is not present, whether it is partially present or whether the description is fully met. A scoring of 30+ is required for a diagnosis of psychopathy (Storey et al 1997). This classification is particularly useful for research purposes and for determining severity. The items are a compromise between what the patient self-reports and what the clinician observes about this behaviour. There are other classifications and typologies of importance and they are discussed in detail in the book by Dolan & Coid (1993).

CARE AND TREATMENT ISSUES

There is little argument that any treatment of personality disorder has to focus on the behavioural repertoires manifested as a result of the disorder. Many of these are antisocial or challenging and

have been well established since early childhood. A number of risk factors have been identified in relation to the development of personality disorder and Moran (1999) discusses these in relation to childhood conduct disorder; childhood hyperactivity; delinquency; childhood temperament; childhood victimization; and coercive child rearing. Dolan & Coid (1993) report that research has demonstrated that those who show conduct disorder in childhood and poor peer relationships and who come from disordered and deprived family backgrounds, with parents displaying mental illness, criminality and abusive behaviour, are more likely to have personality disorder in adulthood. They extensively discuss all these natural history issues and the reader is recommended to read this text.

Treatment in a forensic setting has to focus on the reduction of risk or dangerousness and must aim at reducing this and/or offending behaviour. Melia (1997), discussing 'boundaries and interrelatedness: practice issues within the personality disorder service' within the Ashworth Hospital Authority response to the Fallon Inquiry, highlights a number of behavioural deficits in relation to patient behaviour, all of these relating to personality and dysfunctional relationships:

Often with personality disorders relationships are emotionally intense, with social interaction often occurring in corrupted or exploitative ways. Anger and hostility are high, with the added burden of expecting to be harmed, exploited or let down. Rejection or abuse is anticipated and loyalties are tested. There is preoccupation with the protection of self, with little concern for the feelings of others or concern for future consequences. There appears to be no capacity to experience guilt or to profit from experience, indeed, often they feel justified in having hurt or mistreated others and shift responsibility for own actions, through blame. They constantly invite collusion from others, cross boundaries, use splitting and secrets, or claim specific staff victimization. (Melia 1997)

This description paints a bleak picture yet arises from years of clinical experience working with the most difficult patient group to engage in therapeutic activity.

Links (1996) indicates how the focus of assessment and its related treatment should be on three areas: self-determination; role functioning; and the clinician maintaining hope. Grubin & Duggan (1998) comment that treatment issues should focus on individual functioning, specific symptoms and behaviours or more distant outcomes, i.e. offending. The most comprehensive review to date of the treatment of psychopathy and antisocial personality disorders is by Dolan & Coid (1993). In summary, this concluded that there was little evidence of sufficient methodological quality to suggest that any particular approach to treatment was effective. Isolated pockets of research are now under way but as yet the situation has not changed.

Allnutt & Links (1996: 23) suggest that it is clinically useful to consider behavioural deficits of the personality disorders from the viewpoint of their DSM-IV criteria. First, for antisocial, these are criminal, aggressive, impulsive and irresponsible behaviours. Second, for avoidant, this is the avoidance of any occupational activity which may involve interpersonal contact. This avoids the possibility of their greatest fear, which is of criticism, disapproval or rejection. Third, for borderline, this is their frantic avoidance of either imagined or real abandonment. Fourth is dependent, where others need to be responsible for their major areas of living. Fifth, for histrionic, they may be uncomfortable in interpersonal situations where they are not the centre of attention. Sixth is narcissistic, where there is a grandiose sense of self-importance. Seventh, obsessive-compulsive, where perfectionism is seen to interfere with daily living. Eighth is paranoid, where ideas that others are exploiting, harming or deceiving are apparent. Ninth is schizoid, where there is no desire for or enjoyment of close relationships. Tenth is schizotypal where behaviour, speech, appearance or thinking is eccentric or peculiar.

Guy & Hume (1998) discuss how the DSM-IV general criteria for personality disorders as enduring patterns of inner experience and behaviour manifest in two or more of the following areas: cognition (ways of perceiving and interpreting self, others or events); affect (range of, intensity, lability and appropriateness of emotional response); interpersonal functioning; and impulse control.

Psychotherapeutics and cognitive and behavioural approaches underpin most of the treatment given to personality-disordered individuals. Underpinning psychotherapeutics is the psychodynamic approach to therapy, where emphasis is placed on the individual's personality structure and development and therapy is aimed at developing understanding and insight into feelings and addressing maladaptive defence mechanisms. Dolan & Coid (1993) indicate poor outcome with individual and outpatient psychotherapy and more success with group and inpatient psychotherapy.

Cognitive and behavioural approaches are perhaps the most widely used at present in forensic services. These programmes usually offer a skills- or social skills-based approach to therapy. Behavioural therapy has been shown to be more successful but this only addresses current environmental antecedents and consequences of behaviour. Cognitive-behavioural approaches question an individual's maladaptive irrational thoughts and provide new cognitions to replace these. Cognitive therapy works at a dual level of manifested behavioural problems and inferred schema. Moreover, according to Andrews et al (1990), Antonowicz & Ross (1994), Hollin (1993) and Tennant et al (1999), effective treatment must include:

- a sound theoretical base
- multifaceted programming
- an individualized assessment of need
- targeting of criminogenic needs
- use of active and structured behavioural and social learning techniques
- modelling of prosocial attitudes
- a cognitive-behavioural emphasis inclusive of social cognitive skills training.

Tennant et al (1999) describe a behavioural approach to treating personality disorders, based around developing trust and a therapeutic relationship, employing the multidisciplinary assessment, focusing on symptoms and offending behaviours. More specifically, the approach involves: a functional assessment of problem- and offence-related behaviours; assessment using the Hare Psychopathy Checklist; standardized psychiatric assessment (e.g. impulsivity, empathy, sexual interest, aggression, blame); pre- and posttest intervention psychological measures (e.g. sexual offending, arson, anger management); and monitoring and recording of behaviours.

It is beyond the scope of this chapter to provide comprehensive accounts of the treatment methods currently being tried with personality disorders.

Stowell-Smith (2000) provides insight into psychodynamic psychotherapy, personality disorder and offending; Jones (2000) describes the therapeutic community in a forensic setting; McGuire (2000) covers problem-solving training with secure hospital patients; and Jackson & Martin (2000) report on relating neurological and neuropsychological deficits to antisocial personality and offending behaviour.

Dolan & Coid (1993) report that overwhelmingly, studies have found high recidivism rates for psychopathic and personality disorder and even more so when untreated.

Few studies have examined the situation for people with a personality disorder following discharge. Those studies that do exist report on rates of reconviction (recidivism). Cope & Ward (1993) examined all those discharged from high security hospitals to medium secure units in the West Midlands between 1981 and 1991. Of these, 31% had been returned to a high security hospital and a further 8% had been convicted of offences following community discharge. For men with a personality disorder, the main reasons for return were concern about danger to the public and no evidence of change.

Bailey & MacCulloch (1992a, b) studied discharges from Park Lane high security hospital directly into the community between 1979 and 1984. Reconvictions were examined over a follow-up period which varied for individual cases from 6 months to 14 years. The study reports the rates for both overall reconviction and reconviction for serious offences (which the authors define as murder, manslaughter, attempted murder, kidnapping, abduction, rape, indecent assault, robbery or arson). The reconviction rate for

mental illness was 21% overall and 10% for serious offences. For those with a legal classification of psychopathy, the rates were 55% overall and 26% for serious offences.

Bailey & MacCulloch also reported an association with absolute discharges as opposed to conditional discharges from their detention where for those with a psychopathic disorder, there was a 79% reconviction rate overall and a 36% reconviction rate for serious offences.

It can be seen from these studies that those people with a primary diagnosis of personality disorder are more likely to reoffend following discharge and are particularly likely to do so if not subject to some form of supervision.

CURRENT RESEARCH AND DEVELOPMENT

The High Security Psychiatric Services Commissioning Board (1997) report of the conference entitled 'Into the millennium: the future agenda for research and development into personality disorder' has been the driving force for the national strategy for personality disorder research and development. Within the report, the development of a shared paradigm or framework is considered to be essential to the research agenda, as it will permit some commonality of understanding. The paradigm is specifically underpinned by the recently developed Virtual Institute for Severe Personality Disorder (VISPED). This institute was felt to be critical as one of the key research questions, in relation to assessment and diagnostic criteria, was sufficiently complex to require a group of academics to develop it further.

Specifically, the research prioritized: longitudinal cohort studies; development of instruments for assessment; randomized controlled trials to elicit outcomes on a number of areas, including health/social/quality of life/criminal justice; staff support measures; evaluation of settings where those with severe personality disorder are managed.

More recently, the Home Office & Department of Health (1999) document *Managing dangerous people with severe personality disorder: proposals for policy development* highlighted a number of key research and development issues. It states that there is further work to be done in relation to: risk assessment and management; evidence-based approach; and dissemination and implementation of research. The main problem highlighted is poor research methodologies, which do not allow for comparisons to be made between similar studies. This is partly owing to different definitions and criteria used for personality disorder, small sample sizes and lack of follow-up. Further, it states that not enough is known about: the incidence of anti-social personality disorder; the population prevalence, in primary care, general psychiatric settings and in other settings; protective factors; natural history of the disorder; effectiveness of interventions, outcomes and models of staff support; and the natural history of an individual with antisocial personality disorder. Particular interventions which need to be evaluated are: dialectic behaviour therapy; cognitive therapy for antisocial personality disorder, which focuses on specific behaviours which are directly linked to personality disturbance; and other psychological approaches.

The discussion document highlights research and development priorities as:

◆ research to underpin the development of new service approaches to the assessment, management, follow-up in the community and outcomes
◆ evaluation of applying a systematic battery of assessment and risk assessment tools, and new definitions
◆ research to gauge the effectiveness of interventions through randomized trials
◆ staff support interventions
◆ evaluation of new and current settings where people with dangerous severe personality disorder are managed.

CONCLUSION

Personality disorders manifest in a variety of behavioural repertoires, which challenge the clinician who has to provide care and treatment and determine when risk and dangerousness have diminished. Personality disorder, and the related concept of psychopathy, often defy true assessment and measurement. Although research and development is high on the UK government agenda of public protection through development of more effective ways of managing the more dangerous and severely personality disordered, results of studies will take considerable time to be integrated into practice.

Thus, until such time as either forensic mental health professionals are able to accurately speculate to effectively determine future behaviours or effective methods of treatment are found which actually reduce risk or dangerousness in the long term, personality-disordered individuals will continue to stretch the imagination and resources of forensic mental health services.

REFERENCES

Allnutt S, Links PS 1996 Diagnosing specific personality disorders and the optimal criteria. In: Links P (ed) Clinical assessment and management of severe personality disorders. American Psychiatric Press, Washington, ch 2, pp 21–47

American Psychiatric Association 1994 Diagnostic and statistical manual of mental disorders, 4th edn. (DSM-IV) APA, Washington

Andrews DA, Zinger I, Hodge RD et al 1990 Does correctional treatment work? A clinically relevant and psychologically informed meta-analysis. Criminology 28: 369–404

Antonowicz DH, Ross RR 1994 Essential components of successful rehabilitation programmes for offenders. International Journal of Offender Therapy and Comparative Criminology 38: 97–104

Bailey J, MacCulloch M 1992a Characteristics of 112 cases discharged directly to the community from a new special hospital and some comparisons of performance. Journal of Forensic Psychiatry 3: 91–112

Bailey J, MacCulloch M 1992b Patterns of re-conviction in patients discharged to the community from a special hospital. Journal of Forensic Psychiatry 3: 445–461

Birmingham L, Mason D, Grubin D 1996 Prevalence of mental disorder in remand prisoners: consecutive case study. British Medical Journal 313: 1521–1524

Blackburn R, Crellin MC, Morgan EM, Tulloch RMB 1990 Prevalence of personality disorder in a special hospital population. Journal of Forensic Psychiatry 1(1): 43–52

Blais MA, Norman DK 1997 A psychometric evaluation of the DSM-IV personality disorder criteria. Journal of Personality Disorders 11(2): 168–176

Bowden P 1978 Men remanded into custody for medical reports: the selection for treatment. British Journal of Psychiatry 133: 320–331

Clark L, Livesley WJ, Morey L 1997 Personality disorder assessment: the challenge of construct validity. Journal of Personality Disorders 11(3): 205–231

Cleckley H 1941 The mask of sanity. Mosby, St Louis

Cope R, Ward M 1993 What happens to Special Hospital patients admitted to medium security? Journal of Forensic Psychiatry 4: 13–24

Dell S, Grounds A, James K et al 1991 Mentally disordered remand prisoners: report to the Home Office. Home Office, London

Department of Health 1999 Review of the Mental Health Act 1983: report of the expert committee. Stationery Office, London

Digman JM 1990 Personality structure: emergence of the five-factor model. Annual Review of Psychology 44: 417–440

Dolan B, Coid J 1993 Psychopathic and antisocial personality disorders: treatment and research issues. Gaskell, London

Grubin D, Duggan C 1998 Staff support and interventions. High Security Psychiatric Services Commissioning Board, London

Gunn J, Maden A, Swinton M 1991 Treatment needs of prisoners with psychiatric disorders. British Medical Journal 303: 338–341

Guy S, Hume A 1998 A CBT strategy for offenders with personality disorders: part one. Mental Health Practice 2(4): 12–16

Hamilton J 1990 Special hospitals and the state hospital. In: Bluglass R, Bowden P (eds) Principles and practice of forensic psychiatry. Churchill Livingstone, Edinburgh, pp 1363–1373

Hare RD 1991 Manual for the Hare Psychopathy Checklist Revised. Multi-Health Systems, Toronto

High Security Psychiatric Services Commissioning Board 1997 Into the millennium: the future agenda for research and development into personality disorder. High Security Psychiatric Services Commissioning Board, London

Hollin C 1993 Advances in psychological treatment of delinquent behaviour. Criminal Behaviour and Mental Health 3: 142–157

Home Office, Department of Health 1999 Managing dangerous people with severe personality disorder: proposals for policy development. Stationery Office, London

Jackson H, Martin J 2000 Relating neurological and neuropsychological deficits to antisocial personality and offending behaviour. In: Mercer D, Mason T, McKeown M, McCann G (eds) Forensic mental health care: a case study approach. Churchill Livingstone, Edinburgh, ch 10, pp 279–292

Jones L 2000 Therapeutic community in a forensic setting. In: Mercer D, Mason T, McKeown M, McCann G (eds) Forensic mental health care: a case study approach. Churchill Livingstone, Edinburgh, ch 10, pp 263–268

Links P 1996 Clinical assessment and management of severe personality disorders. American Psychiatric Press, Washington

Livesley WJ, Schroeder ML, Jackson DN, Jang KL 1994 Categorical distinctions in the study of personality disorder: implications for classification. Journal of Abnormal Psychology 103(1): 6–17

Maden T, Curle C, Meux C, Burrow S, Gunn J 1995 Treatment and security needs of special hospital patients. Whurr, London

Maffei C, Fossati A, Agostoni I et al 1997 Interrater reliability and internal consistency of the structured clinical interview for DSM-IV Axis II personality disorders (SCID-II), version 2.0. Journal of Personality Disorders 11(3): 279–284

Mbatia J, Tyrer P 1988 Personality status of dangerous patients at a special hospital. In: Tyrer P (ed) Personality disorders: diagnosis, management and course. Wright, London, pp 105–111

McGuire J 2000 Problem-solving training: pilot work with secure hospital patients. In: Mercer D, Mason T, McKeown M, McCann G (eds) Forensic mental health care: a case study approach. Churchill Livingstone, Edinburgh, ch 10, pp 269–277

Melia P 1997 Boundaries and inter-relatedness: practice issues within the PD service. Ashworth Hospital Authority response to the Fallon Inquiry. Ashworth Hospital, Liverpool

Meux C, McDonald B 1998 Assessment and diagnostic criteria. High Security Psychiatric Services Commissioning Board, London

Moran P 1999 Anti-social personality disorder: an epidemiological perspective. Gaskell, London

Parker G 1998 Personality disorders as alien territory: classification, measurement and border issues. Current Opinion in Psychiatry 11: 125–129

Perry JC 1992 Problems and considerations in the valid assessment of personality disorders. American Journal of Psychiatry 149(12): 1645–1653

Singleton N, Meltzer H, Gatward R, Coid J, Deasy D 1998 Psychiatric morbidity among prisoners in England and Wales. Stationery Office, London

Smith J, Parker J, Donovan M 1991 Female admissions to a regional secure unit. Journal of Forensic Psychiatry 2(1): 95–102

Storey L, Dale C, Martin E 1997 Social therapy: a developing model of care for people with personality disorders. Nursing Times Research 2(3): 210–218

Stowell-Smith M 2000 Psychodynamic psychotherapy, personality disorder and offending. In: Mercer D, Mason T, McKeown M, McCann G (eds) Forensic mental health care: a case study approach. Churchill Livingstone, Edinburgh, ch 10, pp 251–256

Strack S, Lorr M 1997 The challenge of differentiating normal and disordered personality. Journal of Personality Disorders 11(2): 105–122

Taylor PJ, Gunn J 1984 Violence and psychosis. I: risk of violence among psychotic men. British Medical Journal 288: 1945–1949

Tennant A, Davies C, Tennant I 1999 Working with the personality disordered offender. In: Chaloner C, Coffey M (eds) Forensic mental health nursing: current approaches. Blackwell Science, Oxford, ch 6, pp 94–117

Thompson L, Bogue J, Humphreys M, Owens D, Johnstone E 1997 The state hospital survey: a description of psychiatric patients in conditions of special security in Scotland. Journal of Forensic Psychiatry 8(2): 263–284

Turkat ID, Maisto SA 1985 Personality disorders: application of the experimental method to the formulation and modification of personality disorders.

In: Barlow DH (ed) Clinical handbook of psychological disorders. Guilford Press, New York

Watt F, Tomison A, Torpy D 1993 The prevalence of psychiatric disorder in a male remand population: a pilot study. Journal of Forensic Psychiatry 4: 75–83

Widiger TA, Frances A 1994 Personality disorders and the five-factor model of personality. American Psychological Association, Washington

World Health Organization 1992 The ICD-10 classification of mental and behavioural disorders: clinical descriptions and diagnostic guidelines. WHO, Geneva

Zimmerman M 1994 Diagnosing personality disorders: a review of issues and research methods. Archives of General Psychiatry 51: 225–245

FURTHER READING

Blackburn R 1993 The psychology of criminal conduct: theory, research and practice. Wiley, Chichester

Dolan B, Coid J 1993 Psychopathic and antisocial personality disorders: treatment and research issues. Gaskell, London

Links P 1996 Clinical assessment and management of severe personality disorders. American Psychiatric Press, Washington

Moran P 1999 Anti-social personality disorder: an epidemiological perspective. Gaskell, London

Tyrer P, Stein G 1993 Personality disorder reviewed. Gaskell, London

Chapter Seventeen

Women in secure care

Les Storey   Debbie Murdock

INTRODUCTION

The Standing Nursing and Midwifery Advisory Council (1999) cited several reports that have expressed disquiet about the environment in acute psychiatric facilities. *Working in partnership* (DoH 1994) recommended an urgent review of the therapeutic suitability of district general hospital mental health units. Meanwhile, concern exists that patients often do not have sufficient privacy, nor are they guaranteed the therapeutic and recreational facilities that are a necessary part of good care and treatment. There is clear evidence that women are particularly disadvantaged with regard to both privacy and safety.

The Nursing in Secure Environments report (UKCC & University of Central Lancashire 1999) supports these views, recommending that 'there should be due recognition and evaluation of current service provision for clients from all minority groups, particularly those from ethnic minorities and women, to ensure that their health and other needs are identified and met in secure environments'.

Women with mental health problems, learning disabilities or personality disorder are a minority in forensic mental health environments (15–20%) but their voices still need to be listened to. In 1999 the National Health Service Executive commissioned a group to listen to women throughout the United Kingdom, with a view to collating responses and ensuring they shape a strategy for women in mental health services, which includes secure environments. The group was led by Dame Renée Fritchie and addressed a range of pertinent issues. When representatives of the group visited Rampton Hospital, they were told by several women that if services had been different at medium secure level, they did not believe that their psychiatric careers would have led them to high security mental health care.

Thus, a national strategy is urgently required to coordinate action and drive forward change. The absence of a national strategy is significant when examining why recommendations from robust research studies have been left to gather dust on shelves. Local policies are all well and good when applied to local practice but when considering the needs of women in secure settings, a global view of development is essential.

DEMOGRAPHICS

The patients who reside in the range of secure units throughout the country are a very disparate group. Patients with mental health and learning disabilities include adults who:

◆ have not committed an offence but whose behaviour brings them to the attention of the police
◆ have not committed an offence but whose illness or behaviour leads to their being detained under the Mental Health Acts, sometimes in secure facilities
◆ have committed a minor offence but whose primary need is for mental health services and whom it is not in the public interest to detain or prosecute
◆ have committed an offence and will be prosecuted but whose mental health problems are such that a prison sentence would be an inappropriate disposal. They require treatment in a secure psychiatric hospital
◆ have committed an offence and will be prosecuted and may then enter the prison population with a mental health problem
◆ develop a mental health problem whilst in prison.

Other patients are detained because they are 'unfit to plead', 'insane on arraignment' or 'at Her Majesty's pleasure'.

Women in forensic mental health services are predominantly white. In the high security hospitals 88.5% of women are white, 9.6% are Afro-Caribbean and 1.9% are from other ethnic groups. In the medium secure provision within the NHS, 86% of women are white, 12.9% are Afro-Caribbean and 1.1% are Asian (Lart et al 1998).

Female patients made up 20% of the population in forensic mental health settings in Britain in 1996 (Hemingway 1996) and 15% of the detained population in high security hospitals in March 1999 (see Table 17.1). As a group they are a 'heterogeneous collection of women with a wide range of

Table 17.1 Detained patients within high security care. Figures from 31st March 1999 (Source: DoH 1999a: 134)

Hospital	Females	Males
Ashworth	49	369
Broadmoor	79	345
Rampton	65	398
Total	193	1112

ages, personal, psychiatric and forensic histories, who nevertheless share some characteristics and experiences' (Dolan & Bland 1996).

Women patients are different from male patients in a number of ways: they are less likely to have committed serious criminal offences in comparison with men but are more likely to have experienced previous psychiatric admission (Bartlett 1993). However, in high security environments the admission-to-discharge time for women is less than for men. Rampton Hospital Authority (2000) reported that a woman can hope to be discharged within an average of 6 years, whereas the statistics for men indicate a care and treatment time of 8 years.

A higher proportion of women than men in high security care in England and Wales are admitted from within the NHS mental health services, and regarded as difficult to manage within lower levels of security (Lart et al 1998). Maden et al (1995) report that 44% of women and 16% of men are in high security hospitals under civil sections of the 1983 Mental Health Act, rather than those sections which relate to criminal justice. Data suggest that the number of women in medium and low security care are estimated to be 15% of the total beds available (Parry-Crooke 2000).

Women in high security mental health settings are more likely to be admitted owing to damage to property, suicidal or self-harming behaviour or as the result of aggressive behaviour towards staff in mental health hospitals of lesser security (Women in Secure Hospitals 1999). There is a misperception among the general public that the majority of women in high security mental health environments are there because of offences of infanticide or manslaughter. However, 26% of women compared with 9% of men are detained on a civil order but are viewed in the same way as patients detained under part 3 of the Mental Health Act 1983 (Women in Secure Hospitals 1999). Earlier, Women in Special Hospitals (1997) reported that in 1996, 38% of women in high security hospitals had index offences of a violent or sexual nature, compared with 76% of men, whereas 26% of women had an index offence of arson, compared with 7% of men. The statistics from one high security hospital show that 47.8% of women and 79.8% of men within the current hospital population had committed violent or sexual offences, whereas 35.8% women and 4.5% of men had committed arson (see Table 17.2).

DIAGNOSTIC ISSUES

The statistical bulletin on inpatients formally detained in hospitals under the Mental Health Act 1983 (DoH 1999b) reported that the proportion of women detained under part 2 of the Act had declined from 57% to 49% over the previous 10 years. The number of women detained under

Table 17.2 Comparison of male and female index offences at Rampton high security hospital on 13 January 2000

Category of offence	Number of women (%)	Number of men (%)
None	13 (19.4)	26 (6.5)
Murder	2 (3)	34 (8.6)
Manslaughter	9 (13.4)	75 (19)
Attempted murder	0	17 (4.3)
Violence against person	14 (21)	87 (22)
Arson	24 (35.8)	18 (4.5)
Offences against children	0	29 (7.3)
Offences against females	0	34 (8.6)
Other sex offences	0	1 (0.25)
Kidnapping	0	3 (0.75)
Robbery	1 (1.5)	28 (7)
Damage to property	2 (3)	8 (2)
Others	2 (3)	35 (8.8)
TOTALS	67	395

part 3 has always been relatively low; currently 12% of all admissions from court and prison disposals are women. On 31 March 1999, according to the Department of Health census, out of 12 993 detained patients in NHS trust and private hospitals (including high security hospitals), 4514 (35%) were women (DoH 1999b).

The Mental Health Act Commission (1999: 242) suggests that:

Possible explanations for the declining proportion of women is that priority for scarce inpatient beds is being given to patients assessed as dangerous, who are more likely to be men, or there may be a reluctance to admit women to a ward environment where they may not feel safe. Whatever the reason, women will normally be in the minority on psychiatric wards as the vast majority of wards are of mixed gender. This has a number of consequences for the privacy, safety and care of women patients.

Lart et al (1998) reported that women within secure care are more likely to present with a personality disorder (38.8%), most frequently borderline personality disorder. Indeed, 29% of women but only 9% of men are labelled with this diagnosis.

Women in forensic mental health care share a common problem with women in prison. Travers & Aiyegbusi (1998) report that childhood neglect and trauma overlap with self-neglect and self-harm in later life. Both self-neglect and self-harm by patients can be seen as antecedents to significant physical health problems. Complications associated with eating disorders have led to this population experiencing problems ranging from extremes of anaemia and malnutrition to morbid obesity. Chain smoking, which is common, undoubtedly exacerbates respiratory problems such as asthma, which is present in a high percentage of patients. Women patients present with an increased level of endocrine pathology in the form of thyroid, diabetic and reproductive system disorders. Travers & Aiyegbusi (1998) support the view of Van Der Kolk (1996) who suggests a relationship exists between the restricted ability to express emotions verbally and impaired immune system functioning, which in turn relates to physical illness. They also noted that women patients tend to suffer many infections, which lead to antibiotic treatment.

Although ethnic minority women are a minority within a minority, young Asian women have been reported to have a higher rate of suicide and attempted suicide than other groups. There are also somatic health issues, namely diabetes, sickle cell disorder, thalassaemia and high perinatal mortality, which are racial/genetic specific, affecting particular groups (Lart et al 1998).

CARE AND TREATMENT ISSUES

Women in Secure Hospitals (1999) report that in the high security hospitals, care and treatment are provided for women on single gender wards but there is little access to single-gender off-ward activities, such as work, education and leisure. Rampton Hospital has tried to combat this through increasing the number of activities which only women can attend. A high proportion of women patients have experienced childhood sexual abuse and often feel threatened by mixed-sex environments, suffering harassment or abuse when attending mixed gender activities. The majority of medium secure services are mixed gender and male dominated; many women find it difficult to cope in such environments, therefore they either resist transfer to lower levels of security or are recalled back to high security hospitals, after a trial leave of absence in a medium secure unit (Women in Secure Hospitals 1999). The Mental Health Act Commission (1999) suggests that concerns about privacy and safety mean that women may prefer to stay in their bedroom, where they feel safer, particularly when there are few women patients on the ward and where the behaviour of some of the men may be disturbed and possibly violent. The Commission also highlights the 'special concern for Asian women, who may be particularly reluctant to be admitted to mixed accommodation' (Mental Health Act Commission 1999: 245).

If treatment aims are to be successful, women should be enabled to benefit from therapeutic regimes in environments where they feel safe. Humphries & Eaton (1996) provided knowledge of the needs of women patients in forensic mental health environments, together with an understanding of their lives, their views and their hopes for the future. Extensive work has been undertaken, of which an integral part included listening to women (Gallop et al 1998). Challenges have been set in relation to reshaping services to maximize their ability to deliver gender-sensitive care and treatment. Progress has been made in some areas, such as ensuring the provision of female staff on duty, ensuring access to same-gender doctors and the development of services which focus on needs as well as diagnosis. However, key gaps still exist with regard to the effectiveness of different service models, ways of measuring need and in-depth and comparative research (Lart et al 1998).

One particular recommendation that appears regularly on the national agenda, yet seems to be making little impact on services, is that 'wherever possible, mentally disordered offenders which include women should receive care and treatment under conditions of security no greater than is justified by the degree of danger they present to themselves or to others' (DoH & Home Office 1994, Mental Health Act Commission 1999). In September 1999, the National Service Framework for Mental Health was published, reiterating that people should have timely access to an appropriate hospital bed in the least restrictive environment, consistent with the need to protect them and the public (Department of Health 1999c).

In addition to the need for separate facilities for women, the Mental Health Act Commission has identified other key factors as being of particular importance in the care and treatment of detained women patients.

According to the Mental Health Act Commission (1999: 246) women should be able to:

◆ lock doors
◆ have the choice of a female key worker
◆ be in contact with other women
◆ have the opportunity to take part in women-only therapy groups and social activities
◆ engage safely in the full range of activities, even when their number may be small
◆ have physical health checks on admission
◆ have access to a female doctor for medical care

◆ have access to a female member of staff at all times
◆ be reassured that there is adequate staff supervision at night.

Extensive clinical challenges exist for practitioners working with women in forensic mental health environments. These demand a high level of skills and knowledge around working with self-injurious behaviour; approaches to arson treatment; eating disorders; issues of loss and bereavement; behaviour which challenges services; and in particular, supporting people who have been traumatized by experiences of sexual abuse. Reported incidents of sexual abuse were disclosed by 83% of women at Rampton Hospital in a recent survey.

Women with borderline personality disorder find it difficult to cope in forensic mental health settings, in environments where they are surrounded by the distress of others and where they are controlled by disciplined regimes, influenced by the custodial aspects of secure care. The affective vulnerability, lack of self-identity and sense of powerlessness experienced by women with borderline personality disorder can only be exaggerated; this is likely to promote increased impulsiveness, including self-harming and assaultative behaviour (Women in Secure Hospitals 1999).

Deliberate self-harm is a significant clinical issue for women in forensic mental health environments. One approach that has been used with some success to reduce the incidence of self-harm, as well as teach alternative coping strategies, is dialectical behaviour therapy. This is a cognitive-behavioural treatment developed for patients displaying suicidal and parasuicidal behaviour. It follows a hierarchy of treatment goals, which include decreasing suicidal and parasuicidal behaviours, decreasing therapy-interfering behaviour and increasing behavioural skills. Together, these skills aim to reduce emotional instability and problems with anger, learning assertiveness skills and tolerate unpleasant emotions without impulsive behaviour (Shearin & Linehan 1993).

Compared with men in forensic mental health environments, women are more likely to present a risk of violence to current caregivers or fellow patients than to the general public (Travers & Aiyegbusi 1998). Risk of harm to self is high (Leibling et al 1997, Women in Secure Hospitals 1999) and this is likely to be increased by regression associated with detention in a secure environment, where fellow patients and caregivers replicate family dynamics (Travers & Aiyegbusi 1998). Amongst a number of internal and external risk factors, active psychosis seems to be the single most important mediator of risk to others; the more psychotic, the more dangerous an individual patient may be. Dissociation whilst simultaneously experiencing severe command hallucinations, or terrifying flashbacks which can possibly be considered as extreme examples of numbing and intrusion, seem to feature amongst the most dangerous symptoms patients may experience (Travers & Aiyegbusi 1998).

An analysis of over 700 untoward incidents in the women's services at Rampton Hospital during January–November 1999 indicated that self-injury occurs with great frequency, particularly during the afternoon and evening. Further work is currently being undertaken to examine possible causative factors, such as reduced access to activities or reduced availability of staff (see Table 17.3).

Table 17.3 Untoward incidents in the women's services at Rampton Hospital during January–November 1999

Incident type	Time					
	0900–1200	1200–1500	1500–1800	1800–2100	2100–000	Row total
Self-harm	40	44	70	81	86	321
Physical aggression	28	26	34	30	34	152
Verbal aggression	20	30	47	36	17	150
Other	29	10	15	21	21	96
Column total	117	110	166	168	158	719

Working with women who self-harm is difficult; there is a high risk of splitting between those members of the team who work with these patients and other non-ward based professionals, family and friends. A common theme involves professionals, visitors or clinical staff. After being bombarded with projections about neglect and mistreatment, they often feel they have to do something to rescue the patient from their situation. Current caregivers, already feeling persecuted and invalidated, become increasingly guarded against perceived external threat, to the point where scrutiny of any kind is experienced as severely invasive and punishing. All parties then fear collaborative working, owing to their anxieties about identifying with the 'opposition' (Travers & Aiyegbusi 1998). It is only by working together, in consistent integrated teams, that professionals can avoid splitting and attacking each other. The challenge is to provide a care and treatment service for patients but this is difficult when energy and resources are channelled into operating defensively. Defences tend to involve uncoordinated action, rather than focused, considered thought and debate.

Adshead (1994, 1997) discusses how the patients' need for their fantasized, idealized caregiver leads to denigration of less than ideal care, which is in turn perceived as abuse. Verbal, emotional and physical attacks on caregivers, who are usually forced to provide less than perfect care, are commonplace. Both Main (1957) and Menzies Lyth (1988) describe the agony experienced by caregivers when their attempts to 'cure' are thwarted by patients who refuse to get better.

Travers & Aiyegbusi (1998) explain that many of these dynamic processes can be understood in terms of occurring through the transferences and countertransferences which operate within the wards and clinical areas. Rage toward past abusive and neglecting caregivers, which had been dissociated from, is now displaced onto current caregivers, who are then emotionally perceived in the same way. Adshead (1997) points out: 'The clinical team may not be able to deal with the patient's feelings, but they can (and must) make an attempt to deal with their own'.

Herman (1992) states that some of the most astute descriptions of traumatic transference can be found in the literature about clinical encounters involving individuals who are diagnosed with borderline personality disorder, which were written before the traumatic roots of the disorder were known.

It is essential, therefore, that staff are appropriately supported to enable them to contain anxiety that is evoked. Staff experience stressors which cannot always be dissolved and left at the door of the hospital on their way home. Clinical supervision is part of a package of support. All staff in the women's services at Rampton Hospital have the opportunity to meet regularly with a clinical supervisor, yet less than 50% of staff take advantage of this offer. Debriefing is seen as essential after a serious incident and access is available to an independent counselling service. The appointment of a staff support post is seen as a way of helping staff cope effectively in difficult circumstances. More needs to be done, though, as sickness levels currently run at 11% in the women's services. The hospital average is 6.9%, whereas other mental health services run at 5.65% for a comparable period. This level of health deficit cannot be accepted as an occupational hazard; by looking to other services and adapting the best of what they provide, a difference can be made to the lives of staff and, thus, to the lives of women in forensic mental health environments.

Careful attention is required for the rigorous application of protective factors needed to ensure safety: these take the form of goals, rules, boundaries and support systems for caregivers (Herman 1992). In women's services, within both health care and the prison services, these protective factors need to be a key part of the working conditions for staff.

One service which endeavours to address these issues and provide a service tailored to meet the needs of women is Rampton Hospital. The service is delivered to 450 patients, 67 of whom are women with mental illness, personality disorder or a learning disability. The women's service is delivered by approximately 150 clinicians including medical staff, nurses, psychologists, social workers, occupational therapists and teachers. Additionally, administrative, clerical and ancillary staff support them. Together, they aim to provide gender-sensitive care and treatment to the highest standards, with regard for individual rights, available resources and needs. But in conditions of stringent security and the constraints of a patriarchal organizational culture, this aim, though laudable, could be seen as unrealistic.

Whilst it is recognized that every effort is made to take a holistic approach to women, physical health needs are difficult to prioritize. The services would benefit from the establishment of women's health coordinators, in a type of practice nurse role. This person could not only suture wounds but could proactively develop screening programmes for both breast cancer and cancer of the cervix. Health promotion should have a higher profile, to educate women about the advantages of healthy eating and to encourage them to explore ways of coping with stress other than smoking.

CONCLUSION

Action is occurring on a national level to develop training programmes that address gender issues. This includes a national project coordinated by Liverpool University called Women in Secure Settings (WISS). The project is a joint initiative between the University and Women in Special Hospitals and involves training programmes being piloted on a range of sites. A predischarge ward at Rampton Hospital is the designated site in high security care; other sites have been identified in prison, medium secure provision, a community mental health service and an adolescent secure unit. The project arose from the recognition, at national level, that training was an important component in developing dedicated gender-sensitive services. The aim is to develop over a 3-year period training that will increase staff knowledge, skills and confidence in providing improved services for women in secure settings. The training programmes need to fully reflect the needs of not only the patients but also the staff; the content needs to include issues relating to self-harm, the aetiology of borderline personality disorder and coping strategies for

staff. These programmes should also be supported by rigorous implementation of effective clinical supervision, allowing staff to monitor boundaries and receive appropriate mechanisms to protect them.

It is clear that women need higher levels of relational security and lower levels of physical security than is currently provided. The issue of women receiving care and treatment in conditions of security no greater than justified by the degree of danger presented to themselves or others is something that is also supported by Women in Secure Hospitals. They believe that the majority of women are detained in a higher level of security than is necessary. It is estimated that 78% of women in high security environments could receive appropriate care and treatment in medium secure environments if available. In the same manner, 69% of women in secure environments should be offered placements in low secure environments (Women in Secure Hospitals 1999).

The growth in medium secure provision across the country should be used to facilitate changes in the way that women are managed within mental health services at present. When referring to discharge from high security establishments, it might be useful to set this in the context of the average admission-to-discharge period of 6 years. There is a misconception amongst some people that women come into secure environments and stay there forever. The admission-to-discharge period at Rampton Hospital identifies that this is a myth, not a reality.

Women in Secure Hospitals (1999) reports that the current provision of care and physical resources within secure settings does not meet women's relational and physical security needs; they require high intensive care, with a high staff/patient ratio, providing a supportive and safe environment, rather than physical high security care. WISH also suggests that:

The interaction between their mental health needs and the social and economic marginalization experienced by so many of the women, has also to be considered, if the long term objective of secure provision is to rehabilitate women back into the community. (Women in Secure Hospitals 1999)

Many campaigners are calling for a smaller high security component of care (Women in Special Hospitals 1997, 1999, Travers & Aiyegbusi 1998). They suggest this could be facilitated by the development of women-only wards in medium secure units, which would have to be without a 2-year time limit on the admission. One local strategy acknowledges the importance of making progress in this area, owing to the widespread concern about the welfare of women in secure services, where they are a minority in a male-dominated culture (NHSE 1999). It recommends single-site services for women but change in services will only happen with the development of integrated services, which facilitate skill sharing to enable alternatives to admission to be developed and resourced. This must include essential outreach work. Additionally, there needs to be greater opportunity for women ready for discharge from high security care to build on the existing success of discharge work (Murdock & White 1999).

REFERENCES

Adshead G 1994 Damage: trauma and violence in a sample of women referred to a forensic service. Behavioural Sciences and the Law 12: 235–249

Adshead G 1997 'Written on the body': deliberate self-harm and violence. In: Welldon EV, van Velsen C (eds) A practical guide to forensic psychotherapy. Jessica Kingsley, London, ch 14, pp 110–114

Bartlett A 1993 What do we know about the English special hospitals? International Journal of Law and Psychiatry 16(1–2): 27–51

Department of Health 1994 Working in partnership: review of the mental health nursing team. HMSO, London

Department of Health 1999a Inpatients formally detained in hospitals under the Mental Health Act 1983 and other legislation. Department of Health, Statistics Division, London

Department of Health 1999b Statistical bulletin, 1999/25. Department of Health, London

Department of Health 1999c National service framework for mental health: modern standards and service models, executive summary. Stationery Office, London

Department of Health, Home Office 1994 Review of health and social services for mentally disordered offenders and others requiring similar services, vol. 6, race, gender and equal opportunities. HMSO, London, pp 41–49

Dolan B, Bland J 1996 Who are the women in special hospitals? In: Hemingway C (ed) Special women? The experience of women in the special hospital system. Avebury, Aldershot

Gallop R, Engels S, De Nunzio R, Napravrik A, Dorian B 1998 The development of a safe and empowering environment for women hospitalized in psychiatric settings who have a history of abuse. Women's Health Bureau, Ministry of Health, Ontario

Hemingway C 1996 Special women? The experience of women in the special hospital system. Avebury, Aldershot

Herman JL 1992 Trauma and recovery: from domestic violence to political terror. Basic Books, London

Humphries J, Eaton M 1996 Listening to women in special hospitals. Special Hospitals Service Authority/King's Fund, London

Lart R, Payne S, Beaumont B, MacDonald G, Mistry T 1998 Women and secure psychiatric services: a literature review. NHS Centre for Reviews and Dissemination, York

Leibling H, Chipchase H, Velangi R 1997 An evaluation of nurse training and support needs: working with women patients who harm themselves in a special hospital. Issues in Criminological and Legal Psychology 29: 47–56

Maden T, Curle C, Meux C, Burrow S, Gunn J 1995 Treatment and security needs of special hospital patients. Whurr, London

Main TF 1957 The ailment. In: Main TF (ed) The ailment and other psychoanalytic essays. Free Association, London, ch 2, pp 12–35

Mental Health Act Commission 1999 8th biennial report. Stationery Office, London

Menzies Lyth I 1988 Containing anxiety in institutions: selected essays. Free Association, London

Murdock D, White C 1999 Listening to women. Available on the World Wide Web at the Forensic Nursing Resource homepage: http://www.fnrh.freeserve.co.uk/murdoch.html

NHS Executive 1999 Trent regional forensic strategy. NHS Executive, Sheffield

Parry-Crooke G 2000 Good girls – surviving the secure system. WISH and University of London, London

Rampton Hospital Authority 2000 In-patient statistics. Rampton Hospital Authority, Retford

Shearin E, Linehan M 1993 Dialectic behaviour therapy for borderline personality disorder: treatment goals and strategies and empirical support. In: Paris J (ed)

Borderline personality disorder: etiology and treatment. American Psychiatric Press, Washington, pp 285–381

Standing Nursing and Midwifery Advisory Council 1999 The role of the mental health nurse in the provision of modern mental health acute care. Department of Health, London

Travers R, Aiyegbusi A 1998 A clinical paradigm for women's services. Ashworth Hospital Authority, Liverpool

UKCC, University of Central Lancashire 1999 Nursing in secure environments. UKCC, London

Van Der Kolk BA 1996 The complexity and adaption to trauma: self regulation, stimulus discrimination and characterological development. In: van der Kolk BA, McFarlane AC, Weisaeth L (eds) Traumatic stress: the effects of overwhelming experience on body, mind and society. Guilford Press, New York, ch 9, pp 182–213

Women in Special Hospitals 1997 Annual report 1996–97. WISH, London

Women in Secure Hospitals 1999 Defining gender issues: redefining women's services. WISH, London

FURTHER READING

Hemingway C 1996 Special women? The experience of women in the special hospital system. Avebury, Aldershot

Linehan M 1993 Cognitive behavioural treatment of borderline personality disorder. Guilford Press, New York

Linehan M 1993 Skills training manual for borderline personality disorder. Guilford Press, New York

Women in Secure Hospitals 1999 Defining gender issues: redefining women's services. WISH, London

Chapter Eighteen

Dual diagnosis

Colin Dale

INTRODUCTION

(NB: It is acknowledged that the term 'dual diagnosis' is imprecise and its use has been subjected to significant criticism. However, it continues to be the term most commonly used to describe people who have a co-occurring mental health and substance abuse disorder in the UK and has therefore been adopted for this chapter.)

The interaction between psychopathology and substance use disorders is complex. Psychopathology may act as a risk factor for addictive disorders; psychopathology may modify the presentation and treatment of addictive disorders; and many psychiatric symptoms emerge during the course of chronic intoxication and withdrawal (Brady & Roberts 1995).

Carey (1991) describes four challenges that impede research with the dually diagnosed: access to the existing literature; access to the dually diagnosed population; the heterogeneity of the population; and establishment of accurate diagnoses. There is a lack of research into the drug misuse problems in forensic services. Most of the literature has concentrated on the problems of drug misuse in prisons, the community and local psychiatric hospitals. Furthermore, much of this body of work is concerned with drug misuse problems which are qualitatively and quantitatively different from those faced by staff and patients in forensic services. However, these studies offer the potential for adapting useful strategies for a forensic mental health population.

There is a tension between goals of enforcement and those of demand reduction and public health. This can be particularly acute within a closed institution.

DEFINITION

The Diagnostic and Statistical Manual of Mental Disorders (DSM-IV) (American Psychiatric Association 1994) defines a mental disorder as:

A clinically significant behavioural or psychological syndrome or pattern that occurs in an individual and that is typically associated with present distress (a painful symptom) or disability (impairment in one or more areas of functioning).

Substance misuse, according to DSM-IV, is a maladaptive pattern of use, not meeting the criteria for dependence, that has persisted for at least 1 month or has occurred repeatedly over a long period of time. The dual-diagnosis patient meets the DSM-IV criteria for both substance abuse or dependency and a co-existing psychiatric disorder.

The concept of dual diagnosis can be seen as an umbrella term that incorporates a wide range of co-existing problems, including the co-existence of addictive behaviours such as drug, alcohol, gambling or eating disorders with concurrent mental health problems. The use and misuse of psychoactive substances, including alcohol, may result in the patient developing a wide range of psychiatric disorders depending on the drug being used. Carey (1989) states that with dual-diagnosis patients, the psychiatric disorders and the substance misuse are separate, chronic disorders, each with an independent course, yet each able to influence the properties of the other.

DEMOGRAPHICS

Abuse of and dependence on drugs, alcohol and other substances in schizophrenia are being increasingly recognized and well documented in the literature. It has been suggested that up to 60% of patients with schizophrenia use illicit drugs (Addington & Duchak 1997). El-Mallakh (1998) states that recent epidemiological studies conducted by the National Co-morbidity Survey in the USA have indicated that up to 51% of individuals with a serious mental illness are also dependent on or addicted to illicit drugs.

However, only 50% of these clients with co-occurring addictive and mental disorders receive treatment that addresses both issues.

Greenfield et al (1995) state that between 20% and 70% of psychiatric patients have a co-occurring substance use disorder and rates of substance abuse amongst patients with psychotic disorders are especially high. Patients with co-existing psychosis and substance use disorders typically have poorer outcomes than patients diagnosed with either disorder alone. Frequently, treatment services for such dually diagnosed patients are not integrated and organizational barriers may impede the appropriate detection, referral and treatment of these patients.

Dual disorders are especially common amongst prisoners and patients in mental hospitals. The 1991 Epidemiologic Catchment Area Study carried out by the National Institute for Mental Health in the USA (Robins & Regier 1991) found that 56% of prisoners had an alcohol problem, 54% another drug problem and 56% a psychiatric disorder not involving drug or alcohol abuse. Amongst residents of mental hospitals, 34% had an alcohol problem at some time and 16% had other drug problems. Having a psychiatric disorder nearly tripled the risk of having an associated alcohol or drug problem; 39% of alcoholics and 53% of persons with other drug problems had another psychiatric diagnosis. Alcoholics had a 19% lifetime rate of anxiety disorders (1.5 times the average); a 14% rate of antisocial personality (more than 20 times the average); a 13% rate of mood disorders (nearly double the average); and a 4% rate of schizophrenia (more than three times the average). Illicit drug abusers had unusually high rates of anxiety disorders (28%); mood disorders (26%); antisocial personality (18%); and schizophrenia (7%). Other common problems of alcoholics and illicit drug abusers were impulse control disorders, attention deficit hyperactivity disorder and conduct disorders.

Blankertz et al (1993) describe the negative long-term effects of the specific childhood risk factors of sexual and physical abuse, parental mental illness and substance abuse and out-of-home placement in relation to the development of problems of dual diagnosis in adulthood.

CLINICAL PRESENTATION OF DUAL DIAGNOSIS

The heterogeneity of those with co-occurring addictive and mental disorders has only recently been recognized and treatment strategies for different segments of this population are still being developed (Alexander 1996). Drake (1995) explains that those with dual diagnosis have higher rates of clinical relapse, rehospitalization, depression and suicide, violence and legal problems, incarceration, unstable housing and homelessness, HIV infection, non-compliance with treatment and increased family problems.

Shumway & Cuffel (1996) describe the heterogeneity of signs and symptoms of alcohol disorders. A community sample of 1955 persons with either alcohol disorder alone or alcohol disorder plus one of four categories of major mental disorder (antisocial personality disorder, schizophrenia, affective disorder, anxiety disorder) were investigated. When all diagnostic categories were combined, persons with co-morbid mental and alcohol disorder showed evidence of more severe alcohol-related symptoms than did persons with alcohol disorder alone. Distinct symptom patterns distinguished the four diagnostic groups, reflecting heterogeneity in the manifestation of co-morbid alcohol disorder. Most notably, co-morbid antisocial personality disorder and schizophrenia were associated with higher levels of alcohol consumption and more severe social consequences of alcohol use.

Westreich et al (1997) reviewed the charts of all women and a randomly selected sample of men over a 6-month period on two addiction treatment units at Bellevue Hospital Centre in New York. The men were more likely to be admitted with schizophrenia and to have used substances of abuse other than alcohol and the women were more likely to be admitted with affective disorders. Also, the women on the dual-diagnosis ward were more likely to be domiciled (i.e. not homeless) and the women on both units were significantly more likely to report having been crime victims. These findings suggest that dually diagnosed women need a substantially different treatment paradigm from men.

Patients with a dual diagnosis therefore present a complex clinical picture, with problems which are difficult to disentangle. Dual diagnosis worsens the clinical care and outcomes for individuals with mental disorders. It is associated with symptom exacerbation, treatment non-compliance and more frequent hospitalization, family friction and high services use and cost (Bartels et al 1995, Bellack & Gearon 1998, Havassy & Arns 1998, Mueser et al 1997). Furthermore, patients may be jeopardized by the consequences of substance abuse, namely increased risks of violence, HIV infection and alcohol-related disorders (Institute of Medicine 1995). More specifically, dual diagnosis is associated with:

◆ increased rates of suicide and suicidal behaviour (Drake 1995)
◆ higher rates of homelessness (Bassuk 1994). Drake et al (1991) state that people who are dually diagnosed with severe mental illness and substance use disorders constitute 10–20% of homeless persons in the USA
◆ higher rates of violence (Drake 1995)
◆ worsening of psychological and psychiatric symptoms (Drake 1995)
◆ poorer compliance with medication (Drake 1995)
◆ poorer prognosis (Drake 1995, Greenfield et al 1995)
◆ clients not wanting to address abuse (Dale 1999)
◆ management problems in residential settings (McKeown & Leibling 1995)
◆ workers' lack of knowledge and skills (McKeown & Leibling 1995).

REASONS FOR ABUSING DRUGS

Theories to explain dual diagnosis range from genetic to psychosocial but empirical support for any one theory is inconclusive (Kosten & Ziedonis 1997, Mueser et al 1998). In summary, the cause of such widespread co-morbidity is unknown. Several theories have been put forward to explain why some mentally ill patients misuse drugs and alcohol.

Dixon et al (1990) suggest that some patients may self-medicate in an effort to treat their psychiatric symptoms and stimulant-type drugs, such as amphetamines and cocaine, have been used by some patients to counteract distressing extrapyramidal side effects (Schneider & Siris 1987). In the UK, the recent closures of long-stay psychiatric institutions and increasing emphasis on care and treatment in the community have meant that mentally ill patients are perhaps becoming more exposed to a wider range of illicit drugs than previously. Furthermore, some mentally ill patients who are socially isolated may be drawn into a drug-using culture that appears more attractive and less stigmatized for social interactions. Examining the cause and effect in such cases is often difficult. Aside from coincidence, there are three main possibilities.

◆ The psychiatric symptoms and the substance abuse have common causes – biological, psychological or social.
◆ Drug abuse causes acute and chronic psychiatric symptoms.
◆ Psychiatric disorders produce drug abuse and dependence.

A total of 41 subjects who fulfilled DSM-IIIR criteria for schizophrenia and substance abuse or dependence were asked to describe their reasons for using such substances, the reasons why they might stop and the subjective effects of the substances. Drugs were reportedly used to increase pleasure, to 'get high' and to reduce depression. Subjective effects of increased depression and positive symptoms were also reported (Addington & Duchak 1997).

TREATMENT MODELS

Traditional approaches to dual diagnosis have been via either serial (mental health and substance misuse disorders are treated consecutively) or parallel (mental health and substance misuse services liaise to provide the two services concurrently) systems.

The potential weaknesses of the serial model are that treatment in either system is incomplete because of lack of attention to co-morbid conditions; each system can continue to provide a standard form of treatment and resist modification to accommodate co-morbid conditions; and patients tend to leave both systems due to complications related to co-morbidity (Kipping 1999). The potential weaknesses of the parallel model are that there is often no fixed point of responsibility and the burden of integrating two systems falls to the patient; it maximizes potential for miscommunication, contradictory recommendations and non-compliance (Kipping 1999).

In light of the extent of mental disorder and substance abuse co-morbidity, substance abuse treatment is a critical element of care for people with mental disorders. Likewise, treatment of symptoms and signs of mental disorders is a critical element of recovery from substance abuse. Yet decades of treating co-morbidity through separate mental health and substance abuse service systems have proven to be ineffective (Mueser et al 1997, Ridgely et al 1990).

Research over the past 10 years supports a shift to treatment that combines interventions directed simultaneously at both conditions, that is, severe mental illness and substance abuse by the same group of providers (Kosten & Ziedonis 1997). However, access to such treatment remains limited. Most successful models of combined treatment include: case management; group interventions, such as persuasion groups and social skills training; and assertive outreach to bring people into treatment (Mueser et al 1997). Typically, they take into account the cognitive and motivational deficits that characterize serious mental illnesses (Bellack & Gearon 1998), although many providers still need to be educated (Kirchner et al 1998).

Combined treatment is effective at engaging people with both diagnoses in outpatient services; maintaining continuity and consistency of care; reducing hospitalization; and decreasing substance abuse, whilst at the same time improving social functioning (Miner et al 1997, Mueser et al 1997). Although there is little evidence for any particular approach to combining treatments for co-morbidity (Ley et al 1999), recent research suggests that services incorporating behavioural (motivational) approaches to substance abuse treatment are superior to traditional 12-step approaches (e.g. Alcoholics Anonymous) with this population of clients (Drake et al 1998). This may be because the more structured behavioural methods better accommodate the cognitive difficulties that accompany schizophrenia. Others, however, find self-help interventions tailored to dual-diagnosis clients quite useful (Vogel et al 1998). Current research is seeking to tailor combined treatment to the needs and preferences of specific patient subgroups, such as: men; women (Alexander 1996); people with addiction to multiple substances (as opposed to alcohol addiction alone); and people with histories of physical and psychological trauma (Mueser et al 1997).

THE CHALLENGE FOR SERVICES

In a Royal College of Nursing survey of mental health nurses, 68% of 187 respondents reported illicit drug use in their unit and the problem seemed to be as widespread in rural as in urban areas (Sandford 1995). The survey showed that, of the 68% of respondents who reported incidents of illicit drug and alcohol use in their units, almost half had no policy guidelines to assist them in dealing with the problem. The Mental Health Act Commission has consistently expressed concerns over the lack of policy guidelines for staff so that there are no 'well-defined rules governing the management and control of substance misuse' (Mental Health Act Commission 1999: 233). The Mental Health Act Commission lists some of the common failings of guidelines.

◆ They may be unclear or not adhered to consistently.
◆ Patients or even staff may be unaware of their existence.
◆ It is not clear whether the policy applies equally to alcohol.
◆ It is not clear how patients will be informed of the policy.

◆ No advice is given to staff on what action they should take in the event of a refusal by the patient to be searched or to provide a urine test.
◆ There has been no consultation with the local police (the issue of how far confidentiality can and should be protected is subject to wide variations in practice).
◆ There is widespread confusion about the misuse of drugs legislation and especially about the rights of staff to seize and destroy substances.

Kipping (1999) suggests that much could be achieved in changing the way services are provided currently and suggests that attention is given to:

◆ establishing of dual posts with substance misuse teams
◆ provision of information and advice
◆ conducting assessments
◆ training and education
◆ communication/liaison
◆ simplifying access
◆ prioritizing people with mental health problems
◆ flexibility of rules and boundaries
◆ working with clients who do not see their substance use as problematic.

DUAL DIAGNOSIS IN FORENSIC SERVICES

Unsurprisingly, the increasing incidence of mentally ill substance-abusing individuals generally is reflected in the mentally disordered seen in courts, prisons and secure health services as greater attention has been given to the need for diversion and rehabilitation programmes in these settings. These reflect a need to develop specialized treatment interventions for mentally disordered and substance-abusing offenders and non-offenders. Taylor et al (1998) surveyed all 1740 patients resident in Britain's high security hospitals and found that substance abuse before admission to hospital, which was probably under-recorded, had been most common amongst those with psychosis, together with an independent personality disorder. The authors comment that studies seem increasingly likely to find that substance misuse is a significant factor which increases the risk that a person with a mental disorder will be violent.

The diversity of this population in terms of the choice of primary drugs, the aetiology and history of these disorders and related treatment, symptoms and interactive effects of the disorders, history of criminal justice involvement and violent behaviour, level of impairment in psychosocial functioning and level of social support presents significant challenges (Lehman 1996). The latest DSM-IV formulation of mental disorder now differentiates between several types of co-occurring 'substance-induced' mental health disorders.

McKeown & Leibling (1995) describe a survey of staff perceptions of issues related to illicit drug use amongst patients within a UK high security hospital. Findings suggested that staff are largely concerned about issues around the supply of drugs. A significant level of ignorance regarding illicit drugs and their usage was revealed, indicating a need for coordinated training. A review of literature suggested that future management strategies should not be solely directed towards supply restriction. A discussion of the results highlights parallels between staff perceptions of illicit drug problems, media coverage of the same and the findings of earlier sociological studies of deviance, subculture and moral panic.

In the USA, independent screening and assessment of mental health and substance abuse by mental health and criminal justice systems agencies has resulted in inadequate sharing of information, poor communication and non-detection of mental health and substance use disorders. Examples of misdiagnosis, misattribution of the causes of mental health symptoms, inappropriate treatment and referral and poor treatment are reported (Drake et al 1993, Peters & Bartoi 1997, Teague et al 1990). The reasons why this occurs include: negative consequences associated with disclosure of symptoms; lack of staff training; and cognitive and perceptual difficulties associated with severe mental illness or toxic effects of recent alcohol or drug use. The integration of screening,

diagnosis and assessment approaches within the criminal justice system is associated with more favourable outcomes.

SCREENING

This is a precursor stage to formal assessment and its main aim is to detect mental health (in the case of criminal justice settings) and substance use symptoms and to identify any related problem that reflects the need for treatment (e.g. a history of violence, severe medical problems and/or severe cognitive deficits).

The large numbers involved in the criminal justice system will necessitate use of a brief screening instrument, given the limited staff resources and the need for relatively quick processing of offenders. Screenings are often conducted by staff without experience in diagnosis or assessment of mental health or substance use disorders who may be unfamiliar with treatment services and problems therefore can often be overlooked. This is an area where specialized training in detecting dual-diagnosis disorders; use of screening instruments; developing collaborative screening approaches; and initiating referral to assessment and treatment services could prove to be particularly beneficial. Screening is typically used to identify cases that need more extensive assessment of treatment needs.

This screening should be available to all newly admitted or readmitted patients/prisoners at the earliest opportunity following receipt into care. Screening should be ongoing during the individual's time in care and in particular at key changes in circumstances (e.g. moving to lower levels of security), utilizing agreed and standardized instruments, with information from previously conducted screening and assessments being communicated between agencies. It may be necessary to delay screening if it is considered that the individual is still intoxicated, with drug testing being an important component of screening and assessment. Whenever possible, any results from screenings should be supplemented by information obtained from family and friends (Drake et al 1993).

Evidence would suggest that detection of either mental health or substance use symptoms should indicate a need for screening for the other type of disorder, owing to the high rates of dual-diagnosis disorders in forensic settings. Generally, the presence of mental health symptoms is more likely to signal a substance use disorder than the reverse.

Drake et al (1993) recommend using a short self-report instrument to document the frequency of use of drugs and alcohol over the past 30 days, together with one of the brief rating scales for mental health. Key components that should be reviewed in screening for dual-diagnosis disorders include the following.

◆ Mental health information – including acute mental health symptoms (e.g. agitation, depression, hallucinations, delusions), suicidal thoughts and behaviour, prior involvement in mental health treatment, use of psychotropic medication, cognitive impairment and family history of mental illness.

◆ Substance abuse information – including acute signs of drug or alcohol intoxication, withdrawal or tolerance effects, self-reported substance abuse, negative consequences associated with substance use, prior involvement in treatment and family history of substance abuse.

◆ Interaction effects of dual-diagnosis disorders – including the effects of one disorder on the other and patterns of symptom expression.

◆ Motivation and readiness for treatment – including the perceived level of mental health and substance abuse problems.

◆ Criminal justice information – including the criminal history and history of aggressive or violent behaviour.

◆ Infectious diseases.

There are currently no instruments that address both mental health and substance abuse disorders (Osher & Kofoed 1989) so consideration needs to be given to combining independent instruments. Peters & Greenbaum (1996) conducted the most comprehensive study into screening instruments in the criminal justice system in the USA and found that three instruments were most effective in identifying prison inmates with substance dependence problems:

◆ ADS/ASI-Drug – a combined instrument, consisting of the Alcohol Dependence Scale and the Addiction Severity Index – Drug Use section (McLellan et al 1980, Skinner & Horn 1984)
◆ TCU Drug Dependence Screen – DDS (Simpson et al 1997)
◆ Simple Screening Instrument – SSI (Center for Substance Abuse Treatment 1994).

Several brief mental health screens are available that examine a broad range of mental health symptoms (e.g. Brief Symptom Inventory [BSI] (Derogatis & Melisaratos 1983), Referral Decision Scale [RDS] (Teplin & Schwartz 1989), Symptom Checklist 90 – Revised [SCL-90-R] (Derogatis et al 1974)), whilst others focus on symptoms of a single disorder, such as depression (e.g. Beck Depression Inventory [BDI] (Beck & Beamesderfer 1974)).

Several instruments are now available that examine motivation and readiness for treatment, designed primarily to identify individuals who are inappropriate for admission to substance abuse treatment.

◆ Circumstances, Motivation, Readiness, and Suitability Scale [CMRS] (DeLeon & Jainchill 1986)
◆ Stages of Change Readiness and Treatment Eagerness Scale [SOCRATES] (Miller 1994)
◆ University of Rhode Island Change Assessment Scale [URICA] (DiClemente & Hughes 1990, McConnaughy et al 1983)

ASSESSMENT

Assessment of dual-diagnosis disorders is usually carried out after completion of screening and referral to treatment services and provides the basis for the development of an individualized treatment plan. Assessment is an ongoing process and it is important to consider new issues that arise and new information that is obtained over the course of treatment. The residual effects of addictive substances (e.g. withdrawal effects) that may mask or mimic psychiatric symptoms, such as depression, make the accurate assessment of co-existing disorders especially difficult.

Some individuals may benefit from an extended assessment to:

◆ examine the significance and interactive nature of the mental health and substance abuse
◆ determine the length of the current abstinence, with delay of diagnosis if abstinence has not been achieved
◆ re-examine mental health symptoms at the end of 4–6 weeks of abstinence
◆ provide ongoing re-evaluation of mental health symptoms and appropriateness of treatment placement.

The assessment of dual diagnosis should aim to acquire information on the following areas.

◆ Symptoms of dual-diagnosis disorders
◆ Drugs: types, dose (amounts, cost), frequency, duration and mode of use, effects, complications (physical, social and psychological), presence of any withdrawal symptoms
◆ Alcohol: number of units, frequency and duration of use, withdrawal symptoms and complications
◆ Psychiatric history: nature of illness and details of any previous treatment; whether illness was related to drug and alcohol
◆ Interaction between the dual-diagnosis disorders
◆ Family and social relationships
◆ Medical history and current health status
◆ Criminal justice history
◆ Mental state: appearance/behaviour (withdrawals or intoxication), speech (slurred or rapid), mood and thought disorder, suicidal thoughts/intent, sleep, appetite, perceptual disturbances, insight into problem

Other key areas to address include employment/vocational status, educational history and status, literacy levels, IQ and developmental disabilities, interpersonal coping strategies, skills deficits (e.g. related to problem solving or communication).

TREATMENT INTERVENTIONS

The presentation of acute psychiatric symptoms, such as anxiety and depression, may interfere with traditional forms of substance abuse treatment and more often requires hospitalization or participation in intensive mental health services (Evans & Sullivan 1990, Pensker 1983). In informal settings the involvement and retention of offenders with co-occurring disorders in treatment can often be difficult, owing to rationalization and blaming others for their difficulties, distrust of service providers and sudden changes in psychiatric symptoms (Dale 1999).

Given the variety of presentations of this group in terms of mental disorder, substance abuse and functional skills, considerable flexibility is needed in developing treatment programmes (Zweben et al 1991). A range of different types of treatment setting, service configurations and orientations to treatment must be considered.

The substance abuse and mental health professions operate from different theoretical orientations which are reflected in the types of service provided (Evans & Sullivan 1990). One key difference between the professions is the struggle over which disorder is primary. Whilst many self-help programmes in the substance abuse field emphasize the concept of powerlessness, many mental health interventions are based on empowerment. Similarly, many substance abuse programmes focus on spirituality, which is not a major focus of mental health programmes. This theoretical and philosophical dichotomy can make it difficult for services to work together.

The different types of treatment adapted for offenders with dual-diagnosis disorders have typically involved use of integrated care through modification of traditional substance abuse or mental health approaches such as: therapeutic communities; cognitive-behavioural interventions; relapse prevention; and supportive psychoeducational approaches that are combined with 12-step/AA models (programmes may blend two or more of these approaches in the same treatment setting).

With respect to therapeutic interventions with drug misusers, the literature points to cognitive-behavioural interventions as having the most success. This includes harm reduction and relapse prevention work. This should take place in conjunction with rehabilitation into the community through appropriate vocational schemes and dealing with practical issues outside. The value of abstinence as a measure of success of therapy is questionable. More realistic measures are those of behavioural changes, success being measured by movement towards an increased ability to control drug use (Robertson et al 1989). The comparison of different forms of dual-diagnosis treatment services now clearly indicates that treatment must focus on building cognitive and interpersonal skills (whether refusal skills or prosocial skills to overcome boredom or aggressive impulses) to address the individual's specific deficits.

Professionals can expect considerable fluctuations in patients' motivation and commitment to behaviour change during the early phases of treatment, as offenders are not often initially committed to the idea of becoming abstinent (Drake et al 1996a) and require ongoing work to promote motivation. If left unaddressed, these issues are likely to lead to high rates of dropout and non-adherence to treatment regimes. Early treatment should therefore address motivation to commit to treatment and motivation levels should be subsequently monitored over an extended period of time (Griffin et al 1996). Offenders with dual diagnosis are also more likely to have cognitive limitations, such as difficulties in attention and concentration, memory, abstract reasoning, problem solving and planning ability.

Goals of treatment for offenders with dual diagnosis include:

◆ enhancing public and institutional safety
◆ providing ongoing monitoring and surveillance
◆ promoting ongoing involvement and treatment
◆ reducing substance abuse and mental health symptoms
◆ stabilizing medications and detoxification from drugs and alcohol
◆ developing enhanced awareness of the consequences of behaviour, the relapse process and the importance of treatment.

The best hope for achieving symptom stabilization and abstinence will involve a broad range of services available over several years as opposed to shorter periods of intensive care. Whilst an understanding of the interaction between the dual-diagnosis disorders may be an initial focus of treatment, later interventions are likely to deal with complex interpersonal skills and vocational difficulties.

Hills (2000) outlines several key principles that have emerged from the research and clinical literature in providing services to this population.

◆ Dealing with both disorders as primary.
◆ Integration of treatment services.
◆ Individualized programming to address symptom severity and skill deficits.
◆ Treatment comprehensiveness and flexibility.
◆ Phased treatment interventions should be of graduated intensity.
◆ Psychopharmacological interventions should be used when appropriate.
◆ Involvement in peer support and self-help groups.
◆ Modification of treatment services through reassessment.

TRAINING

A recent survey showed that awareness of the problems of dual diagnosis amongst mental health nurses was low and that carers may be reluctant to intervene with substance misuse problems, owing to either lack of knowledge and expertise regarding substance misuse or having negative attitudes towards the substance misuser (McKeown & Leibling 1995). Other studies point to the negative attitude of carers who deal with the issues of self-abusive behaviour, particularly when it involves illicit drugs, in a suppressive and moralistic manner, probably out of a sense of frustration or inadequacy about their ability to effect any change (Gafoor 1985).

At present, however, much professional education and training of health-care professionals reinforces the view that dealing with substance misuse is a specialist's job (Rassool 1993). Conversely, professionals specializing in substance abuse often have significant ignorance of the mental health treatment needs of clients so the development of an integrated service would require education and development initiatives which embrace both sets of professionals.

Given the statistics on levels of substance abuse amongst the mental health population generally, and the forensic psychiatric population in particular, there is an obvious need for mental health professionals to develop their knowledge and clinical expertise in substance misuse in order to meet the needs of this group of patients. Studies have shown that education and training on substance misuse and addictive behaviour can improve attitudes and build confidence and skills in identifying and working with substance misusers (Cartwright 1980, Kennedy & Faugier 1989, Rassool 1993).

Chappel (1993) describes the need for competent, experienced clinician teachers who have had positive experience with the treatment of dual-diagnosis disorders. The training of addiction and mental health professionals must include cooperation, understanding and respect for each other. Cross-training between trainees in psychiatry and substance abuse is needed in chemotherapy, psychotherapy, abstinence from alcohol and other addictive drugs, 12-step programmes, spiritual issues and milieu therapy. Negative attitudes and ignorance must be overcome for this training to take place. The importance of supervised clinical experience in treating dual-diagnosis patients is emphasized (Chappel 1993).

Guidelines for good practice in the education and training of nurses, midwives and health visitors on substance use and misuse are available (English National Board 1996). It will require attention by curriculum planners of both preregistration and continuing professional education programmes to modify and incorporate aspects of substance misuse and mental health problems into the core curricula (Rassool & Oyefeso 1993).

RECIDIVISM

Weiss (1992) considers that this population is also at a greater risk for relapse following release from custody by the self-medicating of uncomfortable emotional states (e.g. depression, mania) through the use of drugs. There may also be impaired

understanding, due to mental illness, of the negative effects of drugs or alcohol on behaviour where even small amounts of alcohol or drugs may precipitate recurrence of mental health symptoms amongst individuals (Drake et al 1996b) and reinvolvement in the criminal justice or health system (Pepper & Hendrickson 1996).

APPLICATION OF RESEARCH FINDINGS TO FORENSIC MENTAL HEALTH SERVICES

McKeown & Leibling (unpublished work, 1995) summarize the key issues for forensic services to consider in tackling the problems of dual diagnosis.

1. Develop links with outside agencies working with people with problems of substance abuse.
2. Concentrating on reduction of the illicit supply of drugs has failed and more successful approaches are policies of normalization and harm reduction.
3. Distributing information about community drug services results in more prisoners using these services once released from prison.
4. A multidisciplinary approach to drug problems is the most effective.
5. Staff training is a priority and should attempt to move towards the harm reduction model rather than abstinence.
6. Education and counselling of patients has been effective in prisons and could be adapted to a forensic mental health service and should include information on communicable diseases.
7. Treatment of individuals with drug problems should include cognitive-behavioural approaches, i.e. harm reduction and relapse prevention strategies. It could usefully include increasing awareness and more positive attitudes towards drug users. Treatment should also include preparing people for community living and linking in with appropriate agencies for support and employment in the future.
8. Attention should be paid to the issue of women who have drug problems and services should be adapted to suit their needs appropriately.

CONCLUSION

Despite the alarmingly high numbers of people with a dual diagnosis in forensic services, there remains a belief in the system that it is still undiagnosed to a large extent (Taylor et al 1998). It certainly does not receive either the resources or the attention that the problem deserves and it is often the direct care staff who bear the brunt of the lack of resourcing.

As street drugs become more complex and widely available, care staff struggle to keep in touch with newer developments (who had heard of Ecstasy a few years ago?) and are fighting a rearguard action in attempting to police a system with traditional ways of thinking, i.e. that the solution lies in stemming the supply (McKeown & Leibling 1995). Security systems only provide part of the answer; the Fallon Report (DoH 1999a) was both naïve and misleading in criticizing services for the existence of illicit drugs. All practitioners working in contemporary services knew that this was not an isolated issue nor a problem that could be eradicated by introducing draconian security measures. If that had been the case, then prison services in the UK and North America would be exemplars of drug-free environments, when we know that the opposite is true. Multiple methodologies are called for with improvements in initial screening and assessment methods and the adoption of instruments with proven efficacy.

The strong message from the literature and clinical practice is for the integration of treatment services, drawing on expertise in both the mental health and substance abuse sectors. Staff need to be supported in developing skills in the area of dual diagnosis and it should not be seen as a separate or specialist area of practice in the future. The extent of the problem is such that it demands integration into preregistration professional education programmes as well as more focused postqualifying training.

The recent publication of the mental health National Service Framework (DoH 1999b) and the ongoing review of the Mental Health Act 1983 (DoH 1999c) provide an opportunity to put into place systems and structures for managing an increasing and complex group of people whose needs transcend traditional service boundaries.

Staff need to be empowered to tackle often reluctant participants in therapy by having available a range of levers and sanctions to ensure that protection of all concerned, including the individual in need of services, is maximized.

REFERENCES

Addington J, Duchak V 1997 Reasons for substance use in schizophrenia. Acta Psychiatrica Scandinavica 96(5): 329–333

Alexander MJ 1996 Women with co-occurring addictive and mental disorders: an emerging profile of vulnerability. American Journal of Orthopsychiatry 66(1): 61–70

American Psychiatric Association 1994 Diagnostic and statistical manual of mental disorders, 4th edn. American Psychiatric Association, Washington

Bartels SJ, Drake RE, Wallach MA 1995 Long-term course of substance use disorders among patients with severe mental illness. Psychiatric Services 46(3): 248–251

Bassuk EL 1994 Community care for homeless clients with mental illness, substance abuse, or dual diagnosis. Better Homes Fund, Newton, MA

Beck AT, Beamesderfer A 1974 Assessment of depression: the depression inventory. In: Pichot P (ed) Modern problems in pharmacopsychiatry. Karger, Basel, Switzerland, pp 151–169

Bellack AS, Gearon JS 1998 Substance abuse treatment for people with schizophrenia. Addictive Behaviors 23: 749–766

Blankertz LE, Cnaan RA, Freedman E 1993 Childhood risk factors in dually diagnosed homeless adults. Social Work 38(5): 587–596

Brady KT, Roberts JM 1995 The pharmacotherapy of dual diagnosis. Psychiatric Annals 25(6): 344–352

Carey KB 1989 Emerging treatment guidelines for mentally ill chemical abusers. Hospital and Community Psychiatry 40(4): 341–342, 349

Carey KB 1991 Research with dual diagnosis patients: challenges and recommendations. Behaviour Therapist January: 5–8

Cartwright A 1980 The attitude of helping agents towards the alcoholic client: the influence of experience, support, training and self-esteem. British Journal of Addiction 75: 413–431

Center for Substance Abuse Treatment 1994 Simple screening instruments for outreach for alcohol and other drug abuse and infectious diseases. Treatment

Improvement Protocol (TIP) Series, #11. US Department of Health and Human Services, Rockville, MD

Chappel JN 1993 Training of residents and medical students in the diagnosis and treatment of dual diagnosis patients. Journal of Psychoactive Drugs 25(4): 293–300

Dale C 1999 Dual diagnosis: the American experience. Mental Health Practice 3(3): 18–21

DeLeon G, Jainchill N 1986 Circumstance, motivation, readiness and suitability as correlates of treatment tenure. Journal of Psychoactive Drugs 18(3): 203–208

Department of Health 1999a The Report of the Committee of Inquiry into the Personality Disorder Unit, Ashworth Special Hospital. Stationery Office, London

Department of Health 1999b Mental health national service frameworks: modern standards and service models. Stationery Office, London

Department of Health 1999c Reform of the Mental Health Act 1983: proposals for consultation. Cm 4480. Stationery Office, London

Derogatis LR, Melisaratos N 1983 The Brief Symptom Inventory: an introductory report. Psychological Medicine 13: 595–605

Derogatis LR, Lipman R, Rickels K 1974 The Hopkins Symptom Checklist (HSCL): a self-report symptom inventory. Behavioural Science 19: 1–16

DiClemente CC, Hughes SO 1990 Stages of change profiles in outpatient alcoholism treatment. Journal of Substance Abuse 2: 217–235

Dixon L, Haas J, Weiden P, Sweeney H, Frances A 1990 Acute effects of drug abuse in schizophrenic patients: clinical observation and patients' self reports. Schizophrenia Bulletin 16(1): 69–79

Drake RE 1995 Research on treating substance abuse in persons with severe mental illness. National Institute of Mental Health, Rockville, MD

Drake RE, Osher FC, Wallach MA 1991 Homelessness and dual diagnosis. American Psychologist 46: 1149–1158

Drake RE, Alterman AI, Rosenberg SR 1993 Detection of substance use disorders in severely mentally ill patients. Community Mental Health 29(2): 175–192

Drake RE, Rosenberg SD, Mueser KT 1996a Assessing substance use disorder in persons with severe mental illness. In: Drake RE, Mueser KT (eds) Dual diagnosis of major mental illness and substance abuse, vol. 2: recent research and clinical implications. Jossey-Bass, San Francisco, pp 3–17

Drake RE, Mueser KT, Clark RE, Wallach MA 1996b The course, treatment, and outcome of substance disorder in persons with severe mental illness. American Journal of Orthopsychiatry 66(1): 42–50

Drake R, McHugo GJ, Clark RE et al 1998 Assertive community treatment for patients with co-occurring severe mental illness and substance use disorder: a clinical trial. American Journal of Orthopsychiatry 68(2): 201–215

El-Mallakh P 1998 Treatment models for clients with co-occurring addictive and mental disorders. Archives of Psychiatric Nursing 12(2): 71–80

English National Board 1996 Substance use and misuse. Guidelines for good practice in education and training of nurses, midwives and health visitors. ENB, London

Evans K, Sullivan JM 1990 Dual diagnosis: counseling the mentally ill substance abuser. Guilford, New York

Gafoor M 1985 Nurses' attitudes to the drug abuser (letter). Nursing Times 81(44): 12

Greenfield SF, Weiss RD, Tohen M 1995 Substance abuse and the chronically mentally ill: a description of dual diagnosis treatment services in a psychiatric hospital. Community Mental Health Journal 31(3): 265–277

Griffin PA, Hills HA, Peters RH 1996 Criminal justice–substance abuse cross-training: working together for change. Center for Substance Abuse Treatment, Rockville, MD

Havassy BE, Arns PG 1998 Relationship of cocaine and other substance dependence to well-being of high-risk psychiatric patients. Psychiatric Services 49: 935–940

Hills A (2000) Creating treatment programmes for persons with dual diagnosis disorders in the criminal justice system. National GAINS Center, Delmar, NY

Institute of Medicine 1995 Development of medications for the treatment of opiate and cocaine addictions: issues for the government and private sector. National Academy Press, Washington DC, pp 193–202

Kennedy J, Faugier J 1989 Drug and alcohol dependency nursing. Heinemann, London

Kipping C 1999 Dual diagnosis: meeting clients' needs. Mental Health Practice 3(3): 10–18

Kirchner JE, Owen RR, Nordquist C, Fischer EP 1998 Diagnosis and management of substance use disorders among inpatients with schizophrenia. Psychiatric Services 49(1): 82–85

Kosten TR, Ziedonis DM 1997 Substance abuse and schizophrenia: editors' introduction. Schizophrenia Bulletin 23: 181–186

Lehman AF 1996 Heterogeneity of person and place: assessing dual diagnosis addictive and mental disorders. American Journal of Orthopsychiatry 66(1): 32–41

Ley A, Jeffery DP, McLaren S, Siegfried N 1999 Treatment programmes for those with both severe mental illness and substance misuse (Cochrane Review). The Cochrane Library, Issue 4. Update Software, Oxford

McConnaughy EA, Prochaska J, Velicer WR 1983 Stages of change in psychotherapy: measurement and sample profiles. Psychotherapy: Theory, Research and Practice 20: 368–375

McKeown M, Leibling H 1995 Staff perception of illicit drug use within a special hospital. Journal of Psychiatric and Mental Health Nursing 2(6): 343–350

McLellan AT, Luborsky L, Woody GE, O'Brien CP 1980 An improved diagnostic evaluation instrument for substance abuse patients. Journal of Nervous and Mental Disease 168(1): 26–33

Mental Health Act Commission 1999 8th biennial report. Stationery Office, London

Miller WR 1994 SOCRATES: The Stages of Change Readiness and Treatment Eagerness Scale. Department of Psychology, University of New Mexico, Albuquerque

Miner CR, Rosenthal RN, Hellerstein DJ, Muenz LR 1997 Prediction of compliance with outpatient referral in patients with schizophrenia and psychoactive substance use disorders. Archives of General Psychiatry 54: 706–712

Mueser KT, Drake RD, Miles KM 1997 The course and treatment of substance use disorders in persons with severe mental illnesses. NIDA Research Monograph 172: 86–109

Mueser KT, Drake RE, Wallach MA 1998 Dual diagnosis: a review of etiological theories. Addictive Behaviors 23: 717–734

Osher FC, Kofoed LL 1989 Treatment of patients with psychiatric and psychoactive substance abuse disorders. Hospital and Community Psychiatry 40: 1025–1031

Pensker H 1983 Addicted patients in hospital psychiatric units. Psychiatric Annals 13: 619–623

Pepper B, Hendrickson E 1996 Working with seriously mentally ill substance abusers. In: Lurigio AJ (ed) Community corrections in America: new directions and sound investments for persons with mental illness and co-disorders. National Coalition for Mental and Substance Abuse Health Care in the Justice System, Seattle, WA, pp 78–93

Peters RH, Bartoi MG 1997 Screening and assessment of dual diagnosis disorders in the justice system. National GAINS Center, Delmar, NY

Peters RH, Greenbaum PE 1996 Texas Department of Criminal Justice/Center for Substance Abuse Treatment Prison Substance Abuse Screening Project. Civigenics Inc, Millford, MA

Rassool GH 1993 Nursing and substance misuse: responding to the challenge. Journal of Advanced Nursing 18: 1401–1407

Rassool GH, Oyefeso N 1993 Substance misuse in health studies curriculum: a case for nursing education. Nurse Education Today 13: 107–110

Ridgely MS, Goldman HH, Willenbring M 1990 Barriers to the care of persons with dual diagnosis: organisational and financial issues. Schizophrenia Bulletin 16(1): 123–132

Robertson JR, Bucknall ABV, Skidmore CA, Roberts JJK, Smith JH 1989 Remission and relapse in heroin users and implications for management: treatment control or risk reduction. International Journal of Addiction 24: 229–246

Robins LN, Regier DA 1991 Psychiatric disorders in America: the Epidemiologic Catchment Area Study. Free Press, New York

Sandford T 1995 Drug use is increasing. Nursing Standard 9(38): 16–17

Schneider FR, Siris SD 1987 A review of psychoactive substance use and abuse in schizophrenia: patterns of drug choice. Journal of Psychiatry 165: 13–21

Shumway M, Cuffel BJ 1996 Symptom heterogeneity in co-morbid alcohol disorder. Journal of Mental Health Administration 23(3): 338–347

Simpson DD, Knight K, Broome KM 1997 Texas Christian University/Criminal Justice Forms Manual: Drug Dependence Screen and Initial Assessment. Christian University, Institute of Behavioral Research, Fort Worth, TX

Skinner HA, Horn JL 1984 Alcohol Dependence Scale: user's guide. Addiction Research Foundation, Toronto

Taylor PJ, Leese M, Willis D, Butwell M, Daly R, Larkin E 1998 Mental disorder and violence: a special hospital study. British Journal of Psychiatry 172: 218–226

Teague GB, Schwab B, Drake RE 1990 Evaluating services for young adults with severe mental illness and substance use disorders. National Association of State Mental Health Programme Directors, Arlington, VA

Teplin LA, Schwartz J 1989 Screening for severe mental disorder in jails. Law and Human Behavior 13(1): 1–18

Vogel HS, Knight E, Laudet AB, Magura S 1998 Double trouble in recovery. Self-help for people with dual diagnoses. Psychiatric Rehabilitation Journal 21: 356–364

Weiss RD 1992 The role of psychopathology in the transition from drug use to abuse and dependence. In: Glantz M, Pickens R (eds) Vulnerability to drug abuse. American Psychological Association, Washington DC

Westreich L, Guedj P, Galanter M, Baird D 1997 Differences between men and women in dual-diagnosis treatment. American Journal of Addiction 6(4): 311–317

Zweben JE, Smith DE, Stewart P 1991 Psychotic conditions and substance use: prescribing guidelines and other treatment issues. Journal of Psychoactive Drugs 23(4): 387–395

FURTHER READING

Drake RE, Mueser KT (eds) 1996 Dual diagnosis of major mental illness and substance abuse, vol. 2: recent research and clinical implications. Jossey-Bass, San Francisco

Lehman AF, Dixon LB (eds) 1996 Double jeopardy. Harwood Academic Press, Churr, Switzerland

Rorstad P, Checinski K 1996 Dual diagnosis: facing the challenge. Wynne Howard Publishing, Kenley

Chapter Nineteen

Clinical supervision

Les Jennings

INTRODUCTION

The starting point or theme for this chapter is the United Kingdom Central Council for Nursing, Midwifery and Health Visiting (1996) position statement on clinical supervision. It identifies a range of key principles thought effective in the establishment of good and effective clinical supervision practice. What is significant is that it does not provide comprehensive detailed actions but identifies a number of themes and issues to be addressed at a local level. However, a key axiom is that clinical supervision will assist patients and clients to receive high-quality, safe care in a rapidly changing care environment. Furthermore, the potential impacts to be gained from the enterprise

of clinical supervision merit a personal, professional and economic investment in clinical supervision. Also, as inferred by Maden (1996), clinical supervision can make a significant contribution to clinical risk assessment and management, an activity which should be at the epicentre of the enterprise described as forensic mental health care.

The services for those with forensic mental health problems have undergone significant and radical changes in recent times. Proposed governmental changes in mental health legislation, the work done by the National Health Service Confederation & Sainsbury Centre for Mental Health (1997), the Department of Health (1999a) through the National Service Framework for Mental Health and the recent debates on mental health practitioner skills (Butterworth 1994, Faulkner 1998) all indicate a shift in consumer expectations and what constitutes best clinical practice.

A growing realization is evident that many practitioners in forensic mental health care will need to extend the parameters of their professional and vocational functions and become more autonomous and responsible for their own practice. This autonomy, and related increase in the scope of practice for forensic mental health workers, although welcomed, suggests a tacit acknowledgement of what Goldberg (1986) describes as a potential for 'increasing isolation and existential exhaustion'. Additionally, the work of Kennerley (1990) offers powerful indicators that many practitioners experience an increase in the level of anxiety and stress in their work.

Contemporary management theory (Torrington & Weightman 1994), if translated into the world of forensic mental health care, would suggest that there is a need for services that both support and facilitate practitioners, whilst attending to the needs of the consumer. Supervision, if undertaken in a coherent, consistent and logical fashion, can offer the infrastructure required to help meet the needs of all parties within a service provision that is continually in a state of flux and change. There will be occasions when this change and complexity can leave the practitioner in a state of alienation and disempowerment which, ultimately, will translate into real working situations.

This is juxtaposed with strong evidence offered by commentators such as Dolan & Coid (1993), who argue that effective treatment of a large proportion of those patients who find themselves subject to the attentions of the forensic mental health services (personality disorders) is inconclusive and that those charged with caring for this group develop negative attitudes towards the patient group and the effectiveness of their interventions. Palmer (1992) claims that a structure to manage such conflict and dynamic is essential. Furthermore, Melia et al (1999), although talking about a fairly discrete client group, those with personality disorder, clearly illustrate much of the work of the forensic practitioner when they describe the relationships with

the personality-disordered patient as being highly charged and emotionally intense with high levels of anger and hostility. This presents a scenario in which it is fair to assume that no 'one' definitive way of expediting clinical supervision in such environments exists.

Based on this assumption it is intended to use actual case materials which have been brought to supervision and to take the reader through some of the suggestions, interventions and processes as they have been played out in the supervisor–supervisee relationship. This is not to claim that this text contains the 'right' answers or describes what to do in supervision, but to use the information to begin to establish the climate for reflection and challenge within the environs of forensic mental health care.

Evidence for these assumptions, and an appropriate starting point, is based upon the work of contemporary writers such as: Briant (1997), Butler & Zelen (1977), Gemma (1989), Pennington et al (1993), Rushton et al (1996) and Totka (1996). They comment from a diversity of perspectives but a *sine qua non* of their assertions is that an exploration of the 'unspoken and silent' tensions within the arena of professional relationships, such as sexuality, what it means to care too much, what it means to care less in a way that might empower and the nature of the professional relationship and friendship, is pivotal. These key aspects of forensic mental health work, although not made entirely explicit, have provided the basis for the establishment of recent inquiry reports (DoH 1992, 1999b) and rested heavily on the forensic mental health practitioner. However, to begin to address the issues described it is imperative that certain questions are asked to help locate the debate for the practitioner in forensic mental health care.

WHAT IS THE ENTERPRISE CALLED CLINICAL SUPERVISION?

A number of definitions have been proposed for clinical supervision. Loganbill et al (1982) defined clinical supervision as: 'An intensive, interpersonally focused, one to one relationship in which one person is designated to facilitate the development of therapeutic competencies in the other person'.

The UKCC (1996) position paper on clinical supervision contends that: 'Clinical supervision brings practitioner(s) and skilled supervisors together to reflect on practice. Supervision aims to identify solutions to problems, improve practice and increase understanding of professional issues'. However, for the British Association of Counselling (1992: 2) the primary purpose of supervision is: 'to protect the best interests of the client'.

The Community Psychiatric Nurses Association (1989) describes supervision as 'the cornerstone of clinical practice'. However, as Butterworth & Faugier (1992) comment, the implementation of clinical supervision in services has been very ad hoc, often developing from practitioners themselves as a desperate response to critical issues and events in their professional life. The lack, until recently, of any framework for clinical supervision has led to varying practices being identified as clinical supervision. This has led to many practitioners being wary of accepting a practice that appears to have many definitions and interpretations.

I would assert that for the forensic mental health practitioner the UKCC (1996) position statement on clinical supervision may go some way to establishing what it is. However, what can be added is that clinical supervision is a collaborative dynamic process, extending beyond, whilst incorporating a pastoral nurturing role, which works positively towards *enabling* the practitioner. To work effectively, it requires all parties involved in the relationship to participate actively in ensuring that the needs of the patient are being addressed and monitored, and that the supervisee becomes a more competent practitioner.

The following case material offers some useful insight into the benefits of supervision for all members of the multidisciplinary team, particularly around the issue of *enabling*. However, reiterating the initial premise of this chapter and acknowledging the support of Butterworth & Faugier (1992), clearly there is no 'one way' for the forensic mental health practitioner to proceed but to build upon what 'experts' indicate is good practice.

ONE CASE, ONE VIEW?

Box 19.1 provides the story of a patient called Colin. A key issue in this case study is to ask why this state of affairs prevailed. How was the situation managed? How did the multidisciplinary team come to terms with their actions and the impact that Colin had upon them?

First, some general comment on the contextual issues in forensic care. The provision of effective

---

Box 19.1   Case study 1

Colin is a 28-year-old man, detained within a secure hospital facility with a diagnosis of paranoid schizophrenia. Colin is an extremely bright man who, unfortunately, grew up in a family with clear evidence of dysfunction. His illness can only be described as severe and it resulted in him making a vicious attack on his mother. Currently, he presents with an extremely severe and enduring mental illness with resultant impact upon his social relationships. He will routinely throw his possessions out of the windows of the ward, buy goods and then destroy them, rub coffee into his hair and swear and shout at staff and patients. He has no friends on the ward, he is isolative, unkempt and dirty if left to his own devices. He is described as arrogant and unfeeling. He is dismissive of staff members and other patients. He seems to purposely reject the advances of others. This was most evident when the multidisciplinary team were discussing his progress at ward level. He would challenge the decisions in a non-constructive fashion, make derogatory comments about team members and interrupt proceedings. This culminated in the team deciding to lock the door to the room in which the meeting was taking place in order to keep Colin out. This, in essence, challenged the main therapeutic stance of the whole team but it was allowed to happen without questioning.

forensic mental health services is a constant challenge. It sits, at times, uneasily with economic constraints, ideological positions and the expectations of society and the general public. The current debates on the most appropriate dispersal of personality-disordered patients and the need to protect the public offer timely reminders of the complexity. However, for practitioners working in this field this can (and often does) represent a mass of contradictions that render their role difficult and the provision of good-quality care complex. The support of professionals undertaking such roles and function is crucial. Additionally, mental health practitioners have a duty to ensure that their practice is competent and the function of clinical supervision is educative as well as supportive and restorative (Hawkins & Shohet 1984).

The UKCC (1992) Code of Professional Conduct makes reference to the links between continuing professional education and the provision and improvement of the quality of patient care by stating that practitioners must:

◆ maintain and improve professional knowledge and competence
◆ acknowledge any limitations in knowledge and competence and decline any duties or responsibilities unless able to perform them in a safe and skilled manner
◆ assist professional colleagues, in the context of your own knowledge, experience and sphere of responsibility, to develop their professional competence and assist others in the care team, including informal carers, to contribute safely and to a degree appropriate to their roles.

A principal medium for forensic mental health care consists of the relationship which practitioners develop with individuals and groups. The initiation, maintenance, development and ending of those relationships can be problematic and stressful and require complicated and demanding skills. Reflection on practice and its effectiveness in meeting the changing health-care needs of clients can lead to these skills being constantly redefined and improved throughout professional life.

Cooke (1992) raises a pertinent point, felt by many nurses working in the field of general mental health, when she highlights that nurses working in this field are required (and have been for many years) to liaise with many professionals and utilize a multidisciplinary approach to care provision. For many this has necessitated working in departments other than nursing and, for some, having line managers other than nurses. Geographical isolation from other nursing colleagues is yet another example of how nurses working in the community with people who have mental health problems have moved away from the traditional hierarchical structure of nursing management. This is, in some sense, similar to the work of the forensic practitioner in which isolation and marginalization are key features of the working day. The forensic practitioner is presented with cases which represent 'dirty work' and can offer little by way of tangible reward for the job done. This position, if juxtaposed with the vicissitudes of societal values and views in terms of the mentally disordered offender, creates the climate for the marginalization process.

It is now accepted, however, that multidisciplinary teamwork and interagency collaboration are essential prerequisites for effective, high-quality service provision to people who have mental health problems and their carers (Mathias et al 1997). Changes in service delivery and service organization have meant that professionals working in this area have a responsibility to develop and maintain good working relationships with all their multidisciplinary colleagues. The advent of care management means that interagency and multidisciplinary practice are even more bound together. It would make sense, therefore, that if a practitioner is used to working alongside another professional on a regular basis, clinical supervision across disciplines can be beneficial both for the practitioners, where there may be an exchange of knowledge and information, and for the client whose care package may be, in the main, organized, developed and maintained by several members of a multidisciplinary team.

However, Thomas & Reid (1995) highlight the causes of problems that can occur between professionals working within a multidisciplinary team. These include: stereotyped views about each professional's role and function; lack of understanding about each team member's role, working from different theoretical and knowledge bases; functional isolation; and hierarchies. One way to combat all of these problems could begin with the understanding of each team member's role, which should lead to less professional rivalry.

In the case of Colin, the work of Watts & Morgan (1994) proved to be of immense value in helping the team to address some of the clinical and emotional aspects of the care delivery. Watts & Morgan delineate some of the issues surrounding patients who are 'hard to like' and in supervision sessions, this emerged as a major theme. Accounting for patient factors, staff factors and environmental factors enabled an opening up of some issues in the delivery of care to Colin. For example, Watts & Morgan identify strategies for preventing malignant alienation. Some proved invaluable, such as equating challenging behaviour with an inability to seek help in other ways; providing insight into staff members' own vulnerabilities and expectations; early identification of the lack of a therapeutic alliance; and allowing the negative feelings of staff to be discussed openly, rather than 'acted out'. It allowed the staff to 'de-institutionalize' their feelings and process issues in ways more beneficial for Colin and for themselves. Interestingly, the locking of the door and the pathologizing of Colin's inability to ask directly for help were unobserved or denied in terms of what the actions may be symbolizing for the care of individuals on the wards and for the collective ward community. With time, through supervision, the team were enabled to explore their actions and behaviour in other ways that may have been more beneficial to Colin and his subsequent management.

OTHER CASES, OTHER VIEWS?

Some writers in forensic nursing imply that the frequency with which nurses make reference to professional approaches in answer to the problems set by patients, as opposed to 'gut reactions' or to explain such reactions, might conceal negative feelings and affective responses (Melia et al 1999, Moran & Mason 1996, Neilson 1991, 1992, Noak 1995, Tennant & Hughes 1998).

They appear to suggest it is natural to have these angry feelings toward patients who may display little remorse for what they have done. However, it must be noted that if such feelings are kept hidden they will, ultimately, subvert nurses' attitudes to their patients.

The work of Lutzen (1998) offers timely reminders of some of the dynamics which can emerge. The notions of subtle coercion, 'hostage taking' of the patient by mental health legislation and the patient's trust within the relationship (Jennings 1997, Lutzen & Nordin 1994, Mason & Jennings 1997) are clear pointers to the emergence of such dynamics. This underlines the need for supervision in such high-pressure, emotional situations and for the exploration of the impact upon the individual nurse and the patient. It is suggested that there is a potential for such impacts to go beyond what has been stated thus far and set up dynamics which are played out in the clinical arena. The case study set out in Box 19.2 offers illustrations. This is an anonymized case brought to supervision.

One of the strategies utilized by the supervisor was to help Jackie in the development of an action plan that looked at career development, mentorship and guidance in the future. However, the issues suggested by Power (1994) do offer the potential for the supervision to have a different trajectory. I feel it is of the utmost importance to examine some of underlying dynamics and 'acting out' behaviours which are evident. For example, it could be argued (and this would be consistent with the work of Melia et al (1999) and Moran & Mason (1996)) that the care of the personality-disordered patient is redolent with status, power, pain and distress issues and these can be reenacted on female staff within such environments. The ward philosophy, if the rendition in Box 19.2 is accepted, presents a particular view of women. This can be of the woman who abuses or the woman who has been abused. Also, the common role for women in such areas is that of mother or housekeeper, which can mirror the role of women in society generally. Once they fulfil that role it can legitimize abuse and punishment by the patients. In a sense, male staff by their actions are reinforcing a common patient view of women,

---

Box 19.2 Case study 2

Jackie is a staff nurse working within an all-male environment. The clinical speciality of the ward is the assessment of young patients with severe personality disorders. Most of the patient group have committed sex offences of a severe nature toward women or children. Much of their pathology can be crystallized around severely dysfunctional relationships with females, for example, mother, sister or spouse.

What Jackie presented at supervision was an issue of not being allowed to 'act up' and being treated differently from male colleagues. An example was not being allowed to give an injection to a male patient. The reason given was that a senior male colleague had said that he would not allow his wife to do the same and he would not have his wife working in such an environment.

---

that they should be denigrated and humiliated. The apparently innocuous request to make the tea can, in fact, ensure that female members of staff are 'set up' to ensure that the deep cultural and institutional patterns of such care environments are perpetuated. If the situation described is accepted, it offers the potential for a new range of therapeutic strategies to work with such patient groups in order to change some aspects of entrenched, institutional behaviour.

Furthermore, in a more general sense, the scenario in Box 19.2 shows that the supervisee can be offered a unique and valuable opportunity to, as Power (1994: 105) suggests, 'explore the often complicated dynamics of their professional, yet personal relationship with their clients, in a safe environment'.

Supervisors can provide the supervisee with new thoughts and insights into the problems or difficulties that are identified within the relationship. That said, and it is worth repeating and summarizing, it is often useful when reflecting upon therapeutic interventions and responses with a client to have the benefit of an 'outside' view. The gains of using clinical supervision in forensic mental health care and listening to the 'outside view' of practice can be identified as:

◆ personal growth
◆ increased job satisfaction
◆ support and sharing of feelings
◆ reduction in staff turnover
◆ reduction of stress and burnout
◆ increased confidence and autonomy of practitioners.

Few people have stated this as well as Melia et al (1999), in their discussions on triumvirate nursing within secure settings. The 'outside view' or third party offers considerable scope in helping to maintain the integrity of intervention when nursing in such settings. Also, it may facilitate the exploration of the following key factors within the supervisory relationship.

◆ The patient's transference
◆ The nurse's countertransference
◆ Ethical issues
◆ Power relationships
◆ Exploitation and other boundary issues
◆ Previous management of the relationship
◆ Future management of the relationship
◆ The patient's feelings
◆ The nurse's feelings
◆ Attachment styles and responses

ANOTHER CASE, ANOTHER VIEW?

Box 19.3 provides an example of supervision. Much of what is described as forensic care is provided with a temporal aspect to it. The temporal markers used to describe success and failure are often disjointed, hidden or blurred.

It could be argued that if the structures of supervision are not put in place, the climate is ripe for the development of posttraumatic stress disorder. This seemed to be a possibility with Jim. However, and this is a key point that indicates the

Box 19.3   Case study 3

Jim is a staff nurse working in a medium dependency ward within a forensic environment. He is a father of two grown-up children, happily married and has been working in the above setting for 18 years, the last 6 of those years on the medium dependency ward. He is the primary nurse for a patient called Bob.

Bob was diagnosed as schizophrenic with a severe personality disorder. His index offence was attempted rape and grievous bodily harm. This resulted in his victim suffering from a severe anxiety state and she has been unable to take up her previous role in society as a teacher. Bob is described as manipulative on the ward and spends most of his time offering challenges to the system in terms of disrupting the pattern of ward life if he does not get his own way. Attempts to control this challenging behaviour by limit setting and establishing boundaries have had little success. This is due, in the main, to a lack of consistency in Bob's care and several staff members attempting to 'buy'

his cooperation with gifts and privileges. The other disciplines in the care team have offered little by way of support and Jim has been left to manage the situation mostly alone. This he had been attempting for the past 6 years.

Jim, until recently, had not attended any type of supervision. He came to supervision upset, worried and agitated. He considered himself a good primary nurse. During supervision, it was suggested that he approach the ward manager. Jim said he was unable to. He considered the ward manager 'very cut off' and unapproachable, a distant figure. During further sessions Jim was asked to describe what it may feel like to go in and see the manager and he began to cry and spoke about his recent sickness record, of being unable to sleep for continually thinking about the problems which Bob was creating for him, of being unable to solve even the simplest of issues at home and work and of how he felt totally alone.

---

trajectory for discussion, post-traumatic stress disorder is usually related to a single experience of great intensity but limited duration whereas in forensic mental health care, as has been described with some eloquence by Ravin & Boal (1989), a sequence of individual, less intense events can also lead to similar symptoms. Similarly, Scott & Stradling (1992) stated that the predominant post-traumatic stress disorder features of avoidance behaviour (absence/sickness) and intrusive imagery may also occur in response to enduring circumstances involving prolonged duress and these authors have coined the term 'prolonged duress stress disorder'. Similar work completed by Friis & Helldin (1994) identified the necessity of having a stable, experienced staff, clear leadership and predictable, clearly structured staff functions so as to reduce the impact of both post-traumatic stress disorder and prolonged duress stress disorder.

Additionally, this is very much linked to the assertions and dynamics described by Melia et al (1999), that a key feature of much of the work

done by forensic mental health professionals now relates to abuse issues. Lyon (1993) observed that staff reactions to patients' accounts of childhood abuse resemble some symptoms of post-traumatic stress disorder. A detailed analysis of the staff reactions reveals the themes of the 'toxic' or 'contaminating' quality of abuse description, feelings of isolation and alienation from other staff and friends and the questions of good and evil. If these observations are linked to the work of Silfin & Ben-David (1993) and issues surrounding work with violent and self-injurious clients, it can be posited that the stresses of the transference and countertransference relationship, and the resultant lowering of the practitioner tolerance threshold, make strong claims for a robust structure of clinical supervision.

In later sessions with Jim, some of the 'toxicity' and 'contamination' he felt within his relationship with Bob were explored. Jim began to understand that his feelings of being out of control with Bob were invading other aspects of his life and his beliefs about his ward manager. Through the use of role play he was able to explore what it would feel like to make an appointment with the manager, set limits for Bob, engage other members of the care team and take more control of his life.

OTHER PURPOSES OF CLINICAL SUPERVISION IN FORENSIC MENTAL HEALTH CARE

Up to this point the discussion has mainly focused on the clinical issues and impact of supervision but supervision has other purposes outside the immediate clinical issues and it is worth making these explicit. For example, it helps to ensure the promotion of competent and accountable work which concerns the patient, the organization and the supervisee. Another purpose is the facilitation of professional and personal development. The case study in Box 19.4 may help in illuminating these assertions.

The supervisor was able to provide practical advice in terms of giving Dave information about:

◆ support groups who might be able to help
◆ the name of another nurse in a nearby town who had had experience in providing this type of support.

The supervisor also emphasized that Dave was not to feel 'alone' in this and that this issue should be raised whenever it was necessary, in supervision sessions. Moreover, the process of supervision closely parallels that of the practitioner–patient relationship. Both should be a learning process that takes place within the context of a relationship that facilitates positive change, at both professional and personal levels. In this respect, the supervisor may examine the level at which Dave is functioning in the relationship with his patient Lynn (Stoltenberg & Delworth 1987). For example, is Dave able to view the patient in the wider context and present an overview that is cognisant of the patient's personal history or life patterns? Is Dave able to remain fully present with the patient despite her life circumstances and social context?

Respect must be the foundation stone for any supervisory relationship, not only for the process of supervision but also for the supervisor, the supervisee, the client and the organization in which supervision occurs. Butterworth (1994) identified that, for nurses, the development of their role as accountable autonomous practitioners has evolved from their movement away from the medical model of health care. This development has left nurses with the need to develop strong 'protective' mechanisms and to accept that with autonomous practice comes accountability. For nurses working in the forensic mental health field, the protection of medics was never as strong as it was for other nursing specialities, yet by developing new roles, the need for support and supervision has never been more important.

For Bishop (1994) the purpose of supervision is the provision of support to nurses but it may also provide a vehicle for stress reduction, reflection and the identification of problem-solving techniques. However, there is a tripartite arrangement in respect of the benefits of clinical supervision: first, the benefits to the patient; second, the

---

Box 19.4 Case study 4

Dave is a community forensic nurse working with people who have mental health problems. One of Dave's more recent patients, Lynn, has told Dave that she is pregnant. Dave is aware that Lynn's first child was adopted as she was unable to look after the child because of her diagnosis of paranoid schizophrenia and her threats to kill her child. Lynn is desperately keen to care for her second child when it is born and is asking Dave for his support in order to do this. Dave has not met this situation before and is concerned that he will not be able to provide the level of support that Lynn will need. In clinical supervision, Dave raised this concern.

benefits to the service; and third, the benefits to the supervisee.

Benefits to patients

◆ Helps in monitoring effective/non-effective practice.
◆ Encourages reflection on and in practice.
◆ Encourages a climate of negotiated care.
◆ Facilitates a coherent response to patient need.
◆ Offers the opportunity to evaluate key issues and episodes of clinical practice.
◆ Helps in meeting the demands made for partnership in care.

Benefits to the service

The service needs to be committed to the provision of clinical supervision, which requires time and energy to be effective. Planning, implementing, monitoring and evaluating a system of professional supervision in mental health service provision is justifiable if it brings the following benefits.

◆ Clinical supervision, as part of a staff development and support programme, could allow a sustained and detailed exploration of professional issues with a view to increasing job satisfaction and enhancing a sense of teamwork and corporate purpose.
◆ The client's needs being met through improvement in the quality of care provision.
◆ It would provide opportunities for valuing colleagues' strengths and of identifying ways in which their professional needs could be met.
◆ It would encourage colleagues at all levels, across disciplines and agencies to become more confident in exploring their professional input at work in an open way, thus helping to build a climate of trust in which professional development could take place.
◆ It would involve practitioners working on a common problem, weakness or issue to create a greater sense of effective teamwork.
◆ It would offer to the supervisee an idea of what constitutes clinical practice, developmental issues, confidentiality and personal issues.

The caveat is that the supervisee is usually less experienced than the supervisor and so structures must be in place to manage the accompanying power relationship tensions.

Benefits to the supervisee

◆ It provides regular space for the supervisee and supervisor to reflect upon the content and process of their work.
◆ It facilitates the development of understanding and skills within their work.
◆ It allows the nurse space and time to receive information and another perspective concerning their practice.
◆ The nurse can be validated and supported both as a person and as a colleague. In a stressful occupation or at stressful times, it helps to ensure that as a person and as a practitioner, the nurse is not left to carry, unnecessarily, difficulties, problems and projections on their own.
◆ It gives the nurse the opportunity to explore and express personal distress, transference and countertransference that have been provoked by their practice.
◆ It may help the nurse to better plan and utilize their personal and professional resources.
◆ It encourages the nurse to be proactive rather than reactive.
◆ It allows the nurse to use self-appraisal to monitor the quality of their work and provides a formal support system in periods of professional stress, crisis and confusion.
◆ Clinical supervision could be professionally empowering for nurses working within multidisciplinary teams.

MODELS AND FRAMEWORKS, ROLES AND STRUCTURES IN CLINICAL SUPERVISION

Although not prescriptive, implicit in what has been presented thus far is that some model or framework of working ought to be established to bring some consistency to the arena of supervision.

Several different supervision structures have been described, one of the most popular being that described by Cooke (1992) which suggests four ways of structuring supervision. Others such as Procter (1986) offer useful representations of the fundamental base upon which supervision is premised. Clearly, there are the normative, formative and restorative elements joined with the express need for a therapeutic alliance.

The UKCC (1996) position statement on clinical supervision is quite definite in its stance on what clinical supervision is. It argues that: 'Clinical supervision is not a managerial control system. It is not therefore: the exercise of overt managerial responsibility or managerial supervision; a system of formal individual performance review or hierarchical in nature'.

The role and function of supervision must therefore be very clearly identified by the practitioners involved in this relationship. The person who undertakes the supervisor role has the main responsibility in ensuring that such a structure is in place. In forensic care the role of the supervisor may be summarized as set out below.

Role of the supervisor

The role of the supervisor is characterized by two key features:

1. commitment on the part of the supervisor to the facilitation of growth, both educational and personal, of the supervisee
2. an acceptance of the voluntary nature of the contract.

These two features are fundamental to effective, safe, supportive clinical supervision, if the three functions of supervision as described by Procter (1986) are to be achieved. Also, it is posited that the 'special and particular uniqueness' of much of forensic provision makes these two features essential. Some of the issues of special importance in the work of the forensic practitioner, such as the exploration of risk and dangerousness and mental illness and crime, are testament to this assertion. Buchanan (1999), Maden (1996) and Wesley & Taylor (1991) offer clear accounts of the requirement for the practitioner to be skilled in the assessment and management of risk but, also, to be adept in managing the tensions inherent in the association between criminal acts and mental illness. This offers a unique challenge to the forensic practitioner in ensuring that the contextual issues inherent in forensic care and the multiplicity of dynamic already referred to remain in the open, for discussion, and not hidden.

The case study in Box 19.5 identifies how a range of models and structures were used to make

---

Box 19.5   Case study 5

John is a gay nurse working with clients diagnosed with personality disorder in a secure rehabilitation setting. John has been the named nurse for Tony, a 24-year-old personality-disordered patient with behaviour frequently described as narcissistic and manipulative and also a series of convictions for sexual offences against young women and children. Les has been in a supervisory relationship with John for the past 9 months. Their relationship has moved through several developmental stages and functions, mainly at stage 3 described by Stoltenberg & Delworth (1987), which indicates a level of maturity in the relationship. However, Les has noticed that John's descriptions of his

relationship with Tony and his therapeutic input have taken on a qualitative difference. John refers to Tony as a close friend and confidant, often with a warm and seductive quality.

In the supervision sessions Les feels he is being drawn into the relationship between John and Tony. He feels a warmth towards John and considers how he may explore those feelings.

The issue is further blurred by the demand of the multidisciplinary team that Tony ought to be prepared for discharge to a facility which offers a greater degree of freedom and choice. It is important to develop the structures necessary to assess and manage the risks that Tony may present.

an attempt at assessing the risk, both open and hidden, of the patient described within the study. This does not provide a correct and wholly inclusive structure for managing this case but describes a number of speculations and hypotheses which may help in the exploration of pertinent issues and in allowing some of the unspoken and often unheard issues and tensions to emerge.

It is argued that to explore a range of issues contained within the case study Les, as supervisor, would need to demonstrate a range of key skills linked to those described by Procter. For example, Tony may need to be open, accepting and challenging in respect of John's feelings but, more importantly, demonstrate those skills in respect of his own feelings. In terms of skill development, Hawkins & Shohet (1984) offer potent guidance in the exploration of the relationship between the supervisee and the supervisor and the content of their sessions. Les could utilize these ideas to explore the tensions at both a conscious and unconscious level within his relationship with John and the dynamics of the relationship between John and his client and Les's place within the dynamic.

This is of importance in exploring the feelings being generated within the supervisory relationship and how they may be parallelled in the relationship that Tony is generating with others. A decision may then be made as to whether or not they are significant risk factors or should be integrated into any risk management strategy. Also, in terms of the decision to increase the choices that Tony may have in his life once he has been moved on, the feelings he is 'pulling out' of staff may be a signifi-cant risk factor. This is of importance considering some of the criteria in risk management which have been described by commentators such as Grounds (1995) and Potts (1995). That said, and to reiterate the earlier assertions, the above does not claim to be the one answer but to suggest some structures and models which may be of benefit in enabling unspoken issues to emerge.

Procter (1986) describes supervision as having several key features. Clinical supervision should be:

◆ enabling, not dominating
◆ encouraging, not judgemental

◆ valuing, not belittling
◆ exploratory, not dogmatic
◆ open, not defensive
◆ developmental, not restrictive
◆ accepting and yet challenging.

Davies (1993) suggests that supervision allows for:

◆ focusing directly on the practitioner caseload
◆ focusing on the skills, interventions and evaluation of clinical and therapeutic interactions with the client and/or their carers
◆ self-evaluation and self-awareness
◆ guidance and advice on clinical practice and interventions
◆ validation of the practitioner's positive clinical and interpersonal practice
◆ discussion of events and how the practitioner coped
◆ exploration of coping mechanisms and how harmful or beneficial these are.

These points offer succinct guidance to practitioners engaging in supervision with such patients. Also, the interventions and guidance all suggest a fluidity in the process which helps create the necessary climate for exploration and the establishment of appropriate risk management strategies. Also, the clear understanding of the process of managing care is evidenced. This is of importance in enabling the practitioner, particularly in forensic mental health care, to establish clear boundaries in terms of responsibility and accountability.

OVERCOMING RESISTANCE IN THE PROCESS

If the points raised by Melia et al (1999) have significant currency, it would be reasonable to suggest that the context of forensic mental health care offers a breeding ground for resistance and suspicion within the system. Farkas-Cameron (1995) has identified with some clarity the concerns nurses raise about clinical supervision. Questions such as 'What is the purpose of clinical supervision?' may indicate feelings that their practices are being viewed in a negative manner. There may also be concern that supervision is about management, which is why it is vital that the clinical supervision relationship is based on trust and is non-judgemental. Fowler (1996) suggests that the first question that needs to be asked when planning clinical supervision, whether at the individual or organizational level, is: What is the aim of the clinical supervision?

Davies (1993: 52) contends that: 'Supervision should be *for* the practitioner. It is not an audit of practice'. The aim of clinical supervision is to support, assist and facilitate the practitioner in the delivery of high-quality care but it is also about helping the practitioner to manage the demands of their professional working life.

The introduction of clinical supervision into a service may meet with some initial resistance owing to lack of understanding about the purpose of clinical supervision; fears about criticism of professional practice; and a resentment that supervision will remove the autonomy of the practitioner. These fears and anxieties have to be allayed by the methods and skills adopted in the introduction and implementation of clinical supervision. For many people, the possibility that their professional practices may be criticized is threatening. However, clinical supervision can assist practitioners to develop existing good practice and learn new skills. Most practitioners informally discuss their clients' needs and ask for advice. Clinical supervision puts this into a framework that supports the practitioner and acknowledges that, in many instances, the work they are undertaking is difficult and that this difficulty needs to be recognized and shared.

KEY SKILLS

Facilitating a supportive, trusting and therapeutic relationship within clinical supervision requires particular skills and a clear understanding of the purpose of the supervision. If supervision is to be supportive, challenging, professional and effective, the supervisor needs to have high levels of key skills that are used consciously in the supervision. The key skills are:

◆ clarification
◆ exploration
◆ progression
◆ appraisal.

Butterworth (1994) has identified the need for supervisor training to ensure that supervisors have a knowledge of and sensitivity to the interpersonal processes that can occur between individuals and groups and which may impede the therapeutic nature of practitioner–client and supervisor–supervisee relationships. Key skills that facilitate effective communication are therefore vital.

Clarification

This involves identifying clearly the style and methods that the practitioner uses in their everyday working life. The supervisee will be encouraged to explore their 'style of work', the effects that it has on clients, carers and colleagues and their understanding of the efficacy of this style. The skills that the supervisor will need to use here include listening, questioning, summarizing, paraphrasing and checking out. Being a good listener is not easy and the supervisor should be aware of the difficulties that may arise. The supervisor also needs to be aware of any skill development they may need in listening to others.

Exploration

This phase of the supervision is a logical progression from clarification. It may involve the supervisor asking: 'Now that your ideas about your practice have been clarified, can we explore one of your ideas that you currently manage the least effectively?'. A possible consequence of exploration is that it may seem threatening and it is therefore vital that this skill is carried out in a supportive manner, which sets the supervisee at their ease and does not make them feel inadequate.

Exploration may well sound neutral but it is in fact difficult and value laden. It involves coping with confusion, exploring options, considering different ways of working, examining the possibility of changing attitudes. This skill also requires the supervisor and supervisee to deal with conflict. The range of options suggested by the supervisee may not be options the supervisor would themselves consider using. Unless this conflict is acknowledged and dealt with, it could affect the relationship. Exploration involves challenging and this can result in the supervisee feeling inadequate. For the act of challenging practice, beliefs, etc. to be positive it must, therefore, be perceived by the supervisee as supportive. Exploration within the supervision session can provide information, identify goals and aspirations, perceived and actual difficulties and can improve skill awareness.

Progression

This is a generic skill which will be used throughout the supervision session. It is about avoiding going round in circles, becoming blocked down blind alleys and working only at the superficial level. This stage of the session involves identifying relevant action. It is necessary to identify and discuss problems; it is essential to discuss goals. This in turn should lead to greater clarity of actions, goals and aspira-tions. Part of identifying actions must include the exploration of resource availability. Learning to use colleagues as resources is important; seeing their skills and knowledge as useful and supportive can be the first break in the barriers that can exist within multidisciplinary teams.

Appraisal

This skill is required in what is perhaps the most sensitive area involved in supervision. Assessment of professional practice can appear very threatening and produce high levels of anxiety. Appraisal is not only sensitive, it is also complicated. This skill involves several subsidiary skills, including the encouragement of self-assessment in which the supervisee analyses their own strengths and weaknesses, aims, criteria, strategies, etc. It involves being critical in a supportive way. Being critical involves making judgements but the way in which those judgements are presented will significantly affect how they are received.

CONCLUSION

What is the benefit of clinical supervision in forensic mental health care? In this chapter the benefits to the service, and to the client with mental health problems, have been identified. The benefits to the practitioner can be numerous and include the following.

◆ Clinical supervision provides space for the supervisee to reflect upon the content and process of their work.
◆ It facilitates the development of understanding and skills within their work.
◆ It allows the practitioner space and time to receive information and another perspective concerning their clinical practice.
◆ The practitioner can be validated and supported both as a person and as a colleague in a stressful occupation. It helps to ensure that as a person and as a practitioner, the supervisee is not left to carry, unnecessarily, difficulties and problems on their own.
◆ It may help practitioners to better plan and utilize their personal and professional resources.
◆ It encourages practitioners to be proactive rather than reactive.
◆ It allows the practitioner to use self-appraisal to monitor the quality of their work.

It would appear, therefore, that the implementation of clinical supervision in services for people with forensic mental health problems would be of benefit to all involved. For practitioners in particular, the implementation of clinical supervision may provide them with the essential support mechanism that they need to care for people with the range of problems found within forensic facilities. It would be well to heed the words of Pyne (1987): 'To care for and about our colleagues is to care for and about standards of patient care. Our consciences should not rest if we renege on that responsibility'.

Acknowledging the potency of Pyne's assertion to ensure quality supervision, certain criteria need to be met. The following section provides a list of actions that will assist in the facilitation of quality clinical supervision. Practitioners working in the arena of forensic mental health care may use this action list to provide a basic structure from which they can devise and implement their own systems of clinical supervision.

Actions to support good clinical practice in forensic care

◆ Ensuring time and place for clinical supervision to take place.
◆ Clinical supervision should be part of the organizational ethos.
◆ The provision of formal arrangements, i.e. the use of contracts to support the clinical supervision process.
◆ Recognition of the importance of safety in the clinical supervision relationship.
◆ Respect and confidentiality.
◆ Opportunity to attend training sessions for clinical supervision.
◆ Clinical supervision arrangements to form part of an individual practitioner's regular review.
◆ Managers should have clinical supervision.
◆ A record of clinical supervision should be maintained.
◆ The part clinical supervision can play in the management of risk should be acknowledged.
◆ The linkage between clinical supervision and clinical governance should be established.

REFERENCES

Bishop V 1994 Clinical supervision for an accountable profession. Nursing Times 90(39): 34–39

Briant S 1997 Too close for comfort. Nursing Times 93(6): 22–24

British Association of Counselling 1992 Code of ethics and practice for counsellors. British Association of Counselling, Rugby

Buchanan A 1999 Risk and dangerousness. Psychological Medicine 29: 465–473

Butler S, Zelen SL 1977 Sexual intimacies between therapists and patients. Psychotherapy: Theory, Research and Practice 14: 139–145

Butterworth T 1994 Preparing to take on clinical supervision. Nursing Standard 8(52): 32–34

Butterworth T, Faugier J 1992 Clinical supervision and mentorship in nursing. Chapman and Hall, London

Community Psychiatric Nurses Association 1989 Clinical practice issues for C.P.N.s. CPNA Publications, London

Cooke P 1992 Mental handicap nursing. In: Butterworth T, Faugier J (eds) Clinical supervision and mentorship in nursing. Chapman and Hall, London, ch 9, pp 121–131

Davies P 1993 Value yourself ... regular clinical supervision can help reduce stress. Nursing Times 89(4): 52

Department of Health 1992 Report of the Committee of Inquiry into Complaints about Ashworth Hospital. HMSO, London

Department of Health 1999a National service framework for mental health: modern standards and service models, executive summary. Stationery Office, London

Department of Health 1999b Report of the Committee of Inquiry into the Personality Disorder Unit, Ashworth Hospital. Volume 1. Cm 4194-II. Stationery Office, London

Dolan B, Coid J 1993 Psychopathic and antisocial personality disorders. Gaskell, London

Farkas-Cameron MM 1995 Clinical supervision in psychiatric nursing. Journal of Psychosocial Nursing 33(2): 31–37

Faulkner J 1998 A head start. Nursing Times 94(43): 39

Fowler J 1996 Clinical supervision: what do you do after saying hello? British Journal of Nursing 15(6): 382–385

Friis S, Helldin L 1994 The contribution made by the clinical setting to violence among psychiatric patients. Criminal Behavior and Mental Health 4(4): 341–352

Gemma PB 1989 Can nurses care too much? American Journal of Nursing 89(5): 743–744

Goldberg C 1986 On being a psychiatric nurse: the journey of the healer. Gardner Press, New York

Grounds A 1995 Risk assessment and management in clinical context. In: Crichton J (ed) Psychiatric patient violence: risk and response. Duckworth, London

Hawkins P, Shohet R 1984 Supervision in the helping professions. Open University Press, Buckingham

Jennings L 1997 Trust and relationships in polluting climates. Mental Health Nursing 17(6): 4–5

Kennerley H 1990 Managing anxiety: a training manual. Open University Press, Buckingham

Loganbill C, Hardy E, Delworth U 1982 Supervision: a conceptual model. Counseling Psychologist 1: 3–42

Lutzen K 1998 Subtle coercion in psychiatric practice. Journal of Psychiatric and Mental Health Nursing 5: 101–107

Lutzen K, Nordin C 1994 Modifying autonomy concept grounded in nurses' experiences of moral decision making in psychiatric settings. Journal of Medical Ethics 20: 101–107

Lyon E 1993 Hospital staff reactions to accounts by survivors of childhood abuse. American Journal of Orthopsychiatry 63(3): 410–416

Maden A 1996 Risk assessment in psychiatry. British Journal of Hospital Medicine 56(2/3): 78–82

Mason T, Jennings L 1997 The Mental Health Act and professional hostage taking. Medicine, Science and Law 37(1): 58–68

Mathias P, Prime R, Thompson T 1997 Preparation for interprofessional work: holism, integration and the purpose of training and education. In: Ovretveit J, Mathias P, Thompson T (eds) Interprofessional working for health and social care. Macmillan, London, pp 116–130

Melia P, Moran T, Mason T 1999 Triumvirate nursing for personality disordered patients: crossing the boundaries safely. Journal of Psychiatric and Mental Health Nursing 6: 15–20

Moran T, Mason T 1996 Revisiting the management of the psychopath. Journal of Psychiatric and Mental Health Nursing 3(3): 189–194

National Health Service Confederation & Sainsbury Centre for Mental Health 1997 The way forward for mental health services. National Health Service Confederation, London

Neilson P 1991 Manipulative and splitting behaviours. Nursing Standard 6(8): 32–35

Neilson P 1992 A secure philosophy. Nursing Times 88(8): 31–33

Noak J 1995 Care of people with psychopathic disorder. Nursing Standard 9(34): 30–32

Palmer T 1992 The re-emergence of correctional intervention. Sage, Newbury Park

Pennington S, Gafner G, Schilit R, Bechtel B 1993 Addressing ethical boundaries among nurses. Nursing Management 24(6): 36–39

Potts J 1995 Risk assessment and management: a Home Office perspective. In: Crichton P (ed) Psychiatric patient violence: risk and response. Duckworth, London

Power S 1994 A unique source of support and advice: the benefits of supervision in clinical practice. Psychiatric Care 1(3): 105–108

Procter B 1986 Supervision: a co-operative exercise in accountability. In: Marken M, Payne M (eds) Enabling and ensuring: supervision in practice. National Youth Bureau, Leicester

Pyne R 1987 Nurse wastage: confronting stress … community nurses. Nursing Times 83(27): 30–31

Ravin J, Boal CK 1989 Post-traumatic stress disorder in the work setting: psychic injury, medical diagnosis, treatment and litigation. American Journal of Forensic Psychiatry 10: 5–23

Rushton CH, Armstrong L, McEnhill M 1996 Establishing therapeutic boundaries as patient advocates. Paediatric Nursing 22(3): 185–189

Scott MJ, Stradling SG 1992 Counselling for post-traumatic stress disorder. Sage, London

Silfin P, Ben-David S 1993 The forensic psychiatric hospital. Analise Psicologica 11(1): 37–47

Stoltenberg CD, Delworth U 1987 Supervising counsellors and therapists. Jossey-Bass, London

Tennant A, Hughes G 1998 Men talking about dysfunctional masculinity: an innovative approach to working with aggressive, personality disordered offender patients. Psychiatric Care 5(3): 92–99

Thomas B, Reid J 1995 Multidisciplinary clinical supervision. British Journal of Nursing 4(15): 883–885

Torrington D, Weightman J 1994 Effective management, 2nd edn. Prentice Hall, London

Totka JP 1996 Exploring the boundaries of paediatric practice: nurse stories related to relationships. Paediatric Nursing 22(3): 191–196

United Kingdom Central Council for Nursing, Midwifery and Health Visiting 1992 Code of professional conduct for the nurse, midwife and health visitor. UKCC, London

United Kingdom Central Council for Nursing, Midwifery and Health Visiting 1996 Position statement on clinical supervision for nursing and midwifery. UKCC, London

Watts D, Morgan G 1994 Malignant alienation: dangers for patients who are hard to like. British Journal of Psychiatry 164: 11–15

Wesley S, Taylor PJ 1991 Madness and crime: criminology versus psychiatry. Criminal Behavior and Mental Health 1: 193–228

FURTHER READING

Carroll M 1997 Clinical supervision: luxury or necessity? In: Horton I, Varma V (eds) The needs of counsellors and psychotherapists. Sage, London

Farrington A 1995 Defining and setting the parameters of clinical supervision. British Journal of Nursing 4(15): 874–875

Raffert M, Coleman M 1996 Educating nurses to undertake clinical supervision in practice. Nursing Standard 10(45): 38–41

Chapter Twenty

Rehabilitation in practice

Pat Abbott

INTRODUCTION

This chapter provides an overview of rehabilitation as a concept and a summary of the development of rehabilitation services, including the increasingly important interface between rehabilitation and forensic mental health services. The approaches which rehabilitation services tend to adopt, within the eclectic management of severely mentally ill people, will be discussed along with a practical model compatible with the care programme approach. An overview of the contribution of work and occupation to the rehabilitation process will be provided.

REHABILITATION AS A CONCEPT

Rehabilitation, a term often poorly understood and used loosely in forensic mental health care, has developed primarily in relation to long-term mental illness sufferers. Thus, within forensic mental health care it is useful to have a practical working definition of rehabilitation which can be adapted for a range of client groups. One way of approaching this is to consider the component parts of established definitions available.

Wing & Morris (1981) defined rehabilitation as 'the process which: aims to identify, prevent and minimize the causes of social disablement associated with mental disorder; helps individuals to develop and use their talents, thus acquiring confidence and self-esteem through success in social roles'. Anthony et al (1990) indicated that 'rehabilitation assists persons with long-term psychiatric disabilities in increasing their functioning so that they are successful and satisfied in the environments of their choice, with the least amount of ongoing professional intervention'. Johnson & Smith (1994: 22) define rehabilitation as 'activities relating to maintenance of an individual's motivation towards realistic short-, medium- and long-term goals'. Repper & Cooney (1994: 427) state that rehabilitation 'literally means treatment, therapy or cure'.

In using these definitions to develop a practical working model, the many causes of social disablement need to be examined. These include:

◆ impairments directly associated with the mental disorder itself, such as both positive and negative symptoms of schizophrenia, clinical features of other disorders

◆ social disadvantages such as deficits in social or occupational skills, educational disadvantages, physical or learning disability, poverty or lack of social support. These may be created or exacerbated by impairments, creating a vicious cycle

◆ adverse personal reactions to these difficulties, including lowered self-esteem and self-confidence and reduced motivation (Wing & Morris 1981).

The first definition (Wing & Morris 1981) has the advantage of providing a basic framework for the classification of needs, with an emphasis on social functioning. Also, it is acknowledged that rehabilitation should be a developmental process, enabling the individual to work towards achieving their potential. The definition provided by Anthony et al (1990) is consistent with the first but it emphasizes the interaction between the individual and their environment, the importance of patient involvement/choice and the importance of maximum independence from services as an ideal goal. The remaining definitions are encompassed within these two. Finally, any definition should also acknowledge that the prevention of deterioration and maintenance of optimal quality of life are also important aims of rehabilitation. Therefore, a practical working definition is as follows.

Rehabilitation is the development of appropriate skills to enable the individual to achieve an optimal level of functioning. Level of functioning depends on the interaction between the individual and their environment. Rehabilitation may therefore involve interventions geared at improving skills and/or modifying the environment. The rehabilitation process encompasses the prevention of additional disabilities and the maintenance of the best possible quality of life.

THE DEVELOPMENT OF REHABILITATION SERVICES

Rehabilitation services within British mental health-care systems have traditionally concentrated upon providing comprehensive care for people who suffer from severe mental illness. Rehabilitation approaches to severe mental illness had their origins in the philosophy of moral treatment in psychiatry, which evolved in the early 19th century. The value of eschewing authoritarian and restrictive measures in favour of social support and occupational activities became evident in terms of improvement in the level of function of mental illness sufferers. In the early days, absence of effective medical treatment for severe mental illness meant that the only available interventions involved the provision of care and meaningful activity. The development of the large mental hospitals in the 19th century demonstrated the recognition of the importance of work and activity.

An important change in momentum in terms of service development, came with the advent of effective physical treatments in the 1940s. This was coupled with changing social patterns, rejecting incarceration for social reasons and reducing the use of compulsory detention, except in those situations in which it was deemed absolutely necessary. The large mental hospitals were no longer seen as therapeutic environments and a wide range of negative effects of institutional living were described (Barton 1959). More detailed studies of the effects of institutionalized living on severely mentally ill people have shown that many adverse effects attributed to institutionalization were more likely to have been negative symptoms of schizophrenia (Johnstone et al 1981). Furthermore, a major effect of prolonged hospital stay upon people with schizophrenia was an increasing reluctance to be discharged (Wing 1962). A brief review of institutional effects is provided by Abbott (1988).

Formal resettlement programmes and retraction of the large mental hospitals began in the early 1960s and continue to this day. Early re-settlement of the 'old long-stay' population was remarkably successful. This population comprised people who had been in hospital for many years. Many were mentally stable and may never have become inpatients in more recent times. They were predominantly resettled into hostels, small group houses or generic residential settings and their outcomes with regard to readmission to hospital tended to be very good (Jones et al 1986). A 13-year follow-up study of 610 long-stay patients discharged into the community between 1985 and 1993 showed good outcome for the majority (Trieman et al 1999).

However, as mental hospital populations declined and a number of institutions actually closed, it became increasingly clear that a small but highly dependent population remained at the end-stage of hospital retraction. This group was characterized by severe treatment-resistant illness, multiple disabilities and sometimes persistent challenging behaviour. This group required provision of resource-intensive services with 24-hour nursing care, whether in hospital or specialized nursing home settings. Additionally, as well as this 'old long-stay' high-dependency population, a 'new chronically ill' population became evident. This group of predominantly young men, with treatment-resistant illness, frequently experienced additional problems such as substance misuse or personality disorder. This group is characterized by prolonged inpatient care, whether of

a continuous or intermittent 'revolving door' pattern, frequent detention under the Mental Health Act 1983 and a range of challenging and/or offending behaviours.

This relatively small number of severely mentally ill people has a major impact upon mental health services, reducing bed throughput in inpatient units, frequently occupying acute inpatient beds for long periods and proving difficult to place in community settings. The inadequacy of planned services for this patient group has been illustrated vividly by a number of high-profile tragedies (e.g. Ritchie et al 1994). Rehabilitation services, particularly in urban high morbidity catchment areas, have progressed from retraction/resettlement services to more specialist treatment and care services for people with severe and enduring mental illness, who require intensive support in both hospital and the community. An overview of the deinstitutionalization programme which has taken place in the UK, along with community service development, is provided by Thornicroft & Bebbington (1989).

THE REHABILITATION AND FORENSIC SERVICE INTERFACE

Inevitably, working relationships between forensic and rehabilitation services have become closer and a more integrated approach to service development for complex high-risk client groups is emerging from this partnership. Particular areas of common interest include:

◆ assertive case management and the development of individual care packages for patients who require intensive supervision on a long-term basis
◆ service models for long-term medium or low secure care, particularly for people who suffer from treatment-resistant severe mental illness
◆ the development of specialized high-dependency residential settings for young high-risk patients.

The future reconfiguration of services currently provided by the high security hospitals provides

Box 20.1 Rehabilitation service

◆ Originally responsible for large mental hospital retraction/resettlement programmes.

◆ Evolved to provide a wide range of hospital and community-based services for people with long-term severe mental illness.

◆ Frequently occupy an interface position between adult mental health services and forensic services.

◆ Have an important contribution to make in the development of comprehensive services for mentally disordered offenders with long-term needs.

an exciting challenge, in terms of the potential development of needs-based services for complex patients with diverse needs in terms of treatment and security. Much can be learnt in this process from the experience of retraction of the large mental hospitals and the development of reconfigured services in a wide range of settings. Box 20.1 provides a summary of rehabilitation services.

REHABILITATION: A MODEL

A more global understanding of the biological, psychological and social dimensions of severe mental illness demonstrates the necessity for a holistic approach to the treatment and care of forensic mental health patients. Coupled with this is the increasing recognition that many severely mentally ill people who come into contact with forensic and rehabilitation services have additional problems such as: learning disability; personality or emotional problems; substance misuse; and social disadvantage. It is essential, therefore, that the treatment and care of forensic patients are based upon a thorough needs assessment and the development of a comprehensive care programme, with regular review and good communication with all parties involved.

The following is a practical rehabilitation model based upon the Boston psychiatric rehabilitation approach (Anthony et al 1990). This

model is highly compatible with the care programme approach (DoH 1990).

Principles of rehabilitation

A detailed breakdown of the theoretical principles underlying an evaluated approach is described by Anthony et al (1990). However, the principles of rehabilitation may be summarized as follows:

◆ It is a holistic approach which takes account of biological, psychological and social dimensions.

◆ It is focused upon meeting the needs of the individual, taking full account of the person's own views and experiences, maximizing their involvement in all aspects of planning and intervention.

◆ The approach recognizes the importance of maintaining hope, whilst focusing upon achievable and realistic goals. Experience of success is important.

◆ Rehabilitation is a long-term enterprise, frequently lifelong.

◆ A culture of formal measurement of change is an important framework for the process, providing useful feedback to the patient, the practitioners and others such as carers, all of whom may otherwise have difficulty perceiving relatively modest changes over prolonged periods of time.

Process of rehabilitation

Needs assessment

Rehabilitation is based upon a sound comprehensive needs assessment of both the individual's current level of functioning and support and that required to achieve a specific goal. Goal planning is an important part of the process. Goals need to be:

◆ realistic
◆ specific
◆ positive (acquisition of positive behaviours and skills rather than focusing on reduction in negative behaviours)
◆ achievable within a reasonable timescale (for example 6 months) and to prevent deterioration (which is a worthwhile goal in itself).

Both the person and their environment must be considered in the process of needs assessment and goal planning, as changes in environment alone may have a major impact upon a person's level of function.

Formulating planned interventions

A series of planned interventions needs to be developed, aimed at addressing identified needs. The planned interventions must be specific in terms of who, what, when and for how long. The review process must be built in with the proviso that needs may change and goals may need to be modified in the light of changing needs or experience of rehabilitation

The person's real-life role and function within living, working or social milieu are the main areas of emphasis in rehabilitation. However, particularly when working with mentally disordered offenders and other high-risk client groups, it is essential that risk assessment and management inform all levels of the process. Consideration of risk may form a major part of the assessment process and may significantly modify goals and interventions deemed to be appropriate, as well as forming a significant aspect of the review process. The spectrum of rehabilitation approaches may contribute towards the reduction in risk, in terms of improving social functioning, improving coping skills and reducing maladaptive behaviours. Figure 20.1 provides an overview of the rehabilitation model.

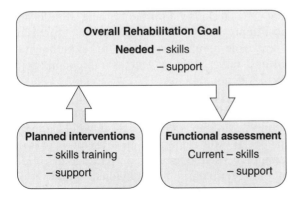

Figure 20.1 A rehabilitation model.

RESEARCH BASIS

A useful review of the literature relating to a range of rehabilitation approaches can be found in Anthony et al (1990). However, it is important to emphasize a number of general points.

1. Behaviour change and improvement in social functioning may not necessarily generalize across all settings.
2. Improvement in a single outcome measure may not necessarily be evident in other measures (it is actually possible for some outcome measures to show inverse trends, e.g. anxiety levels may deteriorate with increased interpersonal contact).
3. Improved level of skills within an experimental 'test' environment does not necessarily reflect an improvement in, in vivo, functioning.

INTEGRATION OF THE REHABILITATION MODEL INTO THE CARE PROGRAMME APPROACH

The care programme approach (DoH 1990) has four main themes:

1. an identified key worker
2. a care plan based upon a needs assessment
3. a system for reviewing the care plan involving all relevant agencies
4. close interprofessional collaboration and active involvement of the patient and carers.

It is clear that the rehabilitation model, with its emphasis upon systematic needs assessment followed by planned interactions on a cyclical basis, is highly compatible with the care programme approach. Figure 20.2 provides a graphical view of this.

REHABILITATION APPROACHES

The early rehabilitation emphasis upon social milieu, training and occupation has remained

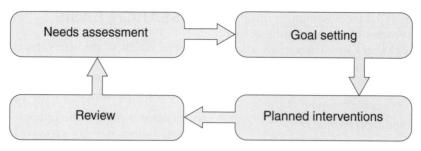

Figure 20.2 Cyclical view of the integrated rehabilitation model and care programme approach.

Box 20.2 Rehabilitation approaches

◆ Work and occupation

◆ Psychosocial interventions – family interventions

◆ Skills training/support packages – social skills training

◆ Assertive outreach and residential provision

---

important within the evolutionary process which has occurred in rehabilitation. Particular spheres of interest have included:

◆ the role of work and occupational therapy
◆ psychosocial interventions
◆ skills training approaches, coupled with the development of support packages
◆ assertive outreach and residential care geared towards meeting individual needs more appropriately.

In parallel with substantial developments in psychosocial spheres, there have been considerable improvements in drug treatments for severe mental illness, coupled with an increased awareness of the importance of cognitive impairment in terms of rehabilitation outcome. This raises the possibility that neurocognitive approaches may be helpful for the severely mentally ill, a potentially fruitful area for future research. Box 20.2 provides a summary of rehabilitation approaches.

A brief summary of current available trends in evidence relating to other interventions of rehabilitation will now be given.

SOCIAL SKILLS TRAINING AND SUPPORT PACKAGES

Social skills training and support packages:

◆ Improve level of functioning, particularly in formal test environment
◆ May improve community outcome
◆ May require ongoing reinforcements to be built into the living environment if improvements are to be sustained.

There is considerable interest in this area of work in the USA where a wide range of literature has evolved. Overall, it is well established that severely mentally ill people may be effectively taught social skills via formal training. Results are most impressive when outcomes are measured by repeat role play assessments in experimental settings, rather than by general improvements in soical functioning.

Evidence exists that skills may decline with time if not subject to long-term reinforcement (Penn & Morgan 1996). Thus, it would appear that social skills training is most useful as part of a comprehensive rehabilitation package delivered on a long-term basis. For individuals who live for prolonged periods in residential or inpatient settings, it is most appropriate to develop social

Box 20.3 Social skills training

◆ Is beneficial for severely mentally ill people, particularly if delivered on a long-term basis in vivo

◆ Is best delivered as part of a comprehensive rehabilitation package

skills training as part of the global therapeutic milieu. This should reinforce appropriate social interaction on a consistent and long-term basis. Box 20.3 provides a summary of social skills training.

FAMILY INTERVENTIONS

Family management models have received considerable attention over the past 20 years. These approaches usually involve a combination of an education package for the family and training for problem-solving and coping mechanisms. Sometimes they involve more specific systemic interventions designed to modify the way in which family members interact with the mentally ill member.

The development of family interventions was based upon the observation that certain characteristics of family interaction would appear to increase the likelihood of mental illness relapse, in the form of increasing positive psychotic symptoms, arousal and behaviour disturbance (Leff & Vaughn 1985). These characteristics of family interactions are known collectively as a *high expressed emotion*, which comprises critical comments, overinvolvement and hostility. Intervention studies have shown that these communication patterns may be modified and risk of relapse reduced (Falloon et al 1985). There is some evidence that improvements may decline with time, suggesting that follow-up and reinforcement may be important (Penn & Morgan 1996). Leff (1994) provides an example of outcomes for family interventions delivered in practice and a practical guide is provided by Kuipers et al (1992).

COGNITIVE-BEHAVIOURAL THERAPY FOR MENTAL ILLNESS SYMPTOMS

Cognitive-behavioural therapy (CBT) is used for treatment of a wide spectrum of conditions including: depressive and anxiety disorders; psychosexual problems; psychoses; and personality disorders. There is considerable interest in these techniques for the treatment of personality-disordered offenders (e.g. Guy & Hume 1998, High Security Psychiatric Services Commissioning Board 1997, Home Office & DoH 1999, Tennant et al 1999). However, these wider applications of CBT will not be considered here, as it is beyond the scope of this chapter (see Chapter 16 for a fuller discussion).

CBT is considered useful in the reduction of psychotic symptoms and is included within the umbrella of psychosocial interventions. Many skills-based psychosocial training programmes incorporate simple CBT techniques. CBT for people with schizophrenia is an area of great interest, particularly in relation to relapse prevention and the treatment of those with residual psychotic symptoms. There is increasing evidence that CBT can reduce the level of symptomatology associated with chronic schizophrenia and medication-resistant psychosis (Kuipers et al 1997, Tarrier et al 1998). A strong case exists for the widespread use of CBT interventions for people who suffer from psychosis, as part of a comprehensive treatment and care package. An overview of the use of these techniques for people with schizophrenia is provided by Kingdon & Turkington (1994).

COMMUNITY SUPPORT SYSTEMS, ASSERTIVE OUTREACH AND HOME TREATMENT PACKAGES

Interventions have been developed and researched which provide mentally ill people in the community with a range of support measures, including crisis treatment (Hoult 1986, Stein & Test 1985). Thus, it is possible to care for the mentally ill in the community, during acute relapses of psychosis, by the provision of intensive support and supervision by a specialist community team. Although sufferers and carers favour this option, there is concern regarding potential impact upon families and the practicability in mainstream services. Therefore, more research work in this area would be fruitful.

WORK AS A MEDIUM FOR REHABILITATION

A range of activities can be used to deliver skills training to forensic patients, including work, recreation and education. Work will be considered in some detail here, owing to its established role within rehabilitation services in the US and UK.

Background

Work-based models of rehabilitation are amongst the most well-established interventions for people who suffer from long-term severe mental illness. Health-giving properties of work were recognized by Hippocrates and Galen but the idea of using work in a positive way, as a therapeutic medium, came to the fore in the 19th and 20th centuries (Morgan 1983). Industrial therapy was a prominent part of mental hospital life and over the past 50 years, community models of sheltered work and cooperative approaches, such as the clubhouse model, have developed. These models are in keeping with the general trend in society, moving away from an industrial base towards a service economy.

Work as a concept is not necessarily easy to define. It is not merely the expenditure of energy for a purpose, as implied by dictionary definitions, as this would encompass many leisure pursuits. Neither is work restricted to paid employment, as much work is unpaid, including caring within families and communities, as well as formal and informal voluntary work. There are a number of ingredients which should be present if a task is to be considered work:

- exertion of mind or body
- designed to produce or achieve something beyond the pleasure of the task itself
- involves a degree of obligation, either within oneself or set by others
- involves a level of arduousness.

Thomas (1999) gives an account of the historical development of work and its role within society, providing a useful context in which to perceive the development of work models within mental health care.

Industrial therapy in the mental hospital

Social and economic reasons existed for developing a wide range of work options within mental hospitals in the 19th century. These hospitals recreated many aspects of society and were virtually self-contained communities, patient work making a significant contribution to subsistence and productivity. This rationale would be ethically unacceptable today. However, the 1940s and 1950s saw a major change in the place of work in the lives of mental hospital patients and those with similar needs within the community. The Peircy Report (1956) acknowledged the positive place which work had in the rehabilitation process and the Ministry of Health (1958) issued guidelines concerning the importance of planned treatment needs, the value of factory work and the need for pay and conditions to reflect those within mainstream society. Industrial therapy units within mental hospitals provided 'piecework' which was simple and repetitive. They provided opportunities for patients to:

- earn small sums of money, enhancing independence and self-esteem
- enjoy opportunities for social contact within a setting which was non-threatening and realistic
- learn basic skills and establish a regular life style pattern which was as close as possible to the mainstream population
- progress to higher level work and activities at a pace appropriate to the individual

◆ reduce the detrimental effects of institutionalization and prepare for resettlement into the community.

The benefits of industrial therapy for patients with chronic schizophrenia were demonstrated by a number of studies. Wing et al (1964) showed that a graded programme of basic skills and work preparation reduced relapse after discharge and increased the likelihood of achieving paid open employment. Wing & Brown (1970) found evidence for improvement in primary handicaps associated with schizophrenia when simple industrial work was provided as an alternative to no activity. A range of descriptive studies, reviewed by Morgan (1983), demonstrated the benefits of industrial therapy for long-stay mental hospital patients. Community units based upon industrial therapy models were established, notably those under the auspices of the Industrial Therapy Organization (Early 1974). The latter originated in Bristol to fill the gap in sheltered work provision within the community for people with schizophrenia, but the movement spread nationwide. An overview of the Industrial Therapy Organization and other sheltered work models is provided by Wansborough (1981).

Overall, the available evidence supports the view that a smooth transition from a hospital-based industrial therapy unit to an industrial therapy unit within the community appeared to benefit long-stay mental hospital inpatients in the course of the resettlement process. These benefits included reducing relapse of illness and increasing level of function. The development of community industrial therapy units and the coordination of their work with that of the mental hospitals was a key feature of the mental hospital closure programmes over the past 30 years. However, the importance of a graded approach to activities and the avoidance of over- or understimulation has been well recognized. Wing & Brown (1970) report how overstimulation increases the risk of relapse of positive psychotic symptoms, whereas understimulation exacerbates negative symptoms and results in a deterioration in the individual's level of function. According to this large study of treatment regimes in three mental hospitals, 'the most important single factor associated with improvement of primary handicaps was a reduction in the amount of time spent doing nothing'.

The provision of structured daytime activity remains one of the most important interventions for severely mentally ill people. The value of industrial therapy may be understood within the context of the importance of the psychosocial milieu for the well-being of people with schizophrenia. Industrial therapy units provided structured activity, usually of a low-key, low-stress type. Many also provide opportunities for non-threatening social interaction, which could be regulated according to the individual's tolerance of face-to-face contact. The extensive body of evidence around the importance of high expressed emotion in families also suggests that such a placement may have had beneficial effects by providing separation from such a family environment. Patients who have experienced long periods of institutionalization may have benefited particularly from the industrial therapy model because it provided an ongoing and structured level of institutional support.

The decline of industrial therapy in the context of social change

The 1980s and 1990s saw a marked decline in the popularity of industrial therapy models of work-based rehabilitation. There are a number of reasons for this.

1. It is congruent with the decline in industrial work within society.
2. Industrial therapy placements were less popular with young people with severe and enduring mental illness than the older patient group.
3. The piecework provided by these units may have appeared boring and unattractive to service developers.
4. These units may have appeared less likely to assist people in developing skills which could lead to paid employment, as the latter becomes increasingly based in the service economy.
5. Alternative models, such as the clubhouse and similar cooperatively based models, became increasingly popular.

The clubhouse model

The clubhouse model is a work-based rehabilitation programme for people with mental illness, which originated in Fountain House, New York, in 1948. The clubhouse movement is now international and there are a number of settings in the UK which are members of the International Centre for Clubhouse Development. There is also a wide range of cooperative-style work settings which are modified from the original clubhouse model.

In essence, work and the 'work-ordered day' are central to the clubhouse model. The clubhouse philosophy is based upon a strong belief in the regenerative effects of work and its value in enabling mentally ill people to 'get their lives back on track' and form meaningful social relationships (Waters 1992).

Features of the clubhouse are as follows.

1. A geographical base.
2. Members cooperatively run the clubhouse (with little distinction between staff and non-staff members).
3. The provision of training, support and advice to members.

4. Specific assistance in obtaining open employment via a transitional employment model.

A transitional employment model involves the development of close links with potential employers, who may then approach the clubhouse directly to fill employee vacancies. This is on the understanding that the clubhouse will provide a worker consistently, regardless of whether an individual member is able to attend. The benefits to the clubhouse members are that it enhances opportunities to gain paid employment, in the knowledge that during periods of incapacity there would be clubhouse support for the job to be done. This therefore reduces the potential for work stress. The benefits to the employer are that the problem of absenteeism is eliminated and there is an assurance that the member will receive support, from staff members if necessary, to ensure the job is done to the required standards. Figure 20.3 provides a summary of the clubhouse model process.

Clubhouse programmes have standards set out with regard to membership; relationships; space; work-ordered day; employment, including

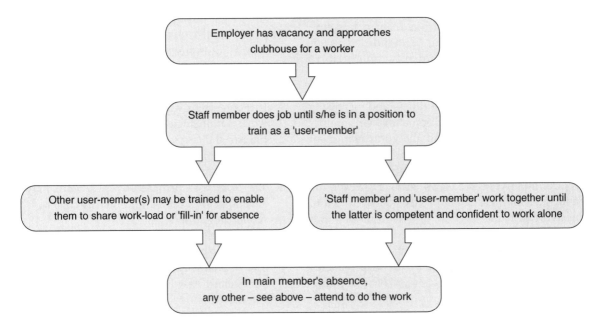

Figure 20.3 Summary of the clubhouse model process.

transitional employment and independent employ-ment; clubhouse functions, including community assistance for members, education and social activity; funding; governance; and administration (Propst 1992). The standards must be adhered to in order for the clubhouse to be certified by the International Centre for Clubhouse Development.

There are a number of descriptive accounts of the operation of these clubhouses, as well as individual accounts of benefits gained in terms of enhancing employment prospects, community adjustment, self-esteem and social relationships. There is evidence that the transitional employment model has limited relation to other consumer outcomes for these services (Blank et al 1996). Moreover, clubhouses have been criticized for providing segregated communities, being too rigid and inducing an unhealthy, almost cult-style fervour amongst their followers (Perkins 1997).

Some of the variations on the formal clubhouse model may address these criticisms. Indeed, it may be that many of the beneficial effects of the clubhouse model are similar to those for industrial therapy, in terms of structured day activity and social contact, which may be modified to suit the service user's need. Additionally, benefits such as their service economy orientated approach to work, the enhancement of paid employment opportunities and their cooperative ethos may have added to their popularity with service developers and made them more acceptable to the younger patient group.

Development of the role of occupational therapy within forensic services

The development of occupational therapy within forensic mental health services has played an important role in promoting rehabilitation approaches within medium secure units and high security hospitals. Occupational therapy provides functional assessment and a systematic approach to meeting identified skills deficits for patients in a range of important areas such as daily living,

social and communication skills. Other areas such as assertiveness, anger and anxiety management may have particular relevance to offending behaviour and occupational therapists, along with other professions, may provide important therapeutic interventions in these areas.

The development of occupational therapy within forensic services has been an important factor in viewing an activity as a medium for assessment and intervention across a range of needs, rather than as an end itself. The diverse patient populations served by secure services, particularly high security hospitals, necessitate a range of rehabilitation approaches, including work, education, recreation and specific skills training interventions. The development of occupational therapy has an important role to play in the assessment of need and prescription of appropriate interventions.

REASONING AND REHABILITATION PROGRAMME

This chapter would not be complete without at least an overview of the reasoning and rehabilitation programme (Ross et al 1988). This programme is the focus of at least one treatment-outcome research study in one of the high security hospitals (Donnelly & Scott 1999). The programme aims to shape the offender's thinking about the consequences of their behaviour, produce alternative ways of behaving and increase awareness of the impact which their behaviour may have on others. The programme involves:

◆ structured learning therapy
◆ lateral thinking techniques
◆ critical thinking
◆ values education
◆ assertiveness training
◆ negotiation skills training
◆ interpersonal cognitive problem solving
◆ social perception training
◆ role playing and modelling
◆ audiovisual presentations, reasoning exercises, games and group discussions.

Donnelly & Scott (1999) report promising results in their high security hospital controlled study. Their programme consists of 54 sessions covering the areas:

- introductory session
- problem solving (9 sessions)
- social skills (3 sessions)
- negotiation skills (3 sessions)
- management of emotions (2 sessions)
- creative thinking (11 sessions)
- values enhancement (10 sessions)
- critical reasoning (5 sessions)
- skills in review (3 sessions)
- cognitive exercises (6 sessions)
- feedback session.

As can be observed, strong emphasis is placed on the future interpersonal skills the forensic patient will need to function in society and ways of enhancing these. If results continue to remain promising and the programme finds more widespread usage in forensic mental health care, reasoning and rehabilitation could be a fundamental building block for the rehabilitation of forensic patients.

CONCLUSION

Rehabilitation approaches make an important contribution to the comprehensive treatment and care of people with serious mental health disorders who come into contact with forensic mental health services. A range of approaches are available although much of the research and rehabilitation practice base is focussed upon the needs of people with severe and enduring mental illness. Systematic needs and risk assessment, care planning and review processes provide the essential structure for the delivery of the comprehensive care of this client group. Rehabilitation approaches are highly compatible with these systematic processes and should be actively integrated into all forensic mental health services, from high security to the community.

REFERENCES

Abbott PM 1988 Institutional effects: a review. British Journal of Clinical and Social Psychiatry 6(1): 15–16

Anthony W, Cohen M, Farkas M 1990 Psychiatric rehabilitation. Boston University College of Allied Health Professions, Boston

Barton R 1959 Institutional neurosis. Wright, Bristol

Blank MB, Jodl KM, McCall BR 1996 Psychosocial rehabilitation programme characteristics in urban and rural areas. Psychiatric Journal 2(1): 3–10

Department of Health 1990 Caring for people: the care programme approach for people with a mental illness referred to the specialist psychiatric services. HC(90)23. Wetherby Health Publications Unit, Department of Health, Wetherby

Donnelly JP, Scott MF 1999 Evaluation of an offending behaviour programme with a mentally disordered offender population. British Journal of Forensic Practice 1(4): 25–32

Early DF 1974 Industrial therapy in Bristol. Nursing Times 70(11): 404–405

Falloon IRH, Boyd JL, McGill CW 1985 Family management in the prevention of morbidity of schizophrenia: clinical outcome of a 2 year longitudinal study. Archives of General Psychiatry 42: 887–896

Guy S, Hume A 1998 A CBT strategy for offenders with personality disorders: part one. Mental Health Practice 2(4): 12–16

High Security Psychiatric Services Commissioning Board 1997 Into the millennium: the future agenda for research and development into personality disorder. High Security Psychiatric Services Commissioning Board, London

Home Office, Department of Health 1999 Managing dangerous people with severe personality disorder: proposals for policy development. Department of Health, London

Hoult J 1986 Community care of the acutely mentally ill. British Journal of Psychiatry 149: 137–144

Johnson FC, Smith LD 1994 Personal and professional roles, skills and behaviours. In: Thompson T, Mathias P (eds) Lyttle's mental health and disorder, 2nd edn. Baillière Tindall, London, ch 2, p 2

Johnstone EC, Owens DGC, Gold A, Crow TJ, McMillan JF 1981 Institutionalization and the defects of schizophrenia. British Journal of Psychiatry 139: 195–203

Jones K, Robinson M, Golightley M 1986 Long-term psychiatric patients in the community. British Journal of Psychiatry 149: 537–540

Kingdon DF, Turkington D 1994 Cognitive therapy in schizophrenia. Guilford, New York

Kuipers L, Leff JP, Lam D 1992 Family work for schizophrenia: a practical guide. Gaskell, London

Kuipers L, Garety P, Fowler D 1997 London–East Anglia randomised controlled trial of cognitive-behaviour therapy for psychosis – effects of treatment phase. British Journal of Psychiatry 171: 316–327

Leff JP 1994 Working with families of schizophrenic patients. British Journal of Psychiatry 164 (suppl 23): 71–76

Leff JP, Vaughn C 1985 Expressed emotion in families: its significance for mental illness. Guilford, New York

Ministry of Health 1958 Rehabilitation in the hospital service and its relation to other services. HM(58)57. MoH, London

Morgan R 1983 Industrial therapy in the mental hospital. In: Watts FN, Bennett DH (ed) Theory and practice of psychiatric rehabilitation. Wiley, London, ch 8, pp 151–167

Peircy Report 1956 Committee of Inquiry on the Rehabilitation and Resettlement of Disabled Persons. Cm 9883L. HMSO, London

Penn DL, Morgan KT 1996 Research update on the psychosocial treatment of schizophrenia. American Journal of Psychiatry 163(5): 607–617

Perkins R 1997 Clubhouses ... no thanks. Open Mind 88: 14–15

Propst RN 1992 Standards for clubhouse programs: why and how they developed. Psychosocial Rehabilitation Journal 16(2): 25–30

Repper J, Cooney P 1994 The provision of care for people with enduring mental health problems. In: Thompson T, Mathias P (eds) Lyttle's mental health and disorder, 2nd edn. Baillière Tindall, London, ch 19, p 427

Ritchie JH, Donald D, Lingham R 1994 Report of the Inquiry into the Care and Treatment of Christopher Clunis. HMSO, London

Ross R, Fabiano E, Ewles CD 1988 Reasoning and rehabilitation. International Journal of Offender Therapy and Comparative Criminology 32(1): 29–35

Stein LI, Test MA 1985 The training in the community living model: a decade of experience. Jossey Bass, San Francisco

Tarrier N, Yusupoff L, Kinney C et al 1998 Randomised controlled trial of intensive cognitive behaviour therapy for patients with chronic schizophrenia. British Medical Journal Clinical Research 317(7154): 303–307

Tennant A, Davies C, Tennant I 1999 Working with the personality disordered offender. In: Chaloner C, Coffey M (eds) Forensic mental health nursing: current approaches. Blackwell Science, Oxford, ch 6, pp 94–117

Thomas K (ed) 1999 The Oxford book of work. Oxford University Press, Oxford

Thornicroft G, Bebbington P 1989 Deinstitutionalisation – from hospital closure to service development. British Journal of Psychiatry 155: 739–753

Trieman N, Leff J, Glover G 1999 Outcomes of long stay psychiatric patients resettled in the community: prospective cohort study. British Medical Journal 319: 3–16

Wansborough SN 1981 The place of work in rehabilitation. In: Wing JK, Morris B (eds) Handbook of psychiatric rehabilitation practice. Oxford University Press, Oxford, pp 79–94

Waters B 1992 The work unit: the heart of the clubhouse. Psychosocial Rehabilitation Journal 16(2): 41–48

Wing JK 1962 Institutionalism in mental health hospitals. British Journal of Social and Clinical Psychology 1: 38–51

Wing JK, Brown GW 1970 Institutionalism and schizophrenia. Cambridge University Press, London

Wing JK, Morris B (eds) 1981 Handbook of psychiatric rehabilitation practice. Oxford University Press, Oxford

Wing JK, Bennett DH, Denham J 1964 The industrial rehabilitation of long stay schizophrenic patients. MRC Memorandum No. 42. HMSO, London

FURTHER READING

Anthony W, Cohen M, Farkas M 1990 Psychiatric rehabilitation. Boston University College of Allied Health Professionals, Boston

Kingdon DF, Turkington D 1994 Cognitive therapy in schizophrenia. Guilford, New York

Kuipers L, Leff JP, Lam D 1992 Family work for schizophrenia: a practical guide. Gaskell, London

Watt FN, Bennett DH 1983 Theory and practice of psychiatric rehabilitation. Wiley, Chichester

Chapter Twenty One

21

Managing the transition from higher to lower levels of security

Chris Skelly

INTRODUCTION

The high security (special) hospitals care for some of the most challenging and disabled patients in the mental health system (Maden et al 1995). These patients have complex treatment needs, not only for their mental disorder but also for their offending behaviours. Many are only partially responsive to treatment and the enduring nature of their mental health problems means that they receive care and treatment for protracted periods; the risk that they present to others ensures that this takes place within an inpatient setting in conditions of high security. As a result they have rehabilitation needs, both to alleviate the residual disablement of a severe mental disorder and also to redress the functional deficits that may result from the treatment episode in the high security 'total institution'.

Following a period of treatment and rehabilitation, most patients will be discharged to lower levels of security. Experience has shown that the transition from high security to lower levels of security can be problematic if the process of rehabilitation, support and aftercare is not actively managed. The failure rate in the past has been high: 31% of ex-high security hospital patients in one medium secure unit were readmitted to high security hospitals (Cope & Ward 1993), whilst one high security hospital readmitted 43% of patients who had been transferred on trial leave to medium secure units (Skelly 1994).

This chapter will examine the high security environment and the skills deficits that result from treatment in this environment; how the transition from higher to lower security is managed; and the range of innovative rehabilitation schemes (some successful and some not) which have emerged within Ashworth Hospital (one of the high security hospitals in the UK). These innovations must be considered within the context of the difficult political background that has resulted from two public inquiries into Ashworth Hospital (DoH 1992, 1999). These dates will be used to demarcate the period to be considered. This perspective is essential in understanding the significance of these clinical initiatives and, indeed, the challenges that confront high security hospitals in rehabilitating and discharging its patients to lower levels of security.

LOWER LEVELS OF SECURITY

The two routes of discharge from a high security hospital are: discharge to the community or transfer to a lower level of hospital security (usually on 6 months trial leave prior to discharge). This excludes those patients who return to the prison system or who are transferred to other high security hospitals. Community placements range from independent living to residential care in a staffed hostel. Furthermore, most patients are usually subject to formal supervision in the community. Medium secure facilities are provided both by NHS and private sector medium secure units. Some patients will be transferred to low secure units, which may offer the security of a locked ward door, or to 'open' wards which may offer no physical security at all.

In 1992, of all patients discharged from high security hospitals, 34% were discharged to the community; 28% to medium secure units; and 22% to other hospital facilities. The remaining 16% were returned to prison (DoH 1994). The discharge pattern appears to have altered considerably in recent years. Of patients discharged from Ashworth Hospital between 1994 and 1999, only 12% were discharged to the community, whilst 43% were transferred to medium secure units.

The preference for a graduated release via lower levels of security arises not only from the need for continuing treatment and rehabilitation but also from the need to test out the patient's level of adherence to socially acceptable norms of conduct. Appropriate social behaviours may not have been internalized and compliance within the high security hospital may only be due to the sanctions and controls available. For the receiving unit, the preference is for the transfer to be initially for 6 months trial leave as this allows for readmission to high security for any patient deemed to be inappropriately placed. It was demonstrated that this route of discharge was successful by Bailey & MacCulloch (1992), who found a significant reduction in the reconviction rates of high security hospital patients discharged to the community via transfer to lower levels of security, compared with those directly discharged.

High security hospitals, however, find it difficult to transfer patients to lower levels of security due to a lack of suitable places. In 1993, of 108 patients awaiting a move, 58% had waited longer than 6 months, with 11% waiting for more than 2 years (DoH 1994). For others, similarly no longer requiring this level of security, no application to lower security was pursued due to the pessimism felt concerning the medium secure unit response to patients requiring long-term care (Dell & Robertson 1988). Many patients, therefore, are detained in conditions of high security unnecessarily, due either to transfer delays or to the absence of an application for transfer due to its perceived futility.

PATIENTS' EXPERIENCES IN A HIGH SECURITY HOSPITAL: TWO PERSPECTIVES

Institutionalization

In creating a safe and therapeutic environment for the treatment of the mentally disordered patient who presents a risk to others, the high security hospital has to impose restrictions on the individual for the safety of others. Patients will have many limitations and controls put upon their freedom of movement, choice and behavioural expression. In this environment patients are often unable to meet their needs by utilizing their own resources and they become reliant on the institution and more resistant to change. Additionally, high security hospitals continue to show many of the cluster of factors which Barton (1959) identified as causing institutional neurosis, particularly: loss of contact with the outside world; poor ward atmosphere; loss of future prospects; and loss of personal friends, possessions and events.

The institutionalizing effects of high security hospitals are apparent from examination of the daily routine. The day may commence with the patient being told when to get out of bed. Toiletries and a razor will have to be requested from nursing staff, where these are considered as security items. The patient may dress in hospital-issue clothing and there may be difficulty in obtaining age-appropriate personal clothing. The day will be punctuated with set times for meals, medication and attendance at therapeutic activities. Housekeeping skills are largely redundant as the hospital has employees to clean and maintain the living environment. Budgeting skills may involve no more than ensuring that less is spent on cigarettes each week than is received in benefits. Money is not allowed and all purchases are completed via paper transactions debited from the patient's hospital account.

There will be little opportunity for the patient to make contact or to develop appropriate relationships with patients of the opposite gender. Attendance at any multiward activity entails the patient being escorted along in a movement which commences at one extremity of the hospital, collecting patients along the way from each ward. The patient is subject to rules and restrictions, often for reasons of security or patient management, and these may appear unnecessary to the patient. All patients will receive a personal search and room search at least once each month, may have to provide urine samples for drug screening on request and may, in some circumstances, have all incoming and outgoing mail read. The day may conclude with the patient being told when to go to bed.

Quality of life

Over a period of time the patient will have learned to temper demands to the institutional realities and adjusted behaviour and expectations accordingly. As a result, at the time of discharge or transfer, the patient may have a quality of life that, apart from community access, is better than that which is available in lower levels of security. The quality of life to be described here applies primarily to male patients (88% of the Ashworth population), who mostly reside on a different site, with different facilities, from female patients.

The patient will have progressed through the hospital wards and is likely to reside on a predischarge ward, where violence is rare and privileges are greater. The external ward doors may be unlocked for most of the daylight hours, giving the patient unsupervised access to the extensive hospital grounds and the facility to visit friends on other wards. Close affections and friendships may have been developed, with both staff and patients, and these may be the only personal relationships which the patient has. The patient may have a television and video in his bedroom, which is fully fitted and has en-suite facilities. Relative privacy may be available on the ward and the patient will have a key to his bedroom and can lock it from the inside to keep out other patients. The patient will have adjusted to the minor inconveniences of ward-based security and security will largely be felt to be at the perimeter level.

During the day the patient can attend a large range of occupational, educational, recreational and psychotherapeutic activities, the resources for which are probably unequalled in any other clinical setting. There are large workshop areas where the patient can be trained in specific work-related skills which include joinery, metalwork, television repairs, upholstery, vehicle maintenance and pottery. There are therapeutic groups for anxiety and anger management, offending behaviours, empathy and relationship development, assertiveness and social skills. During the evening there will be off-ward social activities on at least four evenings during the week and regular access to a large sports hall and swimming pool. Such is the quality of life for many patients prior to transfer from high security; it could be suggested that this is a far cry from the neglectful and brutalizing regime that has been portrayed (DoH 1992).

PROBLEMS ON TRANSFER

Patients experience an increased level of psychological disturbance when moving wards within a high security hospital (Tavernor et al 1996). Greater problems are likely to be experienced when the transfer is to lower levels of security, as the move entails greater changes, and the effects of institutionalization and quality of life issues can impact at this point. In a study to investigate the experience of high security hospital patients who had been transferred to a medium secure unit and then readmitted to the high security hospital following the failure of the transfer, a picture emerged of inadequately prepared patients with unrealistic expectations, who experienced high levels of psychosocial stress in the medium secure unit (Skelly 1993).

Prior to transfer this sample of patients received little information about the medium secure unit and they approached the assessment interview as their opportunity to impress the interviewing team, rather than to assess the suitability of the medium secure unit to meet their needs. Following the assessment, they rarely received any specific therapy or additional rehabilitation, other than that which the medium secure unit recommended. Rehabilitation for these patients tended to equate only with escorted excursions into the community, which were limited in number, rather than to improve their daily living skills. The patients did not expect to engage in further therapy at the medium secure unit, viewing the transfer as just a stepping stone into the community. They often experienced a delay of between 12 and 24 months in the transfer process, which increased their frustration, leading to anger and resentment.

Patients often found that the conditions at the medium secure unit were poorer than at the high security hospital. These patients were generally behaviourally settled and had progressed through the hospital system building up privileges, which they lost on transfer. Many considered the transfer to be a 'backward step'. They had to learn to adjust to the altered demands of the new environment, where their learned responses were no longer appropriate. High security hospital patients experienced a pervasive feeling of threat, that if they were not compliant with the therapeutic programme, they would be returned to the high security hospital. They also felt vulnerable to assault from more disturbed patients, as well as concerned about the consequences if they had to defend themselves. For some, the medium secure unit was a more secure and restrictive environment than the high security hospital.

REHABILITATION NEEDS

Rehabilitation is an integral part of the transition from higher to lower levels of security. Although high security hospital patients have considerable rehabilitation needs, these needs may not receive sufficient priority. Assessments of skills and deficits are poor and are not always relevant to the skills necessary for community living. The high security hospitals are noted to be effective in managing violent behaviour but are less effective in preparing patients for transfer (Maden et al 1995). This problem is not new to the high security hospitals. Norris (1984) investigated the integration of high security hospital patients into the community. It was found that patients reported life skills deficits that had not been addressed, as most high security hospital consultants did not consider rehabilitation to be a function of a high security hospital.

Whilst much can be done within the high security hospitals to rehabilitate patients and prepare them for lower levels of security, there are problems inherent in the high security environment that restrict the extent of rehabilitation. Some deficits cannot be adequately addressed in the high security hospital due to the restrictions imposed by the environment or the inability to test the patient out in a less controlled situation.

Community orientation, for example, proves difficult for the high security hospitals, though this is particularly important in managing the transition to lower levels of security as patients have limited experience of transport, money, crowds, shopping, crossing roads, making purchases and interacting with the public.

Rehabilitation trips into the community are limited in their scope by guidelines emanating from central and local management and from the Home Office. These guidelines are responsive to problems that occur, particularly the absconding of patients, and this has resulted in a restricted list of permitted destinations and in periods when all trips have been cancelled.

Familiarization with monetary transactions is also difficult as patients are not allowed to possess money within the hospital, both for reasons of security and to avoid the financial exploitation of vulnerable patients. A pilot scheme to allow patients on one predischarge ward to hold up to £30 in cash commenced after one public inquiry (DoH 1992) had engendered a feeling of therapeutic optimism. By 1996 and the start of yet another public inquiry (DoH 1999), what had seemed like a good idea at the time had come to look increasingly risky and the scheme was discontinued.

REHABILITATIVE SCHEMES

A number of schemes have been introduced at Ashworth Hospital in recent years to assist in the transition of patients to lower levels of security. The following are some examples.

Independent living scheme

A joint venture between Ashworth Hospital and a housing association in 1993 led to a community-based independent living scheme (ILS). This scheme was purpose built for Ashworth patients who required rehabilitation into the community. Patients referred from Ashworth were assessed by the ILS staff. If the patient was potentially suitable he or she would be offered day attendance for 12 weeks prior to taking up residency. The ILS provided a comprehensive assessment of living skills, social skills and risk. It was able to offer community orientation, confidence building, skills development and individual rehabilitation programmes. As the patient progressed, links would be developed with the home area prior to seeking accommodation there. After the patient

moved on the ILS offered an outreach programme with regular visits.

In 1996, several Ashworth patients absconded from escorted leave and as a result all leave was postponed which prevented the non-resident patients from attending the ILS. By the time leave was reestablished, the potential risks involved in this venture had been reassessed and referrals to the scheme declined. The withdrawal of funding was not far behind and the scheme was abandoned.

Learning disability

It had been recognized for some years that learning disability patients were inappropriately placed within high security care. This situation has been exacerbated for all patient groups by the 'perverse incentive' of health and local authorities bearing no financial responsibility for high security hospital placements and, therefore, these placements are often perceived as a 'free good'. Once the patient is discharged, however, the home authorities become financially responsible for providing what can often be expensive care and supervision which in some circumstances, e.g. learning disabilities and long-term mental illness, span many years.

The legal challenge by an ex-patient of Rampton Hospital, heard in the European courts in 1998, focused on this issue and his unnecessary detention in conditions of high-security care. Whilst this patient suffered from a mental illness the principles laid down by this case may prove true for all diagnostic groups.

The patient's victory in this case may pave the way for increased litigation by patients on this in the future (Mental Health Act Commission 1999: 44–45). Referrals and admissions had been decreasing and the proportion of learning disability patients in the special hospitals was consequently declining (Special Hospitals Service Authority 1995). A steering group was set up at Ashworth Hospital to assess the needs of learning disability patients and to relocate them to more appropriate environments. Health authorities responsible for individual patients were contacted and hospital staff worked with them to identify appropriate placements in lower security. Patients and their relatives were involved in the process and care staff were involved in preparing patients for transfer. Between 1992 and 1998, of 75 learning disability patients leaving the hospital, 59 were transferred to lower security. None required readmission. By 1999 only three patients continued to be detained in Ashworth Hospital under the diagnostic category of learning disability.

Medium secure unit awareness group

Following the realization of the poor outcomes of patients transferred to medium secure units and the need for better preparation, an awareness group was established for patients. The aims were to engender more realistic expectations of the move to medium security; to develop an understanding of the expectations of patients on trial leave; and to teach coping strategies for dealing with potentially stressful situations.

The awareness group was established for male mentally ill patients who were being considered for referral to medium secure units. The programme consisted of 14 sessions, each of 2 hours' duration, with input from both high security and medium security staff. Each session consisted of information giving to raise awareness; the development of positive thinking skills; and the learning of some coping strategies. This was followed by group discussion to develop peer support and the sharing of experiences.

Wordsworth Unit

The Wordsworth Unit is a predischarge unit for male personality-disordered patients located within the secure perimeter of Ashworth Hospital. It offers an alternative model of care based on social therapy, where the emphasis is on teamwork and clinical supervision. It provides day care, as well as residential facilities that can allow for a more independent existence within the high security environment. Since it became operational in 1997 its potential has not been fulfilled as it has been unable to offer this residential aspect of care.

Patients referred to the unit are assessed over a 6-week period. This involves interviewing the patient and the clinical team and reviewing preadmission and inpatient history. The risk assessment that results from this may indicate areas of concern that make the patient unsuitable for a less secure placement. Those patients accepted engage in a range of therapies, both individual and group, with the emphasis on resocialization issues. This includes work on relationships, coping skills, social skills, offence-related work, relapse prevention, managing the change of environment, awareness of the mental health problems of others and individual living skills.

Resettlement team

There are currently two models for the provision of aftercare and support available within different service areas at Ashworth Hospital. Traditionally, the ward-based primary nurse had a responsibility for liaising with the lower secure unit, escorting the patient to visit the unit and, following transfer, offering a contact point for support and advice. This model provides a more seamless service and utilizes the nurse who has the best knowledge of the patient. It has benefits in motivating staff and ensuring that rehabilitation is an integral part of their work. The difficulties, however, are in freeing up time for ward-based staff to adequately attend to this along with their other duties and with the large catchment area involved. It can provide only a reactive, rather than proactive, service which responds to crises rather than preventing them.

More recently, resettlement teams have been developed which provide a focused and responsive service to the lower secure unit and the patient. Liaison with, and knowledge of, the lower secure environment is improved and the patient can be kept better informed. Aftercare and support are enabled as the service is specifically resourced for this and the resettlement nurse, by regular posttransfer visits, can help maintain the patient in the lower secure environment. A similar scheme between Broadmoor Hospital and a medium secure unit reports fewer problems with patients on trial leave and where problems do arise, they are dealt with quickly and effectively (Rooney et al 1995).

PROCESS OF TRANSITION

Preparation

Following a successful period of treatment and rehabilitation that has reduced the risk presented to others, the patient will be referred to a lower level of security. In some cases this may be an initial approach to seek an early input or it may follow a protracted period at the high security hospital, when it is considered that all concerns have been addressed. The lower secure service will send a multidisciplinary team to assess the patient's suitability for transfer. The assessment of high security hospital patients presents greater problems than it does for other patients, with problematic cases receiving several assessment visits over a period of time (Bullard & Bond 1988).

The assessing staff will submit a report and will often suggest further therapy or rehabilitation to resolve deficits, that they believe should occur in high security, before the patient is acceptable for transfer. This 'second opinion' is valuable in ensuring that the referral is not only based on a functional improvement but also that all offence-related interventions have been completed. The patient may initially view this as a rejection but in reality it is a constructive response that gives a focus to the work that needs to be done with, and by, the patient. Following the completion of these interventions, the patient will be referred again.

Once accepted, the patient is then placed on a waiting list for transfer. High security hospital patients are not seen as priorities for scarce medium secure beds as they are already receiving treatment in a secure and therapeutic environment. Medium secure units primarily assess and treat mentally ill remand prisoners and this severely restricts admissions from high security hospitals (Murray 1996). There has also been some anecdotal evidence of other 'unspoken' issues such as the reluctance for lower secure units to accept personality-disordered patients and reluctance to accept some index offences, most notably arson. During this waiting period the primary interventions are continued, with specific preparations that ease the transition to lower security and maintain the patient's morale

in what is often a long wait. Restricted patients will additionally require Home Office approval for the move from high security.

Prior to the transfer the resettlement nurse will visit the lower secure unit to assess the potential problems of this environment for the patient and to provide information about the patient's management. With this knowledge of the receiving unit, the nurse can provide information to better prepare the patient for the change of environment. The patient will be escorted for an initial visit to the unit with the resettlement nurse and his primary nurse, so that he can orient himself to the structure and routine of the new environment and get to know the staff and patients. Further visits may gradually extend the period spent there and the high security hospital staff may gradually withdraw their support as the patient gains confidence. Unfortunately, the distance from high security hospital to lower secure units is often so large (sometimes hundreds of miles) that making frequent visits for the purpose of acclimatization is impractical. Some medium secure units conduct regular visits to the high security hospital to maintain support to all patients accepted by them for transfer.

Aftercare

Prior to the move a systematic assessment of the patient's health and social needs will have been conducted and a plan of care formulated under the care programme approach. The plan of care will address the patient's general care and treatment needs and the specific needs that will arise due to the transfer. It will also address how potentially problematic behaviours can best be managed. Clinicians will have identified predictors of disturbed behaviour and will have developed strategies to best manage this behaviour. This experiential knowledge will be shared with clinicians from the receiving unit. Clinicians will hand over information at a pretransfer meeting and nursing staff will additionally discuss the plan of care in detail on the day of transfer.

Eventually the patient will be transferred to a lower level of security, usually on 6 months trial leave prior to discharge. At the end of 1992 there were 116 high security hospital patients on trial leave (DoH 1994). Some patients may be returned to high security before the end of the 6 months if there is a clinical crisis or if the patient is felt to be unsuitable for a lower level of security. It is important, during this posttransfer period, that both the patient and the clinicians involved are supported by staff from the high security hospital in maintaining the patient within the lower secure unit.

The resettlement nurse will maintain contact with the patient and staff by regular visits and phone calls. The benefits of this for the patient are having someone who can act in a counselling role outside the present care team and with whom he can ventilate any concerns that he may be anxious about addressing directly. The nurse can also take on a social role as someone with whom the patient shares a recent past. The benefits for the staff are that as problems arise they can be discussed early and dealt with proactively, with advice from a nurse with some previous experience of the patient's management. Where crises occur, the resettlement nurse can offer a response within 48 hours. This level of aftercare should ensure that patients are not returned to high security without some attempt to resolve the presenting difficulties in the lower secure unit first.

CONCLUSION

High security hospitals have often failed their patients, through lack of preparation for the transition to lower levels of security. Although management changes over the past decade have allowed the high security hospitals to focus more intently on the clinical agenda, in the politicized environment of these hospitals the balance between security and therapy swings in response to public criticism. This affects the view, at any point in time, of what constitutes an acceptable risk, which has implications for rehabilitation and the route of release of patients from high security.

Although there are some difficulties in providing a community-focused rehabilitation service in a high security hospital, it is clear that there are many areas that can be improved. There is a need for better global assessments to ensure that treatment and rehabilitation address all relevant areas

of therapeutic concern and that risk assessments concentrate on the reoffending risk in the community rather than on inpatient violence. This ensures that the patient is safe for discharge. In addition to treating the original problems there is also a need to redress the problems created by the institution, which requires a facility for more independent living within the high security environment. This ensures that the patient has the necessary skills for discharge.

The transfer of patients from high security to lower levels of security has to be actively managed if it is to be successful. This entails the provision of aftercare and support which should be delivered by a service model that is effective in maintaining the patient at the lower level of security. Regardless of such improvements, some patients will still experience a 'failed' transfer. With the current range of clinical initiatives and examples of good practice, however, there is now more reason to be optimistic for improved patient outcomes on transfer from high security to lower levels of security than there has been in the past.

REFERENCES

Bailey J, MacCulloch M 1992 Characteristics of 112 cases discharged directly to the community from a new special hospital and some comparisons of performance. Journal of Forensic Psychiatry 3(1): 91–112

Barton R 1959 Institutional neurosis. John Wright, Bristol

Bullard H, Bond M 1988 Secure units: why they are needed. Medicine, Science and the Law 28(4): 312–318

Cope R, Ward M 1993 What happens to special hospital patients admitted to medium security? Journal of Forensic Psychiatry 4(1): 13–24

Dell S, Robertson G 1988 Sentenced to hospital: offenders in Broadmoor. Oxford University Press, Oxford

Department of Health 1992 Report of the Committee of Inquiry into Complaints about Ashworth Hospital. HMSO, London

Department of Health 1994 Report of the Working Group on High Security and Related Psychiatric Provision. HMSO, London

Department of Health 1999 Report of the Committee of Inquiry into the Personality Disorder Unit, Ashworth Special Hospital. Stationery Office, London

Maden A, Curle C, Meux C, Burrow S, Gunn J 1995 Treatment and security needs of special hospital patients. Whurr, London

Mental Health Act Commission 1999 Mental Health Act Commission 8th biennial report 1997–1999. Stationery Office, London

Murray K 1996 The use of beds in NHS medium secure units in England. Journal of Forensic Psychiatry 7(3): 504–524

Norris M 1984 Integration of special hospital patients into the community. Gower, Aldershot

Rooney J, Pierson S, Dunn L 1995 Another step forward: improving liaison between secure unit and special hospital. Psychiatric Care 2(2): 55–57

Skelly C 1993 From special hospital to regional secure unit: a qualitative study of the problems experienced by patients. Unpublished MSc thesis

Skelly C 1994 From special hospital to regional secure unit: a qualitative study of the problems experienced by patients. Journal of Advanced Nursing 20: 1056–1063

Special Hospitals Service Authority 1995 Service strategies for secure care. SHSA, London

Tavernor R, Tavernor S, Crispin Z 1996 Life events and psychopathy: influence of sudden ward environmental change on psychosocial functioning in psychopathically disordered special hospital patients. Journal of Forensic Psychiatry 7(2): 393–399

FURTHER READING

Mental Health Act Commission 1999 Mental Health Act Commission 8th biennial report 1997–1999. Stationery Office, London

Skelly C 1994 From special hospital to regional secure unit: a qualitative study of the problems experienced by patients. Journal of Advanced Nursing 20: 1056–1063

Special Hospitals Service Authority 1995 Service strategies for secure care. SHSA, London

Chapter Twenty Two

Supervising the rehabilitated patient in the community

Alan Gilmour   Helen Edment

INTRODUCTION

The final stage of the rehabilitation process for the mentally disordered patient in forensic mental health services, once deemed no longer a risk to society, is their return to the community. This chapter will explore some of the key issues with the follow-up process for this patient group, the complexities of the services required, the legislation, the pitfalls and benchmarks for good practice.

It is a major skill for forensic mental health teams to integrate a patient into a community with the appropriate level of support and to maintain the person within that community, whilst undertaking continuous assessment of risk to maximize the safety of all. Furthermore, in many parts of the United Kingdom, the level of community services tailored to meet the needs of mentally disordered individuals is limited. The forensic mental health-care team who work with these individuals face a particularly uphill struggle to maintain the link with their patient and at the same time operate within very diverse roles in close liaison with other agencies.

One of the major challenges in designing screening and assessment approaches, treatment intervention and supervision strategies for forensic mental health patients is the diversity of this population. Many are likely to have cognitive limitations that affect their community supervision, such as difficulties in attention and concentration, memory, abstract reasoning, problem solving and planning ability. Problems include forgetting critical information regarding their community supervision (e.g. dates of hearings or appointments) and not recognizing the full range of consequences resulting from violations and other criminal behaviour.

GOVERNMENT POLICY AND LEGISLATION

The absence of coordination between the health, local authority and criminal justice services presents difficulties for individuals in accessing services, often owing to lack of awareness, confidentiality issues and waiting lists for treatment services. In the absence of comprehensive and integrated services, there is a danger of individuals repeatedly cycling through treatment, probation and prison and thus being at higher risk of relapse and other behaviours that often lead to more involvement with the criminal justice system.

Following the Reed Report (DoH & Home Office 1991), a number of recommendations were made to improve links between agencies and to develop community services for mentally disordered offenders. Included was the development of liaison services between the health-care services and criminal justice agencies, such as the police, court and the prison service, and also the training and development of the role of the forensic community mental health nurse.

The Reed Report may have been a catalyst for the development of community services but this has been further stimulated by the continuing pressure on general psychiatric services and also by the good practice that is arising across the United Kingdom.

Most of the legislation is based on improved care management, close monitoring and supervision of high-risk individuals in the community. The care programme approach (DoH 1990), supervision registers (NHSME 1994) and supervised discharge (DoH 1995) are the benchmarks for good practice. Wright & Stockford (1999) indicate that combining these with the plethora of guidance available provides the framework for good practice.

Care programme approach

Health authorities were required to introduce the care programme approach by 1991 (DoH 1990) and it was further extended to incorporate risk assessment (NHSME 1994). The care programme approach was said to be the cornerstone of mental health care (DoH 1996). Any patient involved with specialist services who is especially vulnerable or who poses a risk in other ways will receive appropriate mental health and social care in the community. All those patients detained in forensic mental health services will, thus, fall within the scope of the care programme approach.

In direct parallel, local authority Social Services have specific care management responsibilities under the NHS and Community Care Act 1990. Underpinning both approaches to care are:

◆ a systematic and multidisciplinary assessment of need
◆ a documented care plan agreed between all involved agencies, the person and carers
◆ a key worker with coordination responsibilities
◆ a regular review of progress and continued needs.

Following problems with the introduction of the care programme approach, the Department of Health (1996) introduced a three-tier system:

◆ minimal
◆ more complex
◆ full multidisciplinary.

Health authorities should establish formal procedures with Social Service departments and NHS trusts to jointly ensure that the care programme approach is being implemented consistently and appropriately using the audit tool (NHSE 1996), as well as any other policies which concern all agencies. There is a clearly defined process whereby each agency can raise concerns about implementation.

It is important that care programme approach documentation is up to date and implemented; the procedure focuses on the need for and examples of good practice and includes patient and carer satisfaction surveys.

Supervision registers

The supervision register was introduced to identify all those known to services and considered to be at significant risk of committing serious violence, suicide or serious self-neglect as a result of a severe and enduring mental illness (NHSME 1994). The psychiatrist enters the person on the register under one of the three categories following consultation with the multidisciplinary team. The introduction of the supervision register went some way to formalizing multidisciplinary and multiagency risk assessment. The individual should be informed that they have been placed on the register (unless it is deemed detrimental to their health to do so), the reasons why and the criteria for withdrawal.

Supervised discharge

Supervised discharge came into effect on 1 April 1996 (DoH 1995). It ensures that those patients detained in hospital for treatment receive aftercare services provided under section 117 of the Mental Health Act 1983. Risk assessment provides the anchor for which services will be provided.

Under the supervision order the person can be required to reside in a specific place, attend for medical treatment or attend for education or training. The named supervisor has the right to access the person's place of residence and can take the person for treatment, education or training. Present legislation allows that treatment can be reviewed for those who do not comply, allowing for: a change in service provision; a change in requirements placed on the person; discharge from the supervision order; or admission to hospital.

The government has recently introduced a policy booklet to integrate the care programme approach and case management (DoH 2000).

SUPPORTING FORENSIC PATIENTS IN THE COMMUNITY

For mentally disordered offenders to be adequately supported within the community, a diverse range of services is often required. Indeed, Coffey (2000) indicates that the combination of serious mental illness and a forensic history can present a formidable range of needs.

There is little doubt that mentally disordered offenders living in the community give particular cause for concern and community supervision requires careful handling, good supervision and good risk management. Furthermore, mentally disordered offenders face immense problems with social reintegration as many have been in an institution for many years or are even being returned to the area where many still remember their crimes. Care therefore needs to be intensive at times and always collaborative.

There needs to be a shared understanding between all stakeholders in forensic mental health care about their respective contributions to the service and its future pattern, which enables individual agencies to develop their own strategies in partnership with each other. There should be collaborative arrangements to jointly assess and meet training needs to promote multidisciplinary working arrangements for care in the community involving health and Social Services, independent agencies and service users.

Social Services departments and NHS mental health services providers need to have structures and working practices to promote close communication and collaboration between staff and teams working in this field, to ensure that there is no danger of duplication or passing responsibility. This is also the case where health and Social Services boundaries do not overlap. This includes such joint activity as:

◆ induction programmes
◆ monitoring of specific tasks
◆ multidisciplinary team building involving consultants, GPs, hospital and community health and Social Services staff and management
◆ funding
◆ recording
◆ training
◆ audit.

The forensic community mental health nurse

The forensic community mental health nurse usually plays a pivotal role in providing patients with continuity of care from the institution and, as part of a wider multidisciplinary team, supports the patient in a holistic manner in terms of health care, social, vocational and educational needs when in the community.

The forensic community mental health nurse plays a key role in the assertive follow-up of patients discharged into the community. Saggers & McClelland (1999) noted the importance of the community nurse receiving training and information to undertake the role of community key worker for patients. This is further supported by Friel & Chaloner (1996) who recognized that forensic community mental health nurses were increasingly asked to provide reports on patients and that the nurse should be adequately prepared to accept the burden of responsibility that went with this.

Suggestions have been made to share this burden with the involvement of multidisciplinary and multiagency validation of reports but, more importantly, that nurses are given training and support to fulfill their role.

Care and practice issues

There are many care and practice issues in relation to the mentally disordered offender in the community. Highlighted here are some of the more important ones.

Risk assessment and management

The assessment and effective management of risk is high on the agenda within inpatient forensic mental health services. However, it is even more important when the safety net is not a physical wall or door but the support which is given in the community setting. Risk assessment has to be effective in the community setting if tragedies are to be avoided. Further, risks that are identified have to be adequately managed to reduce, as far as possible, the likelihood of the risk occurring.

Good risk assessment and management can only occur if the patient's behaviour can be observed and then reflected on in relation to past knowledge of the patient. Risk markers should be documented, so all those involved in the care can identify when risks are increasing. Good practice would dictate that risk assessment is formally documented and the management plan identifies who is responsible for what and when formal evaluation is to occur.

It should be kept in mind that the vast majority of mentally disordered offenders do not commit offences when returned to the community and are no more dangerous than members of the general population (Wright & Stockford 1999). However, a number of factors need to be considered (Alberg et al 1996, McNeil & Binder 1994).

◆ Past history of violence
◆ Impulsivity
◆ Agitation and excitement
◆ Interpersonal sensitivity
◆ High levels of anger, suspicion or hostility
◆ Active psychotic symptoms (e.g. delusions, command hallucinations, paranoid ideation)
◆ Poor response to or non-compliance with prescribed medication
◆ Failing to maintain contact with support services
◆ Substance misuse

Crisis intervention and relapse prevention

Following on from risk assessment, any effective risk management plan has crisis intervention and relapse prevention measures built into it.

There is a dearth of literature available on the provision of crisis or emergency forensic services, although anecdotally a number of such services can be accessed throughout the United Kingdom, either through accident and emergency or through the health and social care generic crisis teams. The lack of out-of-hours and weekend services has been a frequent source of criticism within the many mental health inquiry reports (Reith 1998). Although these can be high-cost services with low-volume usage, there is certainly the need for every service to determine an appropriate mechanism for patients or relatives to access in the event of an emergency.

Assertive follow-up

Assertive follow-up is, perhaps, the aim of all services with any complex patient group, such as mentally disordered offenders. In terms of managing a caseload, this is particularly important when dealing with offenders with mental health problems or learning disability.

Most mentally disordered offenders or high-risk individuals are subject to statutory coercive control in the community. For instance:

◆ conditional discharge from a hospital order and still subject to Home Office conditions
◆ leave of absence whilst still formally detained under the 1983 Mental Health Act.

Many must reside at a place approved by the Home Secretary and accept mental health and social supervision. Compliance with medication and not returning to the area of the index offence may be just two of the conditions of discharge or leave and if patients are non-compliant they may be recalled back to hospital.

Compliance

A major focus in the management of patients in the community is compliance with medication and treatment programmes. For many patients, this can form the basis of conditions of their discharge and if compliance does not occur, then the individual may relapse and as a result reoffend, thus returning to either the criminal justice service or health-care provision.

Engagement

Knowledge of the patient and the positive therapeutic relationship which exists are important components of caring for mentally disordered offenders in the community. Without such a relationship, the patient is likely to disengage from the service, which could have disastrous consequences.

Comprehensive care

The package of care available to the patient on discharge should be as comprehensive as possible and operate as part of a broad communication process, with the explicit involvement of the patient and their family or carer, as appropriate. The forensic community mental health nurse is a key member of the rehabilitation team and must be involved at the earliest stage possible. The individualized package of care should take account of all aspects of the patient's needs, which could include the following.

◆ *Health needs.* This could include medication, specific treatments related to offences or the continuation of physical health care or health promotion activities.
◆ *Social needs.* Many patients do not mix well and are socially isolated, owing to the nature of the crime that they have committed or the presentation of their mental illness.
◆ *Vocational needs.* For many forensic patients, the chance of employment is extremely limited owing not only to the mental health issue but also their offending behaviour.
◆ *Educational needs.* To maximize the opportunity for employment or to provide personal value for the individual, links with local colleges and libraries can be highly beneficial.

Motivation levels and commitment to treatment can be critical aspects of the individual's recovery or slide into relapse or recidivism. The provision of economic assistance, housing, employment, child care and the removal of other barriers to participation in treatment, and levering involvement in treatment through use of legislation, where appropriate (Griffin et al 1996), can all serve to enhance involvement.

Supervision

One of the key issues for supervision is the level of vigilance required in relation to the surveillance of mental health problems. A balance needs to be struck between care and control, between the service user's rights and welfare and those of the public.

Community supervision of mentally disordered offenders involves monitoring active symptoms and high-risk situations related to both illness and offending, responding to violations, referral for treatment and monitoring involvement in treatment and other services. Goals of supervision include:

◆ enhancing public safety
◆ providing ongoing monitoring and surveillance
◆ promoting ongoing involvement and treatment
◆ reducing mental health symptoms
◆ stabilizing on medications
◆ developing enhanced awareness of the consequences of behaviour, the relapse process and the importance of treatment.

Multidisciplinary and multiagency working

Communication between disciplines is of paramount importance and often it is forensic community mental health nurses who are central to this, given that they will probably see the patient more often than any other professional. The lessons of the past reflect that if communication is ineffective, then tragedy follows (Reith 1998). The care programme approach (DoH 1990) can assist greatly if used as an appropriate framework for care. Working closely with these agencies improves individual care, provides support and assists in reducing risk to the professional staff involved.

Joint training opportunities, and also time spent gaining a better understanding of the role of different agencies, can only be beneficial. The usual difficulties faced by agencies brought together can be minimized by avoiding certain pitfalls in relation to information sharing, language and organizational culture. Each agency will have its own set of abbreviations and jargon; thus, having awareness can only assist in promoting a positive working relationship. There will still be a number of issues which are more difficult to resolve, such as funding and responsibilities, but these can be worked through in terms of contracts, service level agreements, memoranda of understanding, protocols, staff exchanges or agreed procedures. Managers whose staff operate services within other agencies should be aware of the cultural differences and the potential for conflict. Regular review and audit are crucial to identify any difficulties at an early stage.

The process of developing professional relationships with staff from the various agencies should begin with agreement at the most senior level. This agreement should be communicated widely with all levels of staff involved and the service must be actively marketed throughout the organization. Practical experience has shown examples of direct conflict and actual sabotage of service provision where the relationship has not been clarified and the staff have not seen the benefit of the service. This is part of a process of change management and requires a great deal of energy and resilience on the part of all involved.

DISCUSSION

For the patient moving out into the community or attempting to remain in the community, there are a number of challenges that they face if they are to succeed. High-profile cases, which have received huge publicity, stigmatize the patient and create the opportunity for NIMBYism. The creation of stable and appropriate housing solutions is not a difficulty unique to mentally disordered offenders but the public attitude and reaction to offenders can make a significant difference to the success or otherwise of a rehabilitation programme.

Friendship et al (1999) examined the reoffending of patients discharged from a secure unit and concluded that reoffending rates are of limited value in measuring outcomes in forensic psychiatric populations. To the general public, however, one reoffence is one too many! The patient in the community may have spent many years in institutional care, some or all of which may have been in the form of detention against their will. The forensic community mental health nurse must work alongside the patient to break down barriers and to establish a relationship that offers responsibility and trust. Without this, the patient may well see the nurse as part of a negative culture and could rebel by disengaging from services.

In recent years, both as a reaction to tragedy and also due to political pressure, the number of inquiries relating to mental health care has increased significantly and many of these have identified deficits in services. Many of the recommendations within these inquiries have related to the care of violent and criminal individuals, recognizing that, in many areas, services for this patient group are limited or, indeed, do not exist (Reith 1998). It is important that no patient 'slips through the net' and becomes inappropriately disengaged from services, but arguably of more importance is the risk of people who are offenders, or who are at significant risk of offending, being lost to the service. Mentally disordered offenders are more likely to fall between service provision as they tend to be very complex and chaotic at times and are thus difficult to engage. Additionally, owing to the nature of their offence, criminality or the risk of recidivism, they are not embraced warmly by all who come into contact with them.

CONCLUSION

The publication of the National Service Framework for Mental Health (DoH 1999a) and the ongoing review of the Mental Health Act 1983 (DoH 1999b) provide an opportunity to put into place systems and structures for managing an increasing and complex group of people whose needs transcend traditional service boundaries.

Staff need to be empowered to tackle sometimes reluctant participants in therapy by having available to them a range of levers and sanctions to ensure that protection of all concerned, including the individual in need of services, is maximized. It is also evident that community workers involved in treating this group need a firm understanding of the whole range of services that these individuals are likely to be involved with. In the USA, they use the term 'service spanners' to describe those community workers who span service agencies and are involved in putting together a range of community packages aimed at supporting the individual and protecting the public (Dale 1999).

REFERENCES

Alberg C, Hatfield B, Huxley P 1996 Learning materials on mental health risk assessment. Manchester University and Department of Health, Manchester

Coffey M 2000 Developing community services. In: Chaloner C, Coffey M (eds) Forensic mental health nursing: current approaches. Blackwell, Oxford, ch 9, pp 171–190

Dale C 1999 Dual diagnosis: the American experience. Mental Health Practice 3(3): 18–21

Department of Health 1990 Caring for people: the care programme approach for people with a mental illness referred to the specialist psychiatric services. HC(90)23. Wetherby Health Publications Unit, Department of Health, Wetherby

Department of Health 1995 Mental Health (Patients in the Community) Act. HMSO, London

Department of Health 1996 Building bridges: a guide to arrangements for inter-agency working for the care and protection of severely mentally ill people. Stationery Office, London

Department of Health 1999a National Service Framework for Mental Health: modern standards and service models. Department of Health, London

Department of Health 1999b Reform of the Mental Health Act 1983: proposals for consultation. Cm 4480. Stationery Office, London

Department of Health 2000 Effective care co-ordination in mental health services: modernizing the care programme approach: a policy booklet. Stationery Office, London

Department of Health, Home Office 1991 Review of health and social services for mentally disordered offenders and others requiring similar services. Stationery Office, London

Friel C, Chaloner C 1996 The developing role of the forensic community nurse. Nursing Times 92(29): 33–35

Friendship C, McLintock T, Rutter S, Maden A 1999 Reoffending: patients discharged from a regional secure unit. Criminal Behaviour in Mental Health 9: 226–236

Griffin PA, Hills HA, Peters RH 1996 Criminal justice–substance abuse cross-training: working together for change. Center for Substance Abuse Treatment, Rockville, MD

McNeil D, Binder R 1994 The relationship between acute psychiatric symptoms, diagnosis and short term risk of violence. Hospital and Community Psychiatry 45(2): 133–137

NHS Executive 1996 The spectrum of care. A summary of comprehensive local services for people with mental health problems: 24 hour nursed beds for people with severe and enduring mental illness: an audit pack for the care programme approach. HSG (96)6. Department of Health, London

NHS Management Executive 1994 Introduction of supervision registers for mentally ill people from 1 April 1994. NSG (94)5. HMSO, London

Reith M 1998 Community care tragedies: a practice guide to mental health inquiries. Venture Press, Birmingham

Saggers J, McClelland N 1999 How informed are community psychiatric nurses (CPNs) of their role in the implementation of supervised discharge? Medicine, Science and the Law 29(4): 313–318

Wright P, Stockford A 1999 Risk management of mentally disordered offenders in the community. In: Ryan T (ed) Managing crisis and risk in mental health

nursing. Stanley Thornes, Cheltenham, ch 8, pp 105–123

FURTHER READING

Baxter R, Rabe-Hesketh S, Parrott J 1999 Characteristics, needs and reoffending in a group of patients with schizophrenia formally treated in medium security. Journal of Forensic Psychiatry 10(1): 69–83

Chaloner C, Kinsella C 1992 Care with conviction. Nursing Times 88(17): 50–52

Lamb HR, Weinberger EL, Gross HB 1999 Community treatment of severely mentally ill offenders under the jurisdiction of the criminal justice system: a review. Psychiatric Services 50(7): 907–913

Chapter Twenty Three

Security in forensic environments: strategic and operational issues

Colin Dale   Jim Gardner

Chapter Contents

INTRODUCTION

In researching the area of security in forensic mental health services, the most striking yet seemingly obvious result is that there is very little material in the literature or public arena. The material that does exist is in unpublished 'grey literature' by way of reports and inquiries or in confidential documents held by the Home Office and/or Department of Health. The authors were greatly assisted by being able to work alongside key thinkers in the field, such as the architect John Lynch, with whom one of the authors worked on the planning and development of two new forensic residential units and the concept development strategy for high security forensic mental health services. The Special Hospitals Service Authority's work with planners and strategists on a UK-wide basis provided the authors with a distillation of experience, thoughts and ideas from the experts in specialist fields in their subject area.

Swinton (2000: 119–120) states that:

A focus on pathology and control inevitably means that personal needs become subsumed to control and security needs, leading to the disempowerment of the client, the development of models of care which can be oppressive and abusive, and the types of institutional tyranny which Goffman highlighted in his study of mental institutions (Goffman 1991). Within such a situation, therapeutic risk-taking and patient empowerment, two of the central tenets of

251

contemporary forensic mental health nursing practice, cease to be realistic options.

Studies have repeatedly shown that the quality of the environment plays a significant part in reducing aggression and violence. Key factors include the level and type of contact between staff and patients, the ward milieu and how the patients spend their day (Davis 1992).

Within secure environments the heightened level of risk to patients, staff and members of the public means that a wider, more prescriptive range of measures must be employed to control the potential for disruption and violence. These measures are designed to create the optimum environment for the development of any therapeutic alliances and as essential components of therapy (Watson & Kirby 2000).

SAFETY AND ACHIEVING SECURITY

Although forensic mental health services deal with psychiatric patients who need to be detained in circumstances of security, they are hospitals within the ethos of the NHS and are not penal establishments. Their purpose is the care, treatment and rehabilitation of the patients and within that context the needs for physical security must be provided, within the building and site layout design, in a sensitive and balanced way.

Benson (1992), Burrow (1993) and Tarbuck (1994) speak of the 'therapeutic use of security' which they suggest entails the recognition, understanding and resolution of external factors of control against a patient's individual care needs. It is also suggested that a more apt term is a 'controlled environment', as opposed to 'secure', to encompass a wider scope of restrictive phenomena (McCourt 1999). This concept embraces physical security such as the security fence, locked doors, controlled entrances, the design of windows and patient accommodation (Burrow 1993), as well as the accompanying security procedures employed by secure units. It also extends to include the legal restrictions of the

Mental Health Act 1983 (Burrow 1993), the protection of the public (Burrow 1991, Tarbuck 1994), control and restraint and seclusion practices (Topping-Morris 1992), graduated leave systems and the 'relational' aspects of care contained within the professional relationships between staff and patients and the differing elements of the treatment programmes and is consequently a dynamic process (Kinsley 1998). Burrow (1993) states that the 'control of the environment and its degree of restrictiveness can be greatly influenced by nursing staff'.

ETHICS

Some authors suggest that the main distinction between the nurse working in a secure environment and one working in general psychiatry is the ethical dilemma of 'control versus care' (Hopkins & Ousley 2000). Tarbuck (1994) emphasized the clinical application of ethics, placing a significant responsibility on the nurse to act in a manner demonstrating both a beneficence and a fidelity to the patient.

Within health care all professions have adopted codes of practice which have as their basis the principles that the health of the patient will be the first consideration and that human dignity will always be respected. Intentional harm to those seeking help, lack of respect for them as people or action in unnecessary ignorance are all unacceptable and breaches of professional codes (Dale et al 1999).

Working within secure clinical environments presents health-care professionals with a range of issues demanding ethical consideration. An understanding of ethics does not offer a panacea for moral dilemmas but can help to guide effective practice and assist in finding informed responses to ethical decisions (Chaloner 1998).

Singer (1993: 2) points out that '... ethics is not an ideal system that is noble in theory but no good in practice. The reverse of this is closer to the truth ... for the whole point of ethical judgements is to guide practice'.

Ethics provides a framework for examining the morality of human behaviour beyond a somewhat simplistic distinction between 'right' and 'wrong'. Ethics as applied to practice demands an understanding of important ethical concepts (e.g. confidentiality), ethically important decision-making procedures (e.g. deciding when confidentiality should be maintained), the ability to apply such concepts and decision-making procedures to real-life cases, plus effective communication abilities (Gillon 1996).

Problematic ethical questions raised by secure mental health services include: appropriate use of power; justification of appropriateness and cost of treating offenders; and the therapy/security dilemma for staff (Chaloner 1998).

Issues have been raised about the social control aspect of secure mental health institutions: 'The shortening of the periods of detention for treatment, deterrence or retribution have made a live issue of whether (or when) it is justifiable to detain violent and sexual offenders solely for the protection of others' (Walker 1991: 755).

The legal rights of patients are protected by bodies such as the Mental Health Act Commission but their 'moral' rights seem less clear. Whilst it is obviously the case that an individual's physical movements are restricted in a secure environment, this does not necessarily imply that they lack autonomy or lose the 'capacity to think, decide and act on the basis of such thought and decision freely and independently' (Gillon 1985: 60).

The consent of patients is necessary for the majority of health-care interventions (McLean 1989). In secure mental health care, however, an element of coercion may be suggested, as patients may feel compelled to cooperate with treatment programmes for pragmatic reasons in relation to the prospect of earlier discharge or transfer from hospital (Chaloner 1998).

Chaloner (1998) outlines five areas of practical moral issues that nurses face in working in secure environments:

◆ power and control, e.g. the use of restraint including seclusion (Alty 1997, Lehane & Rees 1996)
◆ risk assessment and the prediction of dangerousness (Allen 1997).

◆ consent to treatment (Clarke 1998)
◆ confidentiality
◆ 'unpopular' patients.

Chaloner (1998: 33) suggests that:

> An adherence to professional codes and guidelines can assist in finding a solution to moral dilemmas. However, a strict adherence to such codes, while professionally appropriate, does not provide an adequate replacement for a fully considered ethical appraisal of a particular situation.

POWERS OF STAFF

The Mental Health Act Commission (1999: 221) describes a 'great uncertainty about the extent of the powers of staff to impose rules and enforce sanctions with regard to the behaviour of patients'. It rightly points out that by their very definition, detained patients are involuntary and may therefore resist control, behave inappropriately and break rules (which may of course be the reason they are detained). What then, asks the Mental Health Act Commission (1999: 221):

> ... are the measures that institutions are entitled to take to maintain order and what is the legal, ethical or therapeutic justification for these measures? How are the entitlements and interests of individual patients safeguarded? How can the risk of problem behaviour be minimized?

The Mental Health Act 1983 does not refer to the power to restrain patients, to keep them in seclusion, to deprive them of their personal possessions or to regulate the frequency and manner of visits to them. Apart from the duty of care that staff owe patients and common law powers to act in emergency situations, a few legal cases over the years have shed greater light on some aspects of the powers of staff. The case of Poutney *v* Griffiths (197512 All ER, 888) cited by the Mental Health Act Commission (1999: 223) gives some legal justification for the control and discipline of detained patients. The House of Lords held that treatment necessarily involves the exercise of discipline and control and that, in this case, a nurse was justified in imposing restrictions on the visit of family and friends to the patient, as this was seen as being a necessary part of the patient's treatment (Mental Health Act Commission 1999).

The case brought by three Broadmoor patients (Mental Health Act Commission 1999) may have taken the issue of maintaining order further than that needed for the treatment of the individual patient. The case concerned a challenge by the patients of the hospital's policy to introduce random and routine searches. Previous policy had been to search patients and their belongings only when there had been reason to do so, as indeed was recommended in the 1993 edition of the Code of Practice (DoH & Welsh Office 1993). The change of policy made this a more routine event and the Court of Appeal held that:

> ... it is obvious that in the interests of all in particular the need to ensure a safe therapeutic environment for patients and staff that the express power of detention must carry with it a power of control and discipline, including, where necessary, of search with or without cause and despite individual medical objection. The judge added that it was plain common sense that, on occasion, an individual patient's treatment may have to give way to the wider interest. (Mental Health Act Commission 1999: 223–224)

The justification for the hospital's exercise of its power of control and discipline, in this case, was not in terms of the patient's treatment but because of the need to maintain order for the safety of all.

In discussing the Broadmoor case, Davenport (1999) is concerned that if the interests of security and safety were to override the interests of the patient in every case, it would be difficult to escape the conclusion that the patient's treatment is an irrelevancy. But it is difficult to draw a dividing line between what is permitted in the name of treatment and what can only be justified in the name of detention; often measures to control behaviour involve a mixture of both. Eldergill (1997) points out that it is important not to lose sight of the purpose of the statutory powers, which is that they enable necessary treatment to be given to a patient whose behaviour is putting

himself or others at risk, the aim being to eliminate the risk of harm, or further harm, being done. This is the statutory objective, not the imposition of discipline, control and force for their own sake. It is not possible to complete a necessary programme of hospital treatment unless a disturbed patient can be restrained from leaving the ward or from behaving violently towards himself or others. The patient's recovery, like that of any other patient, depends on the maintenance of a safe, calm, therapeutic environment and this is only possible if medical and nursing staff can control violent behaviour. However, there must be no malice, no ill treatment or wilful neglect and any force used must be reasonable in the circumstances (Mental Health Act Commission 1999).

A SECURITY STRATEGY

Buildings and physical security elements must be designed to comply with the aim of ensuring the safety of the public and to ensure the provision of appropriate treatment for the patients, whilst ensuring a good quality of life for patients and staff. In meeting these aims, a normalized, caring and supportive setting is needed for the hospital or unit. The level of security to be provided is such that patients and staff inside the unit are afforded an appropriate level of protection, with escape being prevented by the physical security measures provided.

It is widely considered that, unlike prisons, patients in forensic mental health services are less likely to act together in an attempt to escape, orchestrate a riot or take hostages (it is also considered less likely that they will receive organized assistance from outside the secure unit). It may be that two or three patients could act together to breach the security system, but the threat is unlikely to be on a scale any larger than that and the main risk will be posed by individual patients working alone and without assistance. This consequently reduces the scale of the risk and, to some extent, the nature of physical protective measures that are needed.

As many of the patients cared for in forensic mental health services are by their admission considered to be dangerous, they can pose a grave risk to others. Therefore, the problem of safety is a significant feature and the safety of other patients and staff is a fundamental feature that needs to be addressed within the physical security measures in a forensic mental health unit.

The buildings and site layout should be designed to promote safe conditions by being planned with good sight-lines and by avoiding blind corners, hidden recesses, dead-ends, isolated and dark areas and difficult-to-observe and supervise spaces. Security can be achieved in a forensic mental health service by the two means of dynamic and passive measures.

Dynamic security may be promoted by:

◆ treatment and care programmes
◆ good interpersonal relationships
◆ effective procedures and operations.

Passive security may be promoted by:

◆ physical and structural elements
◆ technological systems.

The degree of security achieved will rely upon the passive security measures providing a supportive framework to the dynamic security measures. All of these features, however, are interactive and mutually supportive.

DYNAMIC MEASURES

It is considered that the most effective form of security lies in the treatment and care available to the patients, as it is this treatment that will help to reduce the patients' level of dangerousness and lead to stabilization and to their eventual rehabilitation (Kaye & Franey 1998).

Relational security

The primary function of forensic mental health care has been described as providing health care in conditions of special security for mentally disordered offenders and others requiring similar services on account of their dangerous, violent or criminal propensities (DHSS & Home Office 1989).

When the Special Hospitals Service Authority was formed in 1989, it was given two primary objectives (DHSS & Home Office 1989):

1. to ensure the continuing safety of the public
2. to ensure the provision of appropriate treatment for the patients.

Although four further objectives were listed, the maintenance of a proper balance between these two primary objectives inevitably provided the basis for a major conflict: that between security and therapy. Kinsley (1998: 75), who headed security for the Special Hospitals Service Authority at this time, posed the questions: 'Which should come first? How many risks could justifiably be taken in furthering the patient's treatment? How was the public interest best to be served?'

Relational security is concerned with developing good interpersonal and sound professional relationships between the clinical team and the patients, so that there is a build-up of trust that will enable the staff to get to know and understand their patients, their moods and problems, to facilitate interventions before these become major problems or lead to incidents of a security nature (Kinsley 1998).

The most commonly raised issue amongst care staff working in secure environments is that of reconciling the therapeutic needs of patients with the need to ensure that security is maintained (UKCC & University of Central Lancashire 1999). This is not a new phenomenon. In 1794 Philippe Pinel spoke of the need to balance safety requirements with the rights of patients and of the importance of non-punitive approaches and of non-retaliation when patients assaulted staff. Pinel also spoke of the importance of adequate supervision of patients and of sensitive management of any disturbed behaviour (Mental Health Act Commission 1999).

Despite the longevity of the debate on this issue, the therapeutic balance of security and therapy appears to be no nearer resolution or even a satisfactory compromise. Kirby (1999: 300) states that:

Invariably there are cases where security is sacrificed in favour of therapeutic activity and unnecessary and unfortunate incidents occur, or the need for security outweighs the therapeutic value of an intervention or action and the patient makes no clinical progress.

Models of nursing and specific therapeutic approaches in psychiatric nursing have meant that nurses have sanctioned or prohibited certain behaviours which may be viewed as custodial, in an attempt to ensure compliance with treatment or in the promotion of the individual's health (Watson & Kirby 2000). In a forensic mental health setting this suggests that the maintenance of a safe and secure environment is the essential basis for all other psychotherapeutic work, rather than being in opposition to it. Kaye (1991: 8), the then Special Hospitals Service Authority Chief Executive, said: 'Dangerousness is reduced as progress is made towards stabilization and recovery, and treatment is thus part of security'. He went on to suggest that the most effective form of security lay in the treatment of the patient.

In the UK the task of security has always been largely the province of nurses and, as a consequence, they are often viewed by the patients in these services as gaolers as well as carers. A more enlightened view, however, would see security as the responsibility of all staff and each individual member of staff must have a commitment to it.

In some states of the USA and Canada, a different approach has been taken and there is a clear division of responsibility between security staff who manage security and nursing staff who have responsibility for the quality of the environment, advocacy and therapeutic engagement (Scales et al 1993). Kinsley (1998) describes how this North American model was actively considered by the newly formed Special Hospitals Service Authority in 1989; however, it was decided to continue with the combined role for nursing, as it was thought there were inherent dangers in separating the therapeutic and security roles.

There is limited discussion in the literature concerning the impact of the role of the nurse in the creation of a positive or negative culture in secure environments. Burnard (1992), Burrow (1993) and Topping-Morris (1992) assert the importance of avoiding the macho culture and those staff with controlling tendencies,

highlighting the need for a more mature and reflective practitioner.

In the UKCC & University of Central Lancashire (1999) secure environments project, using various survey methods to gain the views of over 1000 nurses in the secure health and criminal justice system, the balance between therapy and security was the most consistently reported dilemma. However, differences in role and responsibility were evident from the responses to individual questionnaires. The health sector respondents saw the physical intervention in situations where there is a breakdown in environment and relationships as a much more significant part of their role than the prison nurses (93.2% and 69.6% respectively). The authors suggested that this finding may reflect the role expectations of nurses in some prison settings, where they would not be expected to become involved with physical intervention. A large difference was also found between health and prison respondents in relation to the creation and maintenance of boundaries. The authors suggest that this may reflect the higher emphasis and use of physical security measures in the prison setting as opposed to the health sector. This reliance on physical security was seen in the high security service before the more liberal policies of the early 1990s (DoH 1999). The realization of the need to develop and enhance deescalation skills has become more evident in the health sector, particularly in relation to people with a personality disorder.

The UKCC & University of Central Lancashire (1999) reported that nurses expressed that difficult patients were easier to manage in a prison setting, with clearer rules in relation to transgressions and a greater array of sanctions available to control behaviour. In these circumstances, the need for psychological skills in relation to boundaries may be seen as less important. One of the solutions put forward by the Fallon Inquiry (DoH 1999) was that patients with a personality disorder should be subjected to more stringent security measures than other forms of diagnosis and that ultimately, means should be sought to segregate this group from the rest of the population.

The UKCC & University of Central Lancashire (1999) reported that escorting patients within and beyond secure settings was a much more highly recognized role within the health service as opposed to the prison setting (90.8% and 53.2% respectively). This finding was also reflected in the level of importance attributed to this by both sectors (88.2% and 61.6% respectively). The authors suggest that this finding may reflect the type of escorting engaged in. In the health sector this would be regarded as a key rehabilitation task that most nurses, particularly primary nurses, would engage in. In the prison service, health staff would not be participating as much in rehabilitative work but would be involved in outpatient accident and emergency events. Unsurprisingly, therefore, they see this as a much less important part of their role.

The experience of forensic mental health nursing, particularly in relation to personality disorders, is that it is not difficult to find examples of staff, usually though not exclusively nurses, who do extraordinary, often dangerous things in providing care and treatment to this group. When boundaries have been eroded, intense personal relationships (including marriages) have occurred, weapons have been supplied and escapes assisted. If organizations respond to these situations as dislocated events carried out by rogue staff members, perhaps they miss the main learning points of these events and how these individual members of staff found themselves in these situations in the first place. The organization is in danger of ignoring the pathology of the patient they are dealing with and deluding themselves that 'getting rid' of the rogue staff member deals with the problem.

Means of overcoming this have been suggested by Melia et al (1999) with a model they refer to as 'triumvirate nursing'. This is described as 'nurses working in a team of three, each with equal responsibility for the care for their patients' (Melia et al 1999: 19). They go on to suggest that this way of working provides a means of relationship formation and of minimizing boundary violation with this particular diagnostic group.

Procedural and operational security

Procedural and operational issues are the methods or means by which patients are managed and safe security maintained and are the most tedious for staff to implement. This concerns the methods and procedures developed by the service for operating and monitoring security effectively, together with the instructions and regulations and practices introduced for dealing with: emergencies; incidents; searching; patrolling; escorts and movements, and training programmes that are needed to maintain up-to-date knowledge, attitudes and responses. These systems must be known, understood and accepted, be as unobtrusive as possible and totally reliable. They should be derived from policy statements and expressed through clearly written operational instructions (Kinsley 1998).

Although the effectiveness of the dynamic measures will largely be determined by the clinical team, as any security system is only as effective as the personnel who operate it, it is the design of the buildings and nature of the site layout that contribute, in a significant way, both to help staff and to promote the efficacy of these measures.

The UKCC & University of Central Lancashire (1999) examined standards in use throughout the secure health and criminal justice system and their impact on nursing. They found that there could be early gain in targeting 'sensitive and problematic' areas for staff and working towards the joint production and implementation of standards utilizing external expertise and guidance where this was indicated.

The production of standards is one task, whilst implementation and monitoring in practice is another. Routine and regular audit activity, training and education, together with a clear expectation of staff reflected in the job descriptions, would all be helpful adjuncts to the visibility of standards in practice. Indeed, this was a key finding of the Fallon Inquiry (DoH 1999).

The UKCC & University of Central Lancashire (1999) found evidence of a wide range of practice standards which had been developed in some aspects of secure care and the prison services. However, there was little coordination across and between services and poor dissemination and uptake of standards. Other findings included:

◆ little evidence of research data within standards, nor of quality control or validation of them

◆ auditing of standards across services was haphazard or minimal
◆ evidence that practitioners were excluded from the development of organizational standards.

The NHSE (1999) issued a circular in relation to the safety and security in Ashworth, Broadmoor and Rampton hospitals. It was produced in the wake of the inquiry into the personality disorder unit at Ashworth Hospital (DoH 1999) which had raised a number of concerns about security within the unit.

In the circular the NHSE (1999: 3) states that:

The directions are issued by the Secretary of State for Health and are mandatory upon the special health authorities which run the high security hospitals. The guidance contains recommendations which are not mandatory, but where the hospital authorities deviate from the guidance they should maintain a written record of the reasons for doing so. The directions and guidance have been drawn up in such a way as to be compatible with the Mental Health Act 1983, other relevant legislation and the Code of Practice and the Mental Health Act 1983.

The direction went on to state that:

The directions and guidance cover minimum physical and operational standards of safety and security. They do not focus on the therapeutic aspects of the work of the special hospital authorities. The intention is, however, that their implementation will, in contributing to the provision of a safe environment for patients and staff, enhance rather than provide a barrier to the therapeutic activities of the hospitals. (NHSE 1999: 3)

The NHSE are not in the same position to prescribe such action on medium and low secure units but it is likely that these 'minimum standards' in high security care will be embraced by units at lower levels of security. The circular offered the advice that:

While it is clearly important that there should be a comprehensive set of policies, efforts should be made to keep the number of them to manageable proportions so that staff are not overwhelmed by paper and have a realistic prospect of being familiar with them. A single page summary attached to each policy, highlighting key principles and instructions for staff, may be useful in this respect. (NHSE 1999: 9)

The NHSE (1999: 9) circular suggests that 'where staff are permitted to use discretion in the exercise of a policy, the reasons for the exercise of that discretion should be recorded' and the special hospital authorities were urged to share copies of their main policies with a view to disseminating good practice and achieving a generally consistent approach. This latter suggestion could be extended to medium and low secure services and was a finding of the UKCC & University of Central Lancashire (1999) secure environments project which found that:

Discussion with participants within the scoping exercise identified a need to determine national minimum criteria for policies and protocols that could be locally developed. These might include policies and protocols in relation to security items, seclusion, leave of absence, and physical health monitoring.

The UKCC & University of Central Lancashire (1999) found that the development of standards in many instances was as a response to incidents or inquiries, rather than being developed proactively to meet the needs of client groups. The NHSE (1999) circular seems one such example of this.

Amongst the many staff that the UKCC & University of Central Lancashire (1999) project contacted, there was confusion between the terms standards, protocols, guidelines and policies. Additionally, there was evidence that practice standards are not made known to clients and that clients have little input into the development of standards.

The specific matters covered by the NHSE (1999) guidance included the following.

Searching

◆ Rub-down searching of patients
◆ Random and routine searching of patients

◆ Searches when patients move around within the secure perimeter
◆ Searches of patients' rooms/lockers
◆ Searches of ward areas and other areas
◆ Written records of certain searches
◆ Searching of members of staff
◆ Searching of contractors, visitors and visiting children
◆ Checks of vehicles

The NHSE (1999: 13) guidance specifically states that:

A hospital authority shall ensure that all patients:

◆ *are subject to a random rub-down search not less than once a month*
◆ *are subject to a rub-down search on any occasion when their rooms or personal lockers located outside their rooms are searched*
◆ *who receive visitors are subject to a rub-down search both before and after seeing any visitor*
◆ *who go on leave of absence from the hospital are subject to a rub-down search before leaving the secure perimeter and on returning from leave.*

Communication

The NHSE (1999: 18–20) gave guidance in relation to:

◆ internal patient-to-patient mail
◆ patients' outgoing telephone calls
◆ patients' incoming telephone calls
◆ patients' incoming mail
◆ patients' outgoing mail
◆ mobile telephones.

Patients' possessions

The NHSE (1999: 17–18) provides guidance on possessions in patients' rooms. It is suggested that these need to be limited to a level and type compatible with the facilitation of searching, the maintenance of security and the reduction of fire hazards. In summary:

◆ limit on number, amount and type of patients' personal possessions
◆ inventory of patients' possessions
◆ items brought into hospital for patients
◆ patients' access to computer equipment etc.

With these objectives in mind, it is recommended that, as far as electrical and related items are concerned, patients should, as a maximum, only be permitted to retain the following in their rooms (NHSE 1999: 7).

◆ A television capable of receiving terrestrial programmes only
◆ A video cassette recorder not capable of copying videos
◆ Either a music centre or a radio, a tape cassette player and a CD player or a mini disc player
◆ Up to 12 audio tape cassettes
◆ Up to five video tapes
◆ Up to 12 CDs but no CD-ROMs
◆ Any other electrical or electronic item which the clinical team, acting on advice from the hospital authority's security department, have agreed that the patient may have

Where videos are concerned, it is recommended that:

Any video brought into the hospital premises should, on arrival in the hospital, be checked by a member of staff to establish that it is what it is purported to be and then be passed to the clinical team for a decision as to whether or not it is suitable for the patient for whom it is intended (bearing in mind that the apparently innocent contents of some videos may be considered inappropriate for some patients). No video should be passed to a patient if it is rated 18R. Patients should not be allowed to loan or exchange videos amongst themselves unless by prior agreement with a suitably qualified member of staff, who should ensure that any necessary amendments are made to the property inventories of the patients concerned. (NHSE 1999: 7)

Other areas to be considered are (NHSE 1999):

◆ patient shops
◆ contractors' vehicles in patient areas

◆ patients' grounds privilege
◆ security of tools.

The development and implementation of policies

The development and implementation of policies needs to be supported within the performance indicators for an organization and subjected to regular audit and update. Care staff should be supported by a robust system of operational policies and procedures, which are known to all, subject to regular monitoring and update and supported and reinforced by management (UKCC & University of Central Lancashire 1999).

From a security perspective contact with a number of high, medium and low secure units revealed that the following were regarded as a minimum range of policies and procedures to have available.

Contingency plans for major incidents

These include: explosive devices/bomb threats; fire; disturbances; escape; and hostage situations.

Emergency communications

These include: categories and means of communication; response to alarm states; use of UHF radio systems; use of telephones; testing of alarms and emergency communication systems.

Searching

These include: authorization; spot checks; ground searches; patient areas; patients' rooms and personal property; missing tool and/or concealed item; searching of patients (rub-down and strip searches); and monitoring systems.

Disturbances

Actions by named wards and departments are necessary together with issues such as authorization and use of control and restraint equipment and personnel and response to rooftop incidents.

Movement of patients around the site

These include: movement of patients around the site to recreational, educational and social events; attendance at off-ward clinics; patients with 'parole' status; and movement of patients during hours of darkness.

Access to secure sites

This includes: the identification and authorization to enter a secure site; issuing and safe keeping of security keys; identification/authorization of vehicles and personnel; identification, reception and entry of visitors and visiting arrangements; security checks on visitors and goods; out-of-hours visiting; high risk – segregated visiting; and children visiting.

Building security

This includes: locking arrangements for wards and departments; routine security checks on all buildings; roof access; window design; and suicide prevention measures.

External escorting of patients

This includes: escort procedure; emergency leave of absence; use of vehicles; use of mechanical restraint; group escorts; escorting of patients to general hospital; and absconding from premises other than secure units.

In evidence to the review team considering new mental health legislation, the Mental Health Act Commission (1999: 224) suggested that attention could be given to:

◆ powers to search patients
◆ powers to withhold property
◆ powers to refuse leave or access to hospital activities
◆ the whole raft of measures considered or taken by service providers to maintain control and discipline in hospitals.

They also felt, however, that 'Equally important is the provision for patients of a form of appeal and redress when they feel they have been subjected to unnecessary, arbitrary or extreme measures' (Mental Health Act Commission 1999: 224).

Operational systems of control

The Mental Health Act 1983 Code of Practice (DoH & Welsh Office 1999) includes guidance on the handling of patients who present particular management problems, which covers the use of physical restraint, seclusion and the locking of doors and the searching of patients and their belongings. Guidance is also given on methods for reducing or eliminating unacceptable behaviour which should take account of the:

◆ need for individual care planning
◆ physical condition of the patient
◆ physical environment of the ward or unit
◆ need to maintain adequate staffing levels.

To these could be added access to advocacy services.

The guidance also points to the need for continuing risk assessment and management where there is a risk of problem behaviour, training by qualified trainers and clear written policies.

The Mental Health Act Commission (1999: 225) believes that there is much more that can be done in addition to individual care plans to prevent the need for restraint, including:

◆ adequate activity space
◆ staff call systems
◆ access to fresh air
◆ pleasant decor and surroundings
◆ non-smoking and quiet areas
◆ staff-to-staff call system
◆ good food and dining facilities
◆ patient control of lighting in own rooms
◆ recreation and visiting rooms
◆ access to a telephone
◆ secure lockers for patients' belongings.

To these could be added patients' access to individual bedrooms and the provision of privacy locks for patients.

The Mental Health Act Commission (1999) also believes that the control of behaviour by medication should only be used in exceptional circumstances after careful consideration and as

part of a treatment plan. Further, physical restraint should be a last-resort measure and is only indicated when other interventions have failed and where: 'actual physical assault, deliberate or accidental self-harm, or, in certain circumstances, the destruction of property (such as where the debris may be used as a weapon or where patients' property is being damaged)' (Mental Health Act Commission 1999: 225). To this criterion could also be added the use of control and restraint to facilitate the administration of medication and to prevent exhaustion of the patient.

The Mental Health Act Commission (1999: 225) also urges caution in the use of physical restraint, making particular reference to the need for a trained three-person team to deal with the situation and warning that higher numbers of staff may exacerbate the situation. The infliction of pain should not form part of the physical intervention and there should be no automatic link with physical intervention and the placing of the patient in seclusion. Where an intramuscular injection is given, consideration should be given to evidence from other tragic incidents, as the rate of absorption of antipsychotic medication may be greatly increased following a violent incident. In all situations the emphasis must be on utilizing deescalation techniques before physical interventions are used.

Seclusion

Seclusion is defined in the Code of Practice (DoH & Welsh Office 1999: 19.16) as: 'the supervised confinement of a patient in a room, which may be locked to protect others from significant harm'. Awareness of the ethical issues in the use of seclusion, as with control and restraint, is essential to good practice. The balance between the rights of a secluded patient to freedom, choice and autonomy and the rights of others to protection from harm needs careful consideration by the multidisciplinary team. The application of seclusion should be regarded as an emergency measure, used only where there is a significant risk of harm to the patient and others. Consequently, it should be an infrequent practice, for the minimum period of time. Its potential for abuse means that it should be subject to the most rigorous control, monitoring and evaluation. The Blom-Cooper inquiry strongly criticized the practice of seclusion and went as far as recommending the 'phasing out and ultimate ending of seclusion' (DoH 1992: 258). This recommendation was the only one from the Blom-Cooper inquiry which was not accepted by the Special Hospitals Service Authority, who regarded it as unworkable.

It is clear that there are harmful psychological effects for the patient in seclusion which the Mental Health Act Commission (1999: 228) lists as: 'feelings of increased despair and isolation, anger, worsening of delusions and hallucinations and the effects of sensory deprivation' and it is not an appropriate intervention for people who are depressed or suicidal. The physical effects on patients can also be marked with the need for nursing staff to assess the patient's level of consciousness, pulse and respiration, noting any physical symptoms or abnormalities, particularly where medication has been administered, including, if indicated and where practicable, recording of blood pressure and temperature levels. Avoiding dehydration is important, as is the monitoring of urinary output. To avoid disorientation of the individual the patient should be able to see a clock, have access to writing material if requested and be encouraged to engage in communication.

The Code of Practice (DoH & Welsh Office 1999) specifies that a secluded patient should always be clothed, although acknowledgement is given to the possibility of self-harm or harm to others and the Code therefore urges vigilance on the part of nursing staff. A small number of patients may need protective indestructible clothing and/or bedding; these patients would normally be in medium and high security services and in these circumstances written approval of medical staff should be evident.

The Mental Health Act Commission (1999) has raised concerns over a practice that it refers to as 'de facto' seclusion, where patients are cared for in a room not specifically designated for seclusion, with the door unlocked and with nursing staff observing from the corridor. The patient is not, however, allowed to leave the room unsupervised and is therefore effectively in a situation of seclusion. The danger of this practice is that the patient does not enjoy the policy safeguards inherent in a seclusion policy (e.g. visiting by a member of medical staff and a senior nurse). The reality for nurses is that patients may present such disturbed and disruptive behaviour that it is necessary to keep them segregated from fellow patients, which may include procedures such as 'time out'. It is important to ensure that patient safeguards are not abrogated during these procedures.

Special observation

The Standing Nursing and Midwifery Advisory Committee (1999) published practice guidance on the observation of patients at risk. It defined nursing observation as:

Regarding the patient attentively, while minimising the extent to which they feel that they are under surveillance. Encouraging communication, listening, and conveying to the patient that they are valued and cared for are important components of skilled nursing observation.

The Standing Nursing and Midwifery Advisory Committee (1999) report listed the possible indicators for increased observation and included:

◆ history of previous suicide attempts, self-harm or attacks on others
◆ hallucinations, particularly voices suggesting harm to self or others
◆ paranoid ideas where the patient believes that other people pose a threat
◆ thoughts and ideas that the patient has about harming themselves or others
◆ specific plans or intentions to harm themselves or others
◆ past problems with drugs or alcohol
◆ recent loss
◆ poor adherence to medication programmes.

The report goes on to recommend and define four levels of observation 'in order to facilitate communication, care planning and training'.

Level I General observation The minimum acceptable level of observation for all inpatients. The location of all patients should be known to staff but not all patients need to be kept within sight. At least once a shift, a nurse should sit down and talk with each patient to assess their mental state. This interview should always include an evaluation of the patient's mood and behaviours associated with risk and should be recorded in the notes.

Level II Intermittent observation The patient's location must be checked every 15–30 minutes (exact times to be specified in the notes). This level is appropriate when patients are potentially but not immediately at risk. Patients with depression but no immediate plans to harm themselves or others or patients who have previously been at risk of harm to self or others but who are in a process of recovery require intermittent observation.

Level III Within eyesight Required when the patient could, at any time, make an attempt to harm themselves or others. The patient should be kept within sight at all times, by day and by night, and any tools or instruments that could be used to harm self or others should be removed. It may be necessary to search the patient and their belongings whilst having due regard for the patient's legal rights.

Level IV Within arm's length Patients at the highest risk of harming themselves or others may need to be nursed in close proximity. On rare occasions, more than one nurse may be necessary. Issues of privacy, dignity and consideration of the gender in allocating staff and the environmental dangers need to be discussed and incorporated into the care plan.

In addition to this, consideration should be given to:

◆ the appropriate level of observation being determined by the senior doctor on the ward and in their absence, the senior nurse
◆ the specified levels of observation including interval observation, continual observation, numbers of staff to be deployed and proximity of staff to the patient (i.e. must stay within arm's length).

Observation levels should not be reduced by junior medical or nursing staff without referring back to senior staff and any change in observation levels should be recorded.

Staff should always be vigilant in identifying times of critical stress for individual patients (anniversaries, birthdays, Christmas) and implement higher levels of observation and support at such times.

The use of CS spray

The Mental Health Act Commission (1999) comments that on occasion the control of disturbances sometimes involves the police. Modern forces have at their disposal CS spray and a number of concerns have been raised with the Commission about its use, including:

◆ the possibility of adverse reactions between CS spray and psychiatric medication
◆ the different effects on patients with different psychiatric disorders (there is anecdotal evidence that CS spray may be less effective on patients in a manic state)
◆ the need for guidance on the mental health assessment of persons who have been sprayed (how long do the effects last?)
◆ whether there are any longer term effects, including psychological as well as physical problems
◆ the use in enclosed spaces and possible crosscontamination, for example of ward staff and other patients (it has reportedly taken up to 48 hours to clear a room of the gas before it can be reused)
◆ the nursing procedures which should be used to mitigate the immediate after-effects of the spray
◆ variations in use between different police forces and the reasons.

In these circumstances, policies for use of CS spray should be agreed between the police and mental health services, both for inpatient units and to assist in conveying patients to hospital. A survey on the use of CS spray on NHS premises revealed that, out of 35 trusts with experience of patients having been sprayed either before admission or as an inpatient, only one trust had produced guidelines on the use of CS spray and two on the handling of patients on whom the spray had been used (Bell & Thomas 1998).

PASSIVE MEASURES

All forensic mental health units have to provide services within an envelope of secure conditions. Consequently, there must be effective physical barriers including walls and fences, possibly both, to agreed standards, good lighting systems and other electronic aids such as closed circuit television cameras (CCTV). The increasingly sophisticated science and technology of the security industry is available to the forensic mental health service and each unit should consider how much of this is utilized alongside other measures.

Passive measures concern the physical barriers and structural and technical systems needed to prevent unauthorized movement and to help control authorized movement. Therefore, secure lines are needed:

◆ around the perimeter of the hospital secure area
◆ around the envelope of buildings lying in the secure area
◆ around the internal parts of certain buildings or sensitive areas.

Physical security is also about the design measures needed to prevent wall scaling and roof stepping to the perimeter and to make concealment of illicit items or contraband difficult. Fixtures and fittings need to be of a specification which renders removal and use as a weapon or escape aid extremely difficult. Secure storage should be provided for dangerous and potentially dangerous items. Areas of passive security requiring consideration would include the following.

A secure perimeter barrier

These are either opaque barriers of brick or concrete or a see-through system using weld mesh panels. Weld mesh is the more commonly utilized system in the UK and has a number of advantages

including cost, speed of construction and the ability for patients to have a view of the outside world and a less claustrophobic feeling than can be the case with opaque systems. Some medium and low security units have utilized weld mesh fences at 3.5 metre heights but in many cases these have proven to be unsatisfactory and have been extended or replaced with 5.2 metre fences. The NHS Medium Secure Unit design guide recommends a weld mesh fence height of 5.8 metres and the Special Hospitals Service Authority standard for medium secure areas is 5.2 metres (NHS Estates 1993).

As part of the risk analysis, consideration should be given to strengthening security by provision of perimeter intruder detection and/or a CCTV system. It is considered more therapeutic to avoid, wherever possible, interior fences between wards and departments, so that there is an open pleasant campus-like environment for patients and staff. Fences may be required, however, to zone off such areas as vehicles, storage and kitchens, entrance area, etc. Landscaping can be utilized to soften the appearance of the perimeter fence but this should not be allowed to compromise security, create observation problems or delay staff response times.

Vehicle access and parking

This includes issues such as vehicle movement in the secure area, car parking and stand-off distance, the approach road, secure vehicle area and inner perimeter road.

Buildings

With the wards and departments themselves, consideration will need to be given to external and internal walls: composition and strength; joints; ground floor slab; and suspended floors and ceilings.

With the internal fixtures and fittings a number of areas need to be covered. *Doors* should be of a heavy-duty standard. Doors for patient-occupied rooms should be made to open outwards, securely anchored into surrounding masonry. Screw fittings should be hidden and screws should have tamper-proof heads. Doorways should be fitted with secure glazed visibility panels. *Windows* should have a secure steel frame and be recessed into robust hardwood or reinforced concrete surrounds. Openings for ventilation should be a maximum of 125 mm with glazing of scratch-resistant polycarbonate. Window catches and hinges should be designed to minimize the possibilities of offering easy ligature points.

Observation panels will be needed within certain subdivisions, partitions and doorways (normally scratch-resistant polycarbonate), with observation over toilet and bathroom areas by a proprietary lens with a swivel cover to the corridor side (there can be problems with these being easy to smear by patients). Good sight-lines will be necessary, especially over those areas where patients will be in groups, such as occupational, social and living areas. *Toilets* should be planned so that it is possible to see if they are occupied and bathroom and shower facilities have tranluscent screens or safety curtaining suspended from antiligature tracking. Override facilities for any privacy locks will also be necessary.

Floor finishes should ensure that they cannot be lifted to provide places for concealment or damage. *Walls* should be chamfered or rounded and metal corner plaster beading avoided. *Loose furniture* should be selected from approved ranges and be of robust construction and securely fitted and fixed, so that it cannot be easily forced apart or dismantled. Care should be taken about places of concealment or anything that makes searching difficult. Bolt-down or fixed furniture may be needed in selected rooms in high dependency or intensive care wards. Shadow boards or cupboards will be needed in rooms where tools or utensils will be used by patients. All furniture will be required to meet the stringent fire retardancy level 7 criteria.

Sanitary appliances will need to be good-quality ceramic earthenware (fire-baked clay) or similar which comply with the Prison Service approved range. Generally, care is needed with WC pans, cisterns, wash basins, baths and mirrors. Stainless steel fittings or glass-fibre reinforced plastic may be specified where the fittings may be subjected to severe force such as intensive care units or seclusion rooms. All *pipe ventilation* and *cablework* should be concealed within secure ducts in patient areas.

Locking technology is a rapidly developing field and advice should be sought from the locking section of the Prison Service, especially if electrical card, magnetic keys or other secure access control is being considered. The aim should be for staff to carry the least number of keys and different key suiting should be kept to a minimum. The procedure in most secure units is for staff from adjoining wards to provide additional support in the event of an emergency. Staff must therefore be able to gain rapid access to any ward, building or room and the locking system must facilitate this.

Finally, areas external to the wards should be planned and laid out so that they are easy to search (DoH 1999). For hard landscaping, materials should be selected that cannot be easily misused or misappropriated for illicit purposes. Care should be taken over the planting of trees and shrubs, keeping clear of buildings, walls, fences and CCTV coverage.

Technological security

Technological security is about the requirements for lighting, CCTV, alarm and communication systems. All of these are specialized, complex and rapidly developing areas of high technology. In addition, there are a large number of system manufacturers and suppliers whose advice will largely centre around the merit of their own particular product.

Therefore, before embarking on design and capital planning work in these areas (and with locking systems), advice should be sought from the Prison Service Security Advisers Unit at an early stage, so as to draw on their experience, trial work and knowledge about the latest developments in these specialized sectors.

The wider implications and possible knock-on effects arising out of technological security, such as staff resource costs, monitoring needs, intervention times, dealing with nuisance alarms, energy, costs, problems from equipment failure, effectiveness in inclement weather, etc. should all be carefully analysed and assessed.

In the first instance, the aim should be for robust passive physical measures with technological security only introduced where there is a shortfall and/or when it is not possible to meet the security standard needed without recourse to electromechanical measures.

These measures will need to be centrally controlled, monitored and recorded from a control room with local registers and controls located in ward offices. These systems are designed to monitor, detect and ensure a quick response to any incident and to record all incidents for later analysis. Their existence should instil a sense of confidence and safety and their very presence will often have a deterrent effect. Some specific technologic considerations would include the following.

Lighting

Good lighting is an important aid to security and may be considered under the following headings.

- ◆ Perimeter lighting
- ◆ CCTV camera lighting
- ◆ General area lighting
- ◆ Entry building lighting
- ◆ Floodlighting
- ◆ Emergency or top-up lighting

Generally, the aim should be to avoid harsh shadows and two-way lighting may be needed in certain areas to achieve this. Glare from mast lighting should be avoided, as this may prove to be a nuisance in patients' rooms. Energy efficiency and low maintenance should be considerations. Lighting should be adequate to support the CCTV system and tamper- and vandal-resistant systems should be considered. Floodlighting would only be used in an emergency or serious incident. Consideration needs to be given to a stand-by generator in case of a mains failure and an uninterruptible power supply.

Closed circuit television (CCTV)

Continuous improvement in CCTV camera technology is taking place and advice from an independent source such as the Home Office Security Advisers Unit should be sought. Cameras capable of transmitting images both day and night are required (housed in weatherproof containers).

Cameras will be needed for security surveillance and control surveillance: separate and dedicated sets of cameras and monitors would be needed for each of these two different surveillance activities. Fixed CCTV cameras will normally be required but some locations, such as sterile areas, may require 360° rotating cameras. The system should have the capability for recording and image assessment and some may be linked to alarm systems in sensitive areas.

CCTV surveillance is usually situated in external areas such as main entrance, grounds and car parks. Within the health service a wide debate is developing on extending the use of CCTV to the direct monitoring of patients. The essence of the debate currently lies in the conflict between possible security opportunities to reduce risk, the privacy of the individual and the clinical potential of TV monitored records (Patterson 1997). Professional nursing journals have raised strong concerns over the spread of 'surveillance' and whether this is an unwarranted invasion of people's privacy or an acceptable way of reducing risk (Nursing Standard 1994).

From the perspective of a secure psychiatric facility, the perceived effects of CCTV appear to mirror the concerns raised in professional journals. Multidisciplinary discussions between high security hospital personnel have raised concerns relating to:

- ◆ privacy and dignity
- ◆ intrusiveness
- ◆ reinforcing paranoia
- ◆ CCTV replacing nurse–patient contact
- ◆ CCTV not necessarily being in the best interests of patients.

A literature search on the use of TV monitoring in a hospital (care) setting revealed very little information. However, a Finnish study described the effects of TV monitoring on a ward atmosphere in a security hospital (Vartiainen & Hakola 1994). The mental health care of offender patients is centralized in two state hospitals. The Finnish study examined the perceptions of staff and patients working and living on a secure ward in Niuvanniemi Hospital, which has 284 beds, 70% of which are occupied by patients with a very serious criminal background. During a ward renovation programme, CCTV was to be installed in two closed wards, in corridors and isolation rooms. These two wards cared for the most dangerous patients, schizophrenia being the predominant mental illness. During the renovation concern was expressed that TV monitoring would have deleterious effects on patients' mental state and violate their privacy. It was decided to conduct a study on the effects of CCTV monitoring but findings showed that contrary to suspicions, there was no increase in paranoid states. The TV cameras used in corridors and isolation rooms, where staff and patients were aware of their location and principles of usage, proved that cameras can be an easily controlled reality even for the sickest patients. During the monitoring period, no cameras were damaged. Violent acts against other patients and personnel decreased markedly in TV-monitored wards

Violent acts often happen quickly and essential features of the incident are not usually observed. CCTV and video recording assist in incident review. The implications of the Finnish study suggest that the perceptions of mental health professionals of the effects of CCTV require a fuller investigation. The assumption of staff that the introduction of CCTV will decrease their security role may have created a 'technological panacea' and a 'seductive myth' that it provides the ultimate answer. For a secure hospital setting, it is essential to understand not only the effectiveness of CCTV but also the threat it can pose to the clinical well-being and privacy of patients.

Crowner et al (1991) describe a study in the USA on a state hospital secure ward where assaultative behaviour by patients was video taped. Using a CCTV camera, the project provided an important insight into the nature of the issues and practical problems in using CCTV. The project concentrated on looking at methods by which assaults, and the circumstances leading up to them, could be analysed in detail. Limitations on staff observations showed they were often unable to relate what happened and why it happened. By videoing the main ward area, the CCTV would provide information to focus on factors which could better describe and classify assaults. The study describes in some detail constraints placed on the use and siting of CCTV cameras. Two years of negotiations and agreements preceded installation, the staff citing concerns about personal privacy and confidentiality. Eventually the cooperation of staff was obtained in the form of guaranteed written agreements.

The limitations imposed on the CCTV included video tape recordings taking place at prearranged times and an indicator light in the nursing station (out of sight of patients) which alerted staff that video recording was in operation. Only tape segments involving patients, not staff, could be stored and analysed. Staff had demonstrated a strong reluctance to take part in what they saw as an intrusive study. Privacy and confidentiality, however, are not absolute rights but can be overridden. Block & Schaffner (1985) describe the ethical principles which provide a basis for exploring more fully the effects of CCTV monitoring in the context of a ward.

The data demonstrating whether or not TV monitoring in a secure environment is effective are not yet available. All that can be stated at present is that TV monitoring offers secure environments a potential way of enhancing levels of care and security. The pace of surveillance monitoring within society and in health-care settings sends out clear messages that it is a powerful medium that requires statutory controls to stop sloppy practice and deliberate misuse. Regulating its use in secure psychiatric wards requires consultation with those who are going to be monitored and, in the case of patients, individual clinical assessment, combined with an appropriate ward placement, will be critical.

Alarms and detection systems

These generally are:

◆ nurse call
◆ fire alarm
◆ general alarm (the push-button alarm will raise the alarm on the ward/department

concerned and indicate the location of an incident, alerting adjacent wards and control room)

◆ tamper alarm (warning that certain doors, gates or cupboards have been opened)
◆ personal alarm (a number of systems exist, from simple stand-alone commercial personal attack alarms through to sophisticated systems linked to a central control room which give information on location).

Other systems include:

◆ perimeter intrusion detector systems (PIDS) may be required either mounted on a fence (geophone) or on a wall (fibre-optic wall sensor)
◆ metal detector portal to check staff and visitors entering and leaving the unit
◆ X-ray machine to check visitors' and staff personal belongings and mail entering the unit
◆ secure access control system such as hand geometry, face recognition, bar-code reader
◆ radio communication to facilitate contact between staff and the unit control room (using a UHF Home Office protected wavelength)
◆ telephones (the hospital control room will require: direct lines to the local police; general internal; internal emergency; and any incident room would require: general internal; direct outside line; and a direct line to the general manager)
◆ entry buildings to allow pedestrian and vehicle access under controlled conditions (keys, sterile areas, control and incident rooms would usually be located here).

Passive measures are an integral part of design and specification and should be considered at an early stage of the design process. Introducing them at a later stage or, worse, after building completion can make them more expensive, less effective and environmentally obtrusive.

The aim should be to concentrate on achieving security protection from passive physical security measures insofar as this is practical and to restrict the introduction of technological measures such as CCTV, alarms and detection sensors to a minimum, as these can be subject to breakdown or lower performance caused by either adverse weather or human error and because they lead to recurring revenue costs.

WARD ACCOMMODATION

Ward accommodation in a forensic mental health unit is normally subdivided into three broad groupings.

High-dependency wards

These wards will be planned as self-contained units with co-located occupations and outdoor exercise facilities. Patient movements off-ward will be limited. A secure line will be needed around the external envelope of the ward and around the occupational facilities and the outdoor exercise area. The detailing and specification should be physically secure and robust with damage-resistant fittings and finishes. Any intensive care facility will need to be made particularly robust and details and finishes should be capable of withstanding severe physical force.

Mainstream wards

These will contain the patients' living accommodation but the patients normally leave the wards for occupations, education, library, shopping and social activities and perhaps daytime dining. The off-ward movements of these patients will normally be under escort. Dedicated garden areas will be provided and these will either be left open and treated as open community gardens or the garden edges will be treated with demarcation fencing or hedging, mainly to give privacy, shelter and separation between wards. A secure line will be required around the external envelope of the ward.

Predischarge and elderly wards

These wards will also contain the patients' living accommodation and a dedicated, open garden will be provided. There should also be a co-located external area where these patients will have freedom of movement to walk and to socialize under the discreet observation of staff. These patients will also have access to central rehabilitation and recreation facilities but in addition they may be allowed access under supervision to occupations and daytime social facilities located outside the secure perimeter.

A secure line will be required around the external envelope of these wards but their internal detailing and finishes, and their spatial designs may be to a more normalized standard. This will mean that these wards can then only be occupied by patient groups who are of a less challenging nature.

None of the above is intended as a prescriptive blueprint but as examples of the various approaches that may be adopted to reflect the specific client group. There may be a number of subsets in these broad groupings and there will also be some gender and age separation.

TRAINING

The UKCC & University of Central Lancashire (1999) comment that:

Induction of staff into a new post or new role should be seen as an investment. The inductee should be confident that they are familiar with policies, protocols and working practices as soon as possible on commencement in the job.

They go on to report, however, that the induction process varies from organization to organization within both the Prison Service and health care.

On one end of a continuum nurses receive a comprehensive on-going structured induction with appropriate mentorship, whilst at the other nurses undertake new roles with minimal preparation and are potentially being put at risk.

A review of the prison inspection reports supports this view, stating that 'In most instances staff, when they had actually received it, felt the induction and/or training was insufficient' (HM

Inspectorate of Prisons 1998: 88–89). One example they cited is of 'newly appointed mental health nurses at … Prison who were left "to sink or swim" because managers failed to set up proper induction programmes'. This situation is less common within hospitals but examples have been given where induction takes place up to 2 months after commencement in post. A further concern of the UKCC & University of Central Lancashire (1999) study involved bank and agency nurses or nurses who were not directly employed by the organization (e.g. CPNs) who provide a specialist service and their lack of knowledge and experience of secure environments.

The topics identified from the UKCC & University of Central Lancashire (1999) study that were regularly mentioned as topics for induction programmes included:

◆ control and restraint, including breakaway techniques and deescalation techniques
◆ management of aggression
◆ 'gaol craft' (for prison nurses)
◆ security training (for health service staff)
◆ boundaries and relationships
◆ custody versus care
◆ risk assessment and risk management
◆ suicide awareness
◆ records and record keeping (appropriate to organization)
◆ organizational policies, procedures and protocols
◆ medications in common usage
◆ legislation
◆ offending behaviour.

The report concluded that:

The availability, length and content of induction programmes are inconsistent. The most effective induction programmes appear to be those where there is a period of time when the inductee is supernumerary, mentorship is in place and initial induction is to the organization and secondary induction to the individual's workplace. (UKCC & University of Central Lancashire 1999)

Control and restraint (C&R) is an area that causes concern to nurses in both sectors. Access to the appropriate training and confusion about the level of involvement in C&R processes are the main issues confronting nurses. Research has been undertaken by the Institute of Psychiatry (Standing Nursing and Midwifery Advisory Committee 1999: 30–31). The Mental Health Act Commission (1999) suggests that training and updating are essential for both qualified and unqualified staff who are likely to face situations of patient aggression and violence. The Commission has previously commented adversely on the 'proliferation of courses of instruction in this area' (Mental Health Act Commission 1997: 168). It was particularly critical of the lack of regulation by a statutory awarding body, which it believed led to 'a divergence of practices which in some instances have been found to be contradictory' (Mental Health Act Commission 1997: 168). It reports that the Department of Health has now responded to this problem by including guidance in the Code of Practice which states that:

Courses should be taught by a qualified trainer and that the trainer should have completed an appropriate course of preparation designed for health care settings and preferably validated by one of the health care bodies (English National Board or Royal College of Nursing Institute). (DoH & Welsh Office 1999: 93)

The Psychiatric Nursing Section of the Institute of Psychiatry (Standing Nursing and Midwifery Advisory Committee 1999: 30–31) carried out a survey on the types of C&R training provided in hospitals in England and Wales, including the variety of techniques taught and the variety of training providers who offer such courses. The survey also sought to ascertain whether the practice of C&R matched trust policies and to describe the subjective experiences of nurses involved in the application of C&R techniques. The survey obtained 294 responses, of which 46% were from females and 54% from males. The highest number of responses (n=104, 37%) were from staff nurses; 80% of the sample had a professional nursing qualification. Only 39% of respondents received C&R training in the first

3 months after starting work on their ward. Thirteen percent of respondents waited more than 2 years for training whilst 41% of respondents did not know to which organization their instructor belonged. Training varied in duration from 5 to 21 days.

The technique most frequently taught was verbal deescalation, followed by restraint using a three-person team, and the third most frequently taught technique was for taking the patient to the ground. The survey revealed that 27% of respondents received an injury whilst training. Questions about the last incident in which the respondent was involved in C&R showed that in 19% of cases, staff were injured and in 11% of cases, patients were injured (n=33). After the incident only 61% of respondents were debriefed and 76% were given documentation for audit procedures. About half of respondents (55%) had a postincident discussion review with the patient.

This survey confirms findings from the focus groups and audits conducted across the UK, in both the health sector and the Prison Service, in the UKCC & University of Central Lancashire (1999) secure environments project. Their report concluded that:

Control and restraint is an issue of concern across both sectors. Nurses have articulated the need to develop national standards for physical interventions when there is a breakdown in relationships that results in physical aggression. Linked to this nurses need to be conversant with the skills and knowledge to identify risk factors and deescalation techniques.

Employers need to consider their expectation of nurses and the findings from the Institute of Psychiatry survey could be used to address the issues identified. The key findings were: staff are not always trained promptly and there is no clear policy about refresher courses. Staff often do not know who trained their trainers or who employs them, which can cause problems of accountability. The meaning of 'control and restraint' varies widely and there is great variation in the duration of training. The content of courses may have inadequate coverage of the theoretical, preventive and defensive aspects of managing violence and aggression and nurses' responsibility for patient safety and dignity may not be given sufficient emphasis. Consequently, staff may lack confidence in their ability to use C&R techniques, which increases the risk of injury to both patients and staff. Postincident debriefing, which should happen in all cases, does not in about a quarter of cases.

The Future Organisation of Prison Health Care report (HM Prison Service & NHSE 1999) has identified that a strategy for the continuing professional development of health-care professionals working in prisons needs to be instigated. The report also suggests that the prison health-care service is isolated from the mainstream of NHS development and that the current training and development of health-care professionals is patchy. From the data captured during the secure environments project, a similar conclusion can be reached about some aspects of education and training of nurses in secure hospital provision (UKCC & University of Central Lancashire 1999).

The main issues that emerged from the UKCC & University of Central Lancashire (1999) study, which were common to both the health and prison systems, were:

◆ clinical supervision
◆ induction
◆ C&R training.

The study found that clinical supervision was sparse in implementation and a significant number of nurses were not aware of the guidance provided by the UKCC on this issue. In the Prison Service, there was some disagreement about whether clinical supervision should be provided by Prison Service nurses or by nurses within the local NHS. The general blockage to the implementation of clinical supervision appears to be lack of resources, in terms of both time and expertise of nurses to provide this service to colleagues.

Watson & Kirby (2000) propose core competencies for working in secure environments which would encompass a number of units and forms of delivery (see Box 23.1).

CONCLUSION

The maintenance of a secure environment in forensic mental health services demands a sophisticated interplay of measures which ensure the safety of patients, staff and the general public yet at the same time promote the therapeutic endeavours of the organization.

This counterdependence of measures can best be illustrated by some of the criticisms of security from the Fallon Inquiry report (DoH 1999), which found the security measures sadly lacking. Examples were given of how patients may have been able to secrete contraband in their rooms. Combatting this would need a room with the physical facilities to support good observation, to minimize hiding places and to ease

Box 23.1	Maintaining patients in a secure environment: core competencies
Title of unit	*Teaching/learning strategy*
Teaching/learning strategy	Computer-assisted learning programme
Fire/hostage management	One-day seminar
Misuse of substances	Half-day seminar/supervised practice
Escorting patients	Role modelling/supervised practice
Visitor control	Role modelling/supervised practice
Observation	Seminar/supervised practice
Communication	Seminar/supervised practice
Preventing and managing aggressive behaviour	Five-day course/supervised practice
Security breaches	Half-day seminar

searching without dismantling the room and its fittings. A clear and unambiguous policy should be available which defines the choice of room to be searched (usually random) and gives guidance on how the search should be carried out. From a relational perspective it is recommended that the patient be present when the search takes place and would ideally involve the patient's primary or associate nurse. Problems in implementing this example can occur if any of these elements are not in place: the room may be difficult to observe or search; the policy or procedure may be unclear and lacking in specificity; and the staff member may simply not carry out their job properly or may conduct themselves in such a way as to antagonize the patient or to invite a complaint.

It is in these circumstances that the role of supervision and monitoring becomes imperative; the saying that a chain is only as strong as its weakest link is most pertinent within this field of practice. Patients, often able and manipulative, have a capacity to observe for weaknesses in systems and individuals and exploit them accordingly.

In relation to policies and procedures it is not enough to have detailed and impressive documents covering all aspects of security and practice if they are not read or understood by the staff who are being asked to implement them. One needs to stand back from the system and consider what is expected from individual members of staff. For some staff, e.g. qualified staff working in an area where there is regular use of, say, seclusion, it would be expected that they would have a thorough knowledge of the procedure; in another area where seclusion was not practised or practised only rarely, then a more superficial understanding may be acceptable. Other seldom-used policies may demand a rudimentary knowledge of their contents and for other, thankfully rare situations (e.g. hostage taking), then knowing that there is a policy and where to access it may be acceptable. In short, knowledge of policies will vary according to the area of practice and level of responsibility but staff do need to be clear about what is expected of them as individuals.

REFERENCES

Allen C 1997 Asylum seekers. Nursing Times 93: 36–37

Alty A 1997 Nurses' learning experience and expressed opinions regarding seclusion practice within one NHS trust. Journal of Advanced Nursing 25(4): 786–793

Bell F, Thomas B 1998 Police use of CS spray: implications for NHS mental health services. Mental Health Care 1(12): 402–404

Benson R 1992 The clinical nurse specialist in forensic settings. In: Morrison P, Burnard P (eds) Aspects of forensic psychiatric nursing. Avebury, Aldershot

Block MR, Schaffner KF 1985 Ethical problems of recording physician–patient interactions in family practice settings. Journal of Family Practice 21: 467–472

Burnard P 1992 Preface. In: Morrison P, Burnard P (eds) Aspects of forensic psychiatric nursing. Avebury, Aldershot

Burrow S 1991 Mental health: special hospitals – therapy versus custody. Nursing Times 87: 64–66

Burrow S 1993 Inside the walls ... work of nursing staff in special hospitals and secure units. Nursing Times 89: 38–40

Chaloner C 1998 Working in secure environments: ethical issues. Mental Health Practice 2: 28–33

Clarke L 1998 What's in a name? Nursing Times 94(22): 38–39

Crowner ML, Douyon R, Convit A, Volavka J 1991 Video-tape recording of assaults on a state hospital inpatient ward. Journal of Neuropsychiatry 3 (suppl): 9–14

Dale C, Wallis E, Taylor P 1999 Professional, contractual and volunteer relationships. In: Taylor P, Swan T (eds) Couples in care and custody. Butterworth Heinemann, Oxford, ch 13, pp 159–187

Davenport A 1999 Random searches of detained patients. Journal of Mental Health Law 1: 59–61

Davis S 1992 Assessing the criminalisation of the mentally ill in Canada. Canadian Journal of Psychiatry 37: 532–538

Department of Health 1992 Report of the Committee of Inquiry into Complaints about Ashworth Hospital. HMSO, London

Department of Health 1999 The Report of the Committee of Inquiry into the Personality Disorder Unit, Ashworth Special Hospital. Volume 2, expert evidence on personality disorder. Stationery Office, London

Department of Health and Social Security, The Home Office 1989 Operational brief for the special hospitals service authority. DHSS & Home Office, London

Department of Health, Welsh Office 1993 Mental Health Act 1983: code of practice. HMSO, London

Department of Health, Welsh Office 1999 Mental Health Act 1983: code of practice. Stationery Office, London

Eldergill A 1997 Mental health review tribunals: law and practice. Sweet and Maxwell, London, pp 59–61

Gillon R 1985 Philosophical medical ethics. Wiley, Chichester

Gillon R 1996 Thinking about a medical school core curriculum for medical ethics and law. Journal of Medical Ethics 22: 323–324

Goffman E 1991 Asylums. Penguin, London

HM Inspectorate of Prisons for England and Wales 1998 Annual report of HM Chief Inspector of Prisons for England and Wales. Stationery Office, London

HM Prison Service, National Heath Service Executive 1999 The future organisation of prison health care: report of the Joint Prison Service and National Health Service Executive Working Group. Department of Health, London

Hopkins N, Ousley L 2000 Clinical psychology and the forensic nursing role. In: Robinson D, Kettles A (eds) Forensic nursing and multidisciplinary care of the mentally disordered offender. Jessica Kingsley, London

Kaye C 1991 Care and confinement. Health Service Journal 101(5265): 8

Kaye C, Franey A 1998 Managing high security psychiatric care. Jessica Kingsley, London.

Kinsley J 1998 Security and therapy. In: Kaye C, Franey A (eds) Managing high security psychiatric care. Jessica Kingsley, London, ch 7, pp 75–84

Kirby S 1999 History and development. In: Chaloner C, Coffey C (eds) Forensic mental health nursing. Blackwell Science, London, ch 15, pp 288–305

Lehane M, Rees C 1996 Alternatives to seclusion in psychiatric care. British Journal of Nursing 5(16): 974–979

McCourt M 1999 Five concepts for the expanded role of the forensic mental health nurse. In: Tarbuck P, Topping-Morris B, Burnard P (eds) Forensic mental health nursing: strategy and implementation. Whurr, London, ch 13, pp 149–161

McLean SAM 1989 A patient's right to know: information disclosure, the doctor and the law. Dartmouth, Aldershot

Melia P, Moran A, Mason T 1999 Triumvirate nursing for personality disordered patients: crossing the boundaries safely. Journal of Psychiatric and Mental Health Nursing 6: 15–20

Mental Health Act Commission 1997 7th biennial report. HMSO, London

Mental Health Act Commission 1999 8th biennial report. Stationery Office, London

National Health Service Estates 1993 Design guide: medium secure psychiatric units. NHS Estates, London

National Health Service Executive 1999 The Safety and Security in Ashworth, Broadmoor and Rampton Hospitals Directions 1999. HSC 1999/150. Department of Health, London

Nursing Standard 1994 Privacy of clients: tags and television. Nursing Standard 8(30): 45

Patterson I 1997 Patient and staff perceptions of TV monitoring on ward atmosphere in a secure hospital. Unpublished MSc thesis, Council for National Academic Awards (sponsoring establishment Leicester University)

Scales C, Mitchell J, Smith R 1993 Survey report on forensic nursing. Journal of Psychosocial Nursing and Mental Health Services 31(11): 39–44

Singer P 1993 Practical ethics, 2nd edn. Cambridge University Press, Cambridge

Standing Nursing and Midwifery Advisory Committee 1999 Practice guidance: safe and supportive observation of patients at risk: mental health nursing: 'addressing acute concerns'. Department of Health, London

Swinton J 2000 Reclaiming the soul: a spiritual perspective on forensic nursing. In: Robinson D, Kettles A (eds) Forensic nursing and multidisciplinary care of the mentally disordered offender. Jessica Kingsley, London

Tarbuck P 1994 The therapeutic use of security: a model for forensic nursing. In: Thompson A, Mathias P (eds) Lyttle's mental health and mental disorder, 2nd edn. Churchill Livingstone, London, ch 27, pp 552–570

Topping-Morris B 1992 An historical and personal view of forensic nursing services. In: Morrison P, Burnard P (eds) Aspects of forensic psychiatric nursing. Avebury, Aldershot, ch 1, pp 2–44

United Kingdom Central Council for Nursing, Midwifery and Health Visiting, University of Central Lancashire 1999 Nursing in secure environments. UKCC, London

Vartiainen H, Hakola P 1994 The effects of TV monitoring on a ward atmosphere in a security hospital. International Journal of Law and Psychiatry 17(4): 443–449

Walker N 1991 Dangerous mistakes. British Journal of Psychiatry 158: 752–757

Watson C, Kirby S 2000 A two nation perspective on issues of practice and provision for professionals caring for mentally disordered offenders. In: Robinson D, Kettles A (eds) Forensic nursing and multidisciplinary care of the mentally disordered offender. Jessica Kingsley, London, ch 4, pp 51–62

FURTHER READING

Department of Health, Welsh Office 1999 Mental Health Act 1983: code of practice. Stationery Office, London

Index